The Big Book
of
Reiki
Symbols

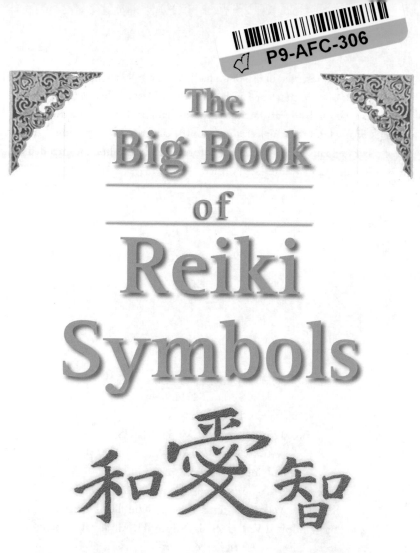

和愛智

The Spiritual Tradition of Symbols and Mantras of the Usui System of Natural Healing

Mark Hosak • Walter Lübeck

LOTUS-PRESS · SHANGRI-LA

The information presented in this book has been carefully researched and passed on to the best of our knowledge and conscience. Despite this fact, neither the author nor the publisher assume any type of liability for presumed or actual damages of any kind that might result from the direct or indirect application or use of the statements in this book. The information in this book is intended for the further education of interested readers.

First English Edition 2006
Reprinted 2011
©by Lotus Press
Box 325, Twin Lakes, WI 53181, USA
website: www.lotuspress.com
email: lotuspress@lotuspress.com
The Shangri-La Series is published in cooperation
with Schneelöwe Verlagsberatung, Federal Republic of Germany
© 2004 by Windpferd Verlagsgesellschaft mbH, Aitrang, Germany
All rights reserved
Translated by Christine M. Grimm
Cover design by Marx Graphik & ArtWork
using a photo by Frank Arjava Petter
and calligraphies by Mark Hosak
Calligraphies, photos, and illustrations:
see Index of Illustrations and Sources on page 651
ISBN: 978-0-9149-5564-1
Library of Congress Control Number: 2006925747
Printed in USA

TABLE OF CONTENTS

PART II –
THE EAST ASIAN SPIRITUAL BACKGROUND OF THE TRADITIONAL USUI SYSTEM
OF NATURAL HEALING WITH REIKI

PART IV –

SPIRITUAL COSMOLOGY AND KNOWLEDGE OF ITS ESOTERIC BACKGROUND

CHAPTER 19

AN SHORT ESSAY ON SPIRITUAL COSMOLOGY 498

INDEX OF EXERCISES AND PRACTICES

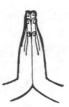

CHAPTER 2
REI KI GONG

CHAPTER 9
THE MEDICINE BUDDHA YAKUSHI NYORAI AND REIKI

CHAPTER 11
KUJI KIRI

CHAPTER 12
DAINICHI NYORAI KIDÔ

CHAPTER 17

THE CR SYMBOL

EXCURSUS

A BRIEF INTRODUCTION TO CALLIGRAPHY

CHAPTER 19

AN SHORT ESSAY ON SPIRITUAL COSMOLOGY

CHAPTER 20

THE SPIRITUAL ENERGY SYSTEM OF THE HUMAN BEING

Preliminary Remarks About Pronunciation

For the spelling of the terms and proper names that are in Japanese, Chinese, and Sanskrit, this book uses a simplified transcription. The long vowels of â, ô, û, and î appear as special signs. These serve as a guide for the correct pronunciation and also generally allow a clear identification of the original word.

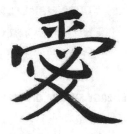

LOVE

Preface

The Search for the Roots of the Reiki System

Writing a book about the traditional Reiki symbols and mantras of the System of Natural Healing established by Dr. Usui is a special challenge—many years have passed since Usui did his work. There is also relatively little written material about his teachings and his life that has found its way to the general public.[1] In particular, we have a very limited knowledge today about what moved Dr. Usui to use the symbols and mantras that have been passed down to us today.

However, since the mid-1990s a great many of Usui's original teachings have been rediscovered by various Reiki Masters, especially Frank Arjava Petter. As a result of his mediation and some fortunate strokes of fate, I (Walter) was able to do the first two degrees of the traditional Japanese Reiki training in Kyoto (Japan) with the Reiki Master Chiyoko Yamaguchi-Sensei. As a young woman, she had learned the traditional Reiki System up to the complete Master/Teacher degree with Dr. Chujiro Hayashi. In 2004, I was fortunate enough to continue studying with her son Tadao Yamaguchi-Sensei, who has carried on the mission of his mother after her death, and complete the first part of the traditional Japanese Reiki Master/Teacher training (*Shihankaku*). This allowed me to resolve many things that had remained unclear in my previous research. It also confirmed important practical and philosophical foundations and provided new, valuable information for the effective orientation of further research.

---

[1] Compare with the following books published by Lotus Press on the life and works of Dr. Mikao Usui and Dr. Chujiro Hayashi by Frank Arjava Petter: *The Original Reiki Handbook of Dr. Mikao Usui*, Petter/Usui, translated by Christine M. Grimm; *The Hayashi Reiki Manual*, F.A. Petter, T. Yamaguchi, Ch. Hayashi; *Reiki Fire*, F.A. Petter; *Reiki—The Legacy of Dr. Usui*, F.A. Petter, translated by Christine M. Grimm.

Spiritual Hands-On Healing Systems in Asia

Through my (Walter's) decades of experiences with various inner martial arts, Asian philosophy and spirituality, as well as various methods of Asian Qi Gong and Nei Gong, I was also able to thoroughly research some of the Reiki System of Healing's origins in theory and practice beyond Japan on the mystical island of Bali and Hong Kong, the threshold to China, as well as extensive journeys to South India. Among other places, my travels took me to the outskirts of the city of Trivandrum where I visited a family who has been passing down the secret of the spiritual hands-on healing from generation to generation for 800 recorded years and still practices it as a profession today. The type of healings, together with the required initiation rituals and the philosophy, are so similar to the Reiki System established by Dr. Usui that I already came to the conclusion at the beginning of the 1990s that there must have been mutual roots here. This was confirmed much later without a doubt by Mark Hosak's scientific research.

This family has books from the early days of the tradition, written in the time-honored manner on palm leaves, which explain the various aspects of this healing art. The current lineage-holder explained to me that the power for the healing that was accomplished by laying on hands came from a ray of the Great Goddess. At that time, I did not yet understand the entire significance of this statement, but the attentive reader will discover that this is just as true of Reiki.

Martial Art and Healing Art

This family had an interesting approach to the training in its tradition of healers: Before a member of the family was permitted to learn healing, he or she first had to attain the degree of Master in the traditional South Indian martial art of *Kalaripayat*. This was because, in their opinion, the only people who could truly heal spiritually even in difficult cases were those who had previously overcome their own fear of death, pain, and injuries.

Various oral sources have also revealed that Dr. Usui and Dr. Hayashi had extensive training and practice in the traditional martial arts. I was fascinated by the story that was later told to me by the Grand Master of *Kalaripayat*, who lived and worked in Trivandrum, about the history of this martial art. Fighting and spiritual healing have always played—and still play—a fundamental role in this martial art on a high ethical level since the beginning of the tradition more than 3,500 years ago. Until the start of colonization, the fighters still learned the methods of energetic healing and the ways to protect themselves from many injuries or heal more quickly from them through a type of Qi Gong.

The initiation into the mantras and special sacred symbols are also part of this discipline.

In Hong Kong, I had the opportunity of comparing notes with experienced representatives of the traditional Chinese Qi Gong systems. I learned from them that almost every school of Qi Gong has initiation rituals in the higher levels of training through which the ability to work with spiritual forces of healing is accessed.

Many of the energetic healing methods differ fundamentally in nature from those of the Usui System of Natural Healing, but I found at least two that show major similarities with Usui Reiki in their essential teachings and approaches.

From the specialists of the native massage traditions on Bali, I learned that there are ancient ways of spiritual healing through the laying-on of hands that are taught in the highest levels of training and come from the original Indian tradition of Hinduism.

Respect and Responsibility Toward the Spiritual Tradition

That fact that this knowledge is treated with the greatest respect and only passed on to especially committed students by means of an intensive and long training in all of the traditions of spiritual hands-on healing that I became acquainted with during my travels put the situation in a new light for me.

According to the information that we now have, Dr. Usui and Dr. Hayashi also demanded that their students come to the teachings on a regular basis and were only permitted to treat others on their own (in their own practice) after thorough theoretical and practical instruction. Because of our own experiences, we also believe that Reiki is too valuable to just become acquainted with it in a quick workshop. As for all good things, it is best to also invest enough time in the Reiki System to have a thorough background in both the theory and the practice.

The End of the Mystery-Mongering

For a long time, the symbols of the Reiki System and their mantras were considered secret, even though the first book that illustrated all of the symbols and briefly described their applications was already published at the end of the 1970s in the USA. Since this time, a constant stream of additional books and many more articles in magazines were published that showed the Reiki symbols. And the knowledge-hungry fan of Reiki can also quickly find a wealth of information on the Internet. Short and simple research in all of the important world languages with the popular search engines presents thousands of websites offering the symbols and their mantras in a vast quantity of variations.

Another Book on the Reiki Symbols?

So the symbols have actually been familiar to the public for a long time, and the question naturally arises: Do we really need another book on the symbols and mantras when there is already so much information about them? Unfortunately, closer scrutiny reveals that there is hardly any solid, verifiable, or more thorough information about them in the abundantly available sources. There is almost nothing published about the spiritual background and the history of the symbols that stands up to an in-depth examination, and the symbols and their mantras usually do not correspond with those used by Dr. Usui and Dr. Hayashi.

In most cases, the information is limited to general applications, possibly channeled messages, and rather amateurish explanations on the basis of superficial knowledge of Buddhism, Taoism, and Hinduism.

It is particularly confusing that the symbols and mantras are shown with a great variety of spelling that sometimes have little similarity with the originals used by Dr. Usui and Dr. Hayashi. So especially laypeople and beginners are very uncertain after an excursion into the world of Reiki because they quickly ask questions like: "So what is right?" "Does it even matter how the symbols are drawn? "Is there some kind of reliable help for properly learning the symbols and mantras?" "Can we write, pronounce, and use the mantras in whatever way we like?" "Are there comprehensible rules?"

This book answers these questions and a great many more in an in-depth approach. However, despite its depth this book obviously cannot replace the personal training and traditional initiation by a qualified Reiki teacher. The symbols and mantras only work for those who have been initiated into their power.

How This Book Was Created

I (Walter) have been carrying the thought of publishing a book about the symbols and their mantras with me since the mid-1990s. But after much deliberation at that point in time, I considered it inappropriate because there was not enough information on the history, spiritual background, and derivation of the sacred symbols that was correct in terms of calligraphy. And I also didn't want to publicly contribute to the abundance of assumptions already existing among the Reikians. However, through many fortunate strokes of fate that led to the possibility combining my own research with that of the Reiki Masters and book authors Frank Arjava Petter and William Lee Rand, who are now my friends, completely new perspectives have arisen since the mid-1990s. Stimulated by the great variety of new information, I began to research again.

Yet, despite the many wonderful advances, which were published in our mutual project *The Spirit of Reiki*, I could not get beyond a certain point in the research. There were many hints between the lines and practical experiences indicating that certain conclusions were obvious, but it was only through the acquaintance with Mark Hosak, at that time a student of East Asian art history, that I received the opportunity to research the Reiki symbols and their mantras in all of their manifold meanings in a truly significant way.

Mark had lived in Japan for a number of years. Because of his course of studies, which he accomplished with a special emphasis on researching the spiritual traditions of Japan and China and much personal commitment, he is especially qualified to create the scientific foundations that are absolutely necessary to truly understand Dr. Usui's heritage in its full meaning. In addition to his academic studies, he learned various martial arts in Japan, some to the degree of Master, and studied classic calligraphy with renowned teachers of this art. He went on pilgrimages to sacred sites and had astonishing experiences with light beings, which completely changed his life. He met people who had delved deeply into the secrets

23

of the mysticism of Japan and learned a great deal from them. Since he had already been initiated into the art of Reiki before his stay in Japan, he naturally also kept his eyes open for everything that could help him better understand this wonderful healing art.

In 2000, Mark began training at my Reiki Do Institute International to become a Rainbow Reiki Master. Now, after four years of intensive learning, he has completed the second level of the three-stage Master training and is therefore one of the most qualified Reiki Masters/Teachers in the world. Rainbow Reiki uses the carefully researched Traditional Usui System of Natural Healing as its foundation for healing and personality-development work. On this basis, a large number of techniques and methods of spiritual energy work with Reiki, as well as important teachings on its spiritual philosophy, have been developed since the end of the 1980s. These are now being transmitted throughout the world by qualified Rainbow Reiki Masters/Teachers and applied by tens of thousands of Rainbow Reiki practitioners.

Because of his familiarity with Japanese history and the spiritual traditions of this country in theory and practice on the one hand and the system of Rainbow Reiki on the other hand, Mark Hosak is the ideal partner as a co-author for this book. Without his extensive and precise research, as well as his comprehensive practical experiences with the material, it would have not been possible produce these texts. As a result of our fruitful cooperation, a great many synergy effects occurred that have opened up new worlds for both of us—and not just in regard to the Reiki System. The thought frequently arose for both of us that we had already done this type of work together in a past life. Who knows?

So this book presents precise scientifically based research results on the symbols and mantras, their references to Asian history and the fundamental spiritual traditions, as well as many (sometimes very personal) experiences with the divine beings that look after the system of healing with Reiki and the people who use it.

We have included in this book many techniques of energy work that are being published for the first time such as Rei Qi Gong and spiritual work with Reiki light beings. Many classic techniques of the energy work with Reiki are being made accessible to a broader public for the first time here. The book also precisely explains the meaning of the traditional Reiki symbols and their mantras in theory and practice. Even a little manual on Japanese and Chinese calligraphy is included because, according to our experience, knowledge of this art contributes a great deal toward a correct—and therefore successful—approach to the Reiki symbols and mantras.

It was often quite difficult for us to draw a line between the topics that we also wanted to include in this book because they are so exciting and useful, yet belong to the larger field of this subject and not what is absolutely necessary for understanding the theme presented here.

It is clear to us that much of this book brings information to the public that extends far beyond what is found in the usual esoteric literature. Following the instructions precisely will bring the opportunity of having the same type of wonderful experiences with the practices as we do, since this is why we decided to also publish this knowledge.

As presented below in the text of this book, the spiritual knowledge, which also includes the knowledge about the Reiki system as a healing art, came in the form of entire shiploads of scrolls from the Chinese temples of Esoteric Buddhism to Japan. These documents are practically impossible for laypeople to understand. Years of studies are necessary to even begin to translate them into practical results, such as applying them for healing, if they are available at all. We would like to make this important knowledge accessible to the modern world in its entirety as it significantly relates to the Reiki system. This is exactly how other authors have also approached spiritual wisdom through the millennia. This enables anyone to learn who wants to do so, thereby honoring the gift of Reiki as a healing art and using it in the best-possible form for the blessing of all sentient beings.

It is important to us to give the millions of committed Reiki friends throughout the world the possibility of precisely understanding what the symbols and mantras mean, which divine beings are connected with them, and how to reach them on a personal level. In our opinion, this will offer each person the same opportunity to have the very important possibilities of spiritual healing and the kinds of experiences that Dr. Usui probably had. We have also been blessed by these experiences.

Because there has been inadequate information about the symbols and mantras belonging to Reiki System created by Dr. Usui up to now, there is hardly a publication today that explains more than the very basic meanings and possibilities of application. As a result, many very effective applications have not been used. However, in our current times it is more important than hardly ever before in the history of humanity that we have powerful tools available for spreading the divine powers in this world. We believe this is the only way that we can truly solve the enormous problems and harmonize the difficulties that people have created for themselves, causing all of us to suffer more and more. If we do not find the way out of the spiral of environmental destruction (Planet Earth) and the destruction of the inner world (the human body), in a few centuries there will probably no longer be a human culture in which people can live good lives or perhaps not even be any human beings left. We do not want a future like that! With love and understanding and the "help from above" so often experienced by spiritual people, it will be possible to radically change the course.

We hope that this book will make a contribution toward giving a tool to those who want to transform the world back into a paradise in which the people, animals, and plants live happily with each other. May it help them do the work necessary to achieve this goal.

The Reiki system is, as this book proves, spiritual light work in the truest sense of the word. Reiki promotes living processes. It arises from the source of all life and is sent to us from there through Dai Marishi Ten, the Great Goddess, and Dainichi Nyorai, the Great God[2], the two highest individual spiritual beings, on behalf of the Creative Force. Love and light, the feminine and the masculine aspects of the Creative Force, the Divine, are included in the Usui System of Natural Healing, which can easily be recognized in the form of the Master symbol.

Whether or not we make use of what the light beings, the messengers of the Creative Force, place in our hands is up to us. Whether or not we are prepared to assume responsibility and eliminate the difficulties that the human race has brought into this beautiful world is up to us. Whether or not we understand that we are divine according to our nature and that

---

[2] These two divine beings appear under many names throughout the world, for example: Isis and Osiris; Ishtar and Tammuz; Shiva and Shakti; Freya and Frey; Metatron and Sandalphon; Holy Spirit (Divine Mother) and Heavenly Father.

it is therefore possible for us to also master the greatest challenges if we call upon this sacred legacy is also up to us.

The sacred beings, the gods and angels, will stand at our side when we no longer know what to do and when we need help. However, the work will not get done without our own efforts. The Creative Force helps those who help themselves. Because the Creative Force assumes the responsibility—a truly divine quality—and is motivated by a love for life and the sentient beings of this world—another divine quality—this creates good. What our striving cannot achieve will be given to us when we send our prayers to the divine beings.

Reiki can help us to become aware of this legacy and it available in a practical manner.

It is our express wish that the knowledge published in this book is spread and becomes integrated in Reiki training and the Reiki practice. Furthermore, we are always very happy to receive feedback. Our contact information is included at the end of the book.

It is much easier to master the tasks at hand through discussions and exchanges of experiences with other Reiki friends. It also feels good to immerse ourselves in the power of love that develops when people come together to serve in the sense of the Creative Force.

We hope you enjoy reading our book. It may be necessary to read one line or the other more than once. Reflecting or meditating quietly helps our heart and mind find an access to this knowledge. Using this time is a good investment. Such new perceptions can help us make quantum leaps in our development and grasp Reiki in a depth that opens up completely new paths of healing and spiritual personal development. Light and love are waiting for us here…

May the blessings of the Creative Force always be with you on your path and as you read this book.

Mark Hosak   Walter Lübeck

PART I –

INTRODUCTION TO THE SYMBOLS AND MANTRAS IN THE TRADITIONAL USUI SYSTEM OF NATURAL HEALING WITH REIKI

CHAPTER 1

Symbols and Mantras
as Tools of Spiritual Energy Work

Starting with the 2[3]ⁿᵈ degree of the Usui System of Natural Healing, three symbols and mantras[4] are used. They enable us to use techniques such as distant treatment and making contact with all types of other beings, as well as with situations beyond the boundaries of time and space (HS), intensification and spatial orientation of the Reiki flow of power (CR), and mental healing (SHK).

They were introduced by Dr. Mikao Usui, the founder of this system, to make the advanced forms of the spiritual healing energy work accessible to his students even without years of intensive practice and personal development.

At the same time, all of the symbols—the three of the 2ⁿᵈ Degree, the Master Symbol, and the *old* character for Reiki[5]—contain a wealth of pro-

---

[3] This statement applies for the Western Usui Reiki. During the time of Usui and Hayashi, Reiki students who had already been practicing the 1ˢᵗ Degree over a longer period of time had the Power-Intensification Symbol transmitted to them per initiation. However, the overall division of the degrees was different back then since the training contents taught today in the form of three degrees were distributed over six levels. And since the training itself was also different in that it was imparted less frequently in the form of seminars than in meetings that took place on a continuous basis, there were considerably more individual differences in relation to the contents imparted within a training level. This system has advantages and disadvantages: The type of training offered at that time was cohesive, containing much practice and a close teacher-student relationship. The type of training we usually find today is much more flexible in terms of the time frame. This makes it easier for a person who would like to learn Reiki but does not live where it is taught. In my experience, if the person attends seminars time and again over a longer period of time and diligently does the "homework," the success of the training is quite comparable.

[4] When we talk about "symbols" we mean the three signs of the 2ⁿᵈ Degree and the one sign of the 3ʳᵈ Degree. With their help, Reiki can be used simply in a great variety of ways. "Mantras" refers to the words that are associated with the symbols and make them effective or activate them.

[5] All of the symbols and mantras are described in detail in the corresponding chapters of this book. See the Contents and Index.

found perceptions on spiritual philosophy, ideas, and precise instructions for a rich variety of spiritual energy work. In addition, they are precise statements about the divine beings who direct Reiki as a flow of power from the heavenly worlds to the beings of the material world, supporting the tradition called the Usui System of Natural Healing.

Studying these symbols can clarify the roots of the healing system founded by Usui and support the seekers in discovering completely new, powerful applications for the energy work. For the first time, this book makes all of this knowledge accessible to a wide audience for self-study. We hope and believe that this will make a contribution toward giving the Reiki System the recognition due to it in the holistic-medical professional world. Only on the basis of secured, practice-oriented knowledge can the entire potential of the healing powers found in the Reiki System be revealed. Anyone who has taken thorough advantage of this impressively large „tool box"" will no longer want to be without it.

Symbols and Mantras—Misconceptions and Confusion

There are many stories, ideas, and assumptions related to the symbols and mantras. For example, that solely the knowledge of the symbols and mantras could already impart access to Reiki and that the initiations would then be unnecessary—which, incidentally, is not true since the corresponding Reiki seminars would have become superfluous since the people would have found out at some point that they could also do it without an initiation. However, the training, which is still necessary for the effective use of the "tool box" would then be missing. And, if this was possible, the many spiritual traditions would certainly not have been passing on the keys to spiritual powers by means of initiations for thousands of years. After all, a lot of time could be saved if this was possible. And it has not just been in short supply in our current era!

Another idea that we frequently encounter is that it basically doesn't matter how the symbols are drawn or the mantras are pronounced, as long as we feel good about it. This is also incorrect. As everyone knows, it is not possible to open a lock when the key does not fit. This also applies to the symbols and mantras that are used within the scope of practical energy work. Incidentally, it would otherwise also be possible to make some random motions that make us feel good and then achieve the same results as with a Reiki distant healing.[6] As the worldwide success of the Reiki method since the introduction of the Usui System proves, there must be some truth to the results of the initiations, symbols, and mantras that has convinced people and continues to convince them to do this instead of just „something." It is important to call such facts to mind now and then in order to not lose sight of the fantastic possibilities found in the Reiki method and drift into wishful thinking.

This chapter provides a general explanation of what symbols are in the spiritual sense, why and under what circumstances they work as tools for the practical energy work, and what makes them an element of a spiritual tradition. This basic knowledge is important in order to understand the special statements about the Reiki symbols in this book.

What Is a Symbol from the Spiritual Perspective?

A symbol is an experience (for example: opening the heart), which is translated into a very abridged and simplified depiction in an abstract form. It can also be an instruction (for example, for directing the spiritual powers of healing) or insight (for example, our personal divine nature or our own vision for our path in life).

There are two major groups of symbols. The first includes all of the symbols taken from nature such as: the moon, the sun, the light, the darkness, the stars, the water, the tree, the snake, a rock or mountain, a lake, people, and animals. The second group includes artificially created symbols like: the letters of the alphabet, mandalas, the yin/yang sign, the Reiki symbols and mantras, as well as stories that illustrate a spiritual principle.[7]

---

[6] A similar approach applies to the sacred geometry, which is used in traditions like Feng Shui (China), Vastu (India), and geomancy (Europe). Specific proportions, layouts, and symbolic elements, as well as materials, are selected because they are appropriate for the spiritual purpose, in order to create a building that corresponds to the Divine Order and can fulfill the respective tasks.

[7] It is very interesting and revealing to look at the oracles that work with images such as the Tarot or the *I Ching*, and see where natural and where artificially created symbols are used to depict spiritual wisdom.

Symbols often serve in the spiritual context as archetypal images of the highest reality, the experiencing of the Divine, that can be attained by expanding our consciousness—for example, during meditation or a visionary experience. They can also serve as mediators of insights, experiences, and contents of sacred knowledge that cannot be depicted and imparted in any other way because it is not possible to find them within everyday experiences in a way that is this comprehensive and interconnected with other life themes.

A symbol can stimulate the process of understanding both in the creative, intuitive, and/or the analytical-intellectual sense on all levels when we open up to it in a sincere way and with the appropriate expertise. Good literature about the *I Ching* and the *Tarot,* as well as some of the works by Carl Gustav Jung on this topic, can help us to better comprehend the symbols on the different levels of understanding and translate them into practically applicable realizations. Related recommended reading can be found in the Commented Bibliography of the appendix.

Of course, a sacred symbol cannot be explained and understood just by the powers of the logically working mind—but also not just through intuition and feeling! **Both portions** of the human spirit must work together harmoniously—i.e. function holistically—in order to grasp a spiritual symbol and use it in every possible way. This is why all major spiritual traditions give instructions in the use of sacred symbols from a mentally oriented, rational approach that includes logical reflection, studying the appropriate texts, and informative conversations about a systemized depiction of the Divine Order[8] on the one hand; on the other hand, they adopt an approach that can use inspiration, creativity, intuition, the personal emotional world, and the mystical experience. In the latter case, for example, meditations on symbols are practiced that develop the intuition and promote a stronger ability to resonate with the

---

[8] Every depiction of the divine order is necessarily false and incomplete. Nevertheless, something like this is very important to: a.) help the mind open up to spiritual topics; b.) translate spiritual teachings into everyday life in a practical and constructive way; and c.) be able to impart comprehensible ideas about spirituality to others who are not familiar with these topics. In addition, we should not forget that there are more or less false depictions of the Divine Order. So it certainly makes sense to look for the version that functions better and exchange ideas about it with like-minded people.

source of wisdom using the techniques of spiritual energy work. Initiations are frequently also given to create a close relationship between the student and the divine being that is appropriate for him/her (called *Yiddam* in Esoteric Buddhism) in order to promote his/her understanding and personal development.

Rational instruction is necessary, for example, to make students aware of the special meaning of the essentially very ambiguous symbols for the spiritual tradition in which they are involved, as well as its references to their personal experiences, interests and qualities, and their momentary learning process. Without the assistance of the cognitive mind, a responsible approach to the symbol in practical applications, but also in teaching the following student generations, is not possible. The mind often lets us easily identify and correct the false interpretations of a symbol that are based on neurotic patterns, fears, and egotistical strivings that have not yet been processed.

Of course, the mind requires intensive training in order to be a match for these tasks. In addition to the generally applicable rules of clear thinking, students must also learn to integrate the intuitive perception and spiritual inspirations that exceed and complement their capacities, as well as their true feelings[9]. This makes it possible for the circle to be squared, the extension of practical perception into the divine truth.

The Different Meanings and Levels of Meaning of Symbols Using the Example of the Cross

The same symbol can contain very different messages in the various spiritual traditions. For example, a cross can have the basic meaning of a harmonious, constructive union of the opposites in a spiritual tradition. In addition, it can point toward the historical occurrences that have a great meaning for the tradition and also to people who have made important contributions to this tradition. In the different areas of a tradition, the cross can have various meanings that, may perhaps initially appear to not

[9] True feelings come from the personality of a human being. They are powerful, spontaneous, caused by and directed at the present moment. The so-called secondary feelings are behavior programs similar to feelings that have been created through the necessity of social adaptation and unprocessed traumas.

be related when seen superficially but reveal and illuminate a fundamental structure of the spiritual teaching when it is understood in a profound sense.

A Selection of the Spiritual Meanings of the Cross

Within this context, the cross can show the relationship between the four archangels *Michael, Gabriel, Raphael,* and *Uriel* or illustrate the four sacred elements of fire, water, air, and earth together with their relationships and functions. It helps to understand that, for example, life can always be created when the conceiving influences of the feminine and the masculine primordial deities—the Great Goddess and the Great God—come together in the sexual union of man and woman. The cross explains the separateness of all types of beings, as well as the possibility of overcoming the separation. This enables us to understand that the constant exchange of all participants in the life process is what makes the so-called four-dimensional[10] time/space continuum possible (length–height–width–time). Its psychological significance explains the different processes in the striving of a human being: toward the *spiritual* (life), toward the *material* (death), toward the *feminine* (yin) themes, and toward the *masculine* (yang) themes of life in the world. The cross shows the union of the sacred powers for conceiving an individual being—but also the process of death in which the individual components separate. It shows the state of suffering that occurs if we do not take responsibility for our own path. An example of this is getting lost in the helper syndrome and, as a result of refusing to use our lives in a way that has true spiritual meaning and joy, suffering, being unable to move, and being virtually nailed to the cross.

If we do not want to use the many opportunities for experiencing happiness, meaning, fulfillment, and love in a physical body, we will obviously vegetate in suffering, helplessness, pain, fear, and meaninglessness. Instead of using the good gifts of the Creative Force in this world, those who reject the physical life indulge in complaints against those who understand the message of the Divine and do their best to also realize

---

[10] In more precise terms, the universe is not four-dimensional. However, such a greatly simplified perspective is completely adequate within this context. A more detailed description regarding the structure of Creation is provided in the chapter on "Spiritual Cosmology."

meaning and love in the material life that has been given to them by the Creative Force.

Yet, the cross also shows the happiness that arises from the dance of relationships, the infinite Tantric dance of desire, longing, hope, and separation on the one hand and union, fulfillment, love and ecstasy on the other hand. This is what makes it possible for us to experience the divine meaning of earthly existence.[11]

We can rest at the center of the cross in the equilibrium of the forces. We can regenerate and keep or attain an overview. Or we can suffer because we cannot do everything at the same time, cannot have continually intensive relationships with everything and everyone, and because we have the habit of looking off into the distance instead of perceiving what is close to us. This results in a chronic poverty and misery consciousness.

Suum cuique—to each his or her own!

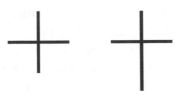

The Meanings of the Cross Related to the Individual

On a personal level, the cross can help us understand and meaningfully integrate experiencing the death of a beloved friend. It can reveal the necessity to make a clear decision of our own instead of waiting for someone else to make it and thereby fill the vacuum of power created by the indecisiveness. The cross can explain the process that is necessary to call forth creativity when it is needed. It can explain the causes of personal suffering through jealousy, greed, dogmatism, and envy and describe the possibilities for the healing of these problems.

Through the classification with the four elements, the cross helps us recognize and compensate for imbalances created by an overemphasis

---

[11] Please compare this with the chapter on Spiritual Cosmology—A Brief Explanation of the Structure of Creation and Existence.

on or neglect of certain elements in everyday life in due time. It shows the relationships of the elements with each other—for example, there is definitely a reason why fire and water are directly opposite each other!

Anyone who wants to master a challenge in life can use the four qualities with which the four elements correspond and which are depicted by the four arms of the cross to make progress. For example, with the power of the fire we can dynamically assert ourselves, motivate others to help us by igniting their feelings, and find (invent) a path with enthusiasm and creativity. Or, through meditative absorption, we can go into our own center where the Divine and the human self touch and let ourselves be guided through the jungle of problems by the mystical insights gained in this manner.

Of course, the symbol of the cross—which, incidentally, was an emblem of the Great Goddess's sacred power in vast portions of the Orient and Occident in ancient times—can be interpreted on a much deeper and more profound level, but we will not continue beyond these examples in order not to lose sight of our objective, the general understanding of spiritual symbols.

Learning to Use a Symbol in a Practical Way

In order to make a symbol useful in a practical way, the mind must be stimulated to experience the abstract meaning of the symbol through the concrete problems and occurrences of everyday life. A spiritual symbol describes a structure in a very concise, precise, and holistic form. A spiritual symbol is a type of shorthand for the philosophy of the sacred.

Through the examples taken from everyday life, it becomes possible to understand the abstract structure of the sign. The conscious mind can recognize similarities in the patterns of the examples until it acquires the ability to independently discern the structure and content depicted by the symbol in the world and naturally also within itself. When we practice regularly, it becomes possible to have a creative approach to the symbol. As a result, this in turn supports personal insight and the applications of the principles represented by the symbol for solving problems in the inner and outer worlds.

Only when we have a comprehensive understanding of where to find the abstract message of the symbol in **concrete experience** can creativity and intuition begin to do their work. Rational probing on the basis of practical experience is like a planting stick or trellis in the garden, upon which the living, proliferating tendrils of intuition, creativity, and inspiration can grow.

In brief: The abstract, boundless potential of the yang needs the concrete, limited, and restrictive (!) structure of the yin in order to manifest and have a practical effect. So when the masculine urge for freedom rebels against the feminine wishes for a home, family, and orderly life, this is very easily understood—even though it is precisely the limitations placed on the man by the feminine structure that helps him truly open up to his potential. As a result, this leads him to accepting responsibility, relationship, and ultimately himself. Without a concrete task, it is not possible to observe the effect of power—because it does not happen. There is no sense in having freedom from something. Having the freedom for something results in responsibility, relationship, love, the realization of visions, and much more ...

The proper approach to the spiritual symbols sets in motion inspiration, creativity, and intuition—which ultimately lead to direct spiritual realization on the basis of paying attention to what we experience. The mind could never accomplish this process without the help of symbols since it would see the experiences in the world that it has been shown as separate from each other and unrelated. Consequently, a spiritual symbol reveals a basic pattern of life that always shows the same essence despite its many forms. Symbols point to the laws and processes behind the directly perceivable occurrences on the surface.[12] In doing so, they give us the possibility of orientating ourselves in our decisions and actions toward the truths of the hidden, esoteric reality.

What Is the Difference
Between Secular and Spiritual Symbols?

Spiritual symbols are different from secular ones because they depict basic patterns of life in an abstract, concise form. For example: The yin/yang symbol. Secular symbols use an abstract, brief form to describe an instruction (stop sign; plus sign in mathematics) or an experience that is perceived through the five senses—seeing, hearing, physical sensation, smelling, and tasting—such as a letter that stands for a certain sound; the word "caress"; a number that describes an amount. Of course, symbols that many people consider to be secular, without any deeper meaning, are very capable of concealing within themselves an extensive philosophy from the eyes of the unknowing.

Numbers, for example, are used by practically everyone on a daily basis for doing arithmetic. In addition, each number can also be associated with a spiritual, cosmic principle. This is done in the venerable art and science of *numerology*. If we have not been trained to also recognize the numbers as spiritual symbols, we will not be able to use them for numerology. This is a further example of how the mind, as the precondition and "water-bearer" for spiritual consciousness, very much has a right to sacred training.

An additional level in the activity of spiritual symbols opens up when we achieve the ability to work with spiritual powers beyond the subjective states, as a practical means of power, through an initiation that may take place in various manners. This can occur through a ritual by a representa-

---

[12] So this means: esotericism—the truth behind the scenes.

tive who is empowered in the spiritual sense and appropriately trained in the respective tradition (for example: Reiki initiation, Kriyâ Yoga initiation, or TM initiation).

Another path involves acquiring a deep understanding of the symbol's essential meaning through learning on all levels of human existence and a ritual of the tradition to which the symbol belongs. The ritual creates a lasting union with the symbol's spiritual essence within the scope of the appropriate tradition. This occurs through personal commitment at a suitable time (the right astrological constellation for the practitioner) and by means of the appropriate techniques of spiritual opening through calling upon the light beings that are in resonance with the symbol, mantra work, suitable music, and symbolic actions (rituals) for increasing the personal resonance with the essence of the symbols and the associated light beings (for example: the self-initiation of Dr. Mikao Usui into the power to work with Reiki; Kûkai's self-initiation into the mantra of knowledge).

What Exactly Happens at an Initiation into the Power of a Symbol?

It is important to understand here that there is not actually an initiation into the power of a **symbol itself.** The symbol is like a radio receiver. Depending on the characteristics of the symbols and our degree of initiation, we can use it to listen to music in a telephone quality or in hi-fi stereo[13]. We can receive just the medium-wave stations or also very-high frequency, short wave, and other bands that may or may not change the sound, and so forth. We either buy a radio (initiation through another person)—or build it ourselves from the individual pieces (self-initiation, as explained above). A radio offers many possibilities, but we need a long time and intensive theoretical and practical learning to understand how to properly use the great variety of functions. A person who sits in front of a radio transmitter in the cockpit of a jumbo-jet without having been trained in how to use it will not benefit from the many great features of the hi-tech device, except through some possible chance results. This

---

[13] It just occurred to me that there has been an intense change in the quality of time when I think back to the distant past of my youth: If you like, you can replace "hi-fi stereo" with "Dolby 7.1 Surround Sound."

metaphor may make it easier to understand why **training and initiation** are inseparable.

As little as a radio can function without a source of power and a transmitter that can receive the messages that it has sent, symbols cannot fulfill their purpose without a source of power and the assistance of a Divine Being. This is an important reason why this book goes into detail about the various light beings that are associated with the Usui System of Natural Healing with Reiki!

As tools of objective energy work (see below) spiritual symbols are always part of a specific spiritual tradition, including the related techniques and divine beings responsible for them. Within this framework, they function in an effective, predictable, and reliable manner as long as we are initiated into them and know how to use the potential because of our training.

What Happens When a Symbol Is Used in a Number of Different Spiritual Traditions?

When a certain symbol is used in a number of spiritual traditions, an initiation within one tradition basically cannot make the functions of this symbol available to all of the traditions where it appears. If one spiritual tradition has evolved from another, a journey to the roots of the initial one can occur through an initiation and training in the first tradition, in addition to studies, experience, and mystical perception. This will eventually reveal more and more of the secret powers of the symbol that were or is accessible in previous traditions. Such a process has many parallels with the above-mentioned approach of self-initiation. This book has been written with the intention of enabling readers initiated into the Usui System of Reiki to experience this kind of deepening and expansion of their knowledge and skills.

What Is a Mantra?

A mantra consists of one word, sentence, or several sentences, usually in a sacred language like Sanskrit or translated from such a language into another. A mantra can generate healing influences on all levels in a

41

specific or general way. We can use mantras for healing, promoting the development of the personality, evoking a specific spiritual influence, harmonizing fear, calming an animal, activating a symbol such as one of the Reiki signs, cleansing healing stones, and much more.

In most cases, the literal significance of a mantra can only be approximated. Because of its direct relationship to divinity, the meaning of each mantra is so complex that an entire library of explanations could be written for some of them, especially since there are often several levels of effects that have various meanings.

The Derivation of the Word "Mantra"

The syllable *man* comes from the Sanskrit word *Manana* (thinking). The syllable *tra* is derived from *Trâna* (liberation from the shackles of the world of appearances = spiritual awakening). Each mantra is an aspect of the Great Goddess in its deepest being, which in turn manifests in reality through the practice of the mantra. Accordingly, each of the mantra practices is a worship of the Goddess. When we experience spiritual awakening through the practice of a mantra, we hear the First Word with which the Great Goddess created the universe, the plane of existence of the material world with all of the related light worlds, in her manifestation as *Vâc*. Each mantra contains *Devatâ*, the Highest Consciousness. But just repeating a mantra is not a spiritual practice and does not result in an effect. We must devote ourselves to the spiritual power in word, thought, and deed—and be prepared to unconditionally realize it and allow the sacred power of the Goddess to flow through us out into the world and take form.

The lips and tongue, with which a mantra is expressed, are reflexology points of the 2nd chakra. The larynx and the vocal cords belong to the 5th chakra, which in turn receives its power from the 2nd chakra. Because of this, it is important to have a strong, balanced 2nd chakra that is well connected with the other energy centers, in addition to a well-functioning 5th chakra.

What Is the Proper Way to Pronounce and Use Mantras?

The proper pronunciation of a mantra is less important than a correct energetic and spiritual relationship to its meaning and its spiritual source, as well as the sincere decision to realize its significance in a way that is positive and serves the highest good of the whole.

Mantras function in the quickest and best way when the practitioner has been appropriately initiated by a competent teacher.

Repeating a mantra every day for at least 108 times results in a general effect. In order to receive a specific effect, a correspondingly positive request should be thought or spoken before each session of mantra work.

Before beginning the mantra practice, we can call upon the respective deity or the Goddess for help in general or in relation to a specific topic. This intensifies the effect of the mantra work like a burning glass. At the conclusion of every practice, we should pray for a blessing and give our thanks.

The minimum repetition of 108 times releases especially strong spiritual healing powers. The Indian spiritual tradition has 108 sacred names of the Creative Force and 108 is the number of the main energy channels (*Nadis*) that run from the major chakras.

Through regular practice—at best on a daily basis—of at least 108 repetitions of a mantra or a multiple of this number, we can become increasingly resonant for the messages, effects, and healing powers of the angel or the deity that protects the respective mantra. As a result, this light being can do increasingly more for us, effecting healing on all levels and helping us change our life pattern in a constructive way. At the same time, the mantra also directly releases the healing processes within us that promote health and well-being and positively influence the psyche.

However, in order for a mantra to even develop an effect, whether direct or indirect, a basic resonance must first be created. This occurs through regular repetition, as described above, or a corresponding initiation that opens a channel to the light being responsible for the respective mantra.

In order to attain a distinct effect, a mantra should be practiced 108 times daily for at least 40 days. A multiple of the 108 repetitions per day considerably intensifies the effect.

When we practice about 125,000 repetitions of a mantra during the approximate period of 3 months, this often (but not inevitably) results in a type of spiritual quantum leap in our development. In addition, we often also receive the ability to initiate others into the mantra.

The Appropriate Use of a Mâlâ (Prayer Beads)

The so-called mâlâs, chains with 108 beads plus one, are generally used for practicing mantras. Beginning with the individual bead, also called the Guru Bead or *Meru* (Sacred Mountain), count each repetition of the mantra, bead by bead, using the thumb and middle finger, until you reach the Guru Bead on the other side. Hold the Guru Bead for a moment between your thumb and middle finger, then continue the practice by counting the beads one by one in the opposite direction. Never cross over the Guru Bead when practicing a mantra. It stores the spiritual power and therefore increasingly intensifies the practitioner's mantra work over time like a lever.

One way to greatly support the effect is by wearing the mâlâ on your body and placing it under your pillow or close to your head at night. Because the mâlâ is a personally imprinted sacred object, it should not be loaned to another person or even handed to someone else unless there is a truly important reason.

There are various types of mâlâs that can intensify the respective specific types of mantras. For example, a *Rudraksh* mâlâ is especially good for Shiva mantras, a basil mâlâ (tulsi wood) supports all of the goddess mantras. However, any mâlâ is suitable for any mantra.

A mâlâ should be kept in a special place like an altar when it is not being used. If a mâlâ is blessed, this intensifies its effect.

What Is the Meaning of the Mantra Endings Namahâ and Svâhâ?

Namahâ means "I offer!" (spiritual offering). This ending is neutral. *Namahâ* is basically used as the ending for mantras until we have reached the age of 29-30 years. *Svâhâ* means: "I offer to the spiritual realms!" This ending is feminine. *Svâhâ* is basically used as the ending for mantras after we have reached the age of about 29-30 years.

The Word Mahâ

This word is often used in a mantra before the name of a deity. It can strengthen the effect of the mantra and create an especially harmonious and holistic attunement of the desired healing.

How Do Symbols Actually Work?

Symbols and mantras are used throughout the world in all of the spiritual traditions for meditation, personal development, mystical experiences, healing, and energy work. They basically have two different types of effects.

Symbols and Mantras that Can Make Subjective Changes

Modern examples of these are things like affirmations and the conscious use of symbolically meaningful objects (the cross, yin/yang symbol, circle), forms, and colors to evoke certain moods and associations. These types of symbols are frequently used within the esoteric context. A good example of this is Chinese Feng Shui—the art and science of designing working and living spaces, as well as gardens, in a way that is supportive of life and healing.

Any arbitrary sign or image, any word, and practically any object can be used in this way by anyone for the purpose of initiating a subjective experience. The one precondition is that we have a certain intense emotional association because of factors like our education, cultural background, affiliation with a religion, or an impressive personal experience that is somehow related to it.

The effects achieved in this way are very different and in no way comparable to the experience of any random, unprepared person who uses them. How we personally and emotionally evaluate what we perceive essentially depends upon the type, length, and intensity of the effect.

These effects appeal to the feelings, moral and ethical values and standards, chains of associations, and memories. We create an attitude of expectation and, in addition to evoking a more or less complex mood, emotional or rational insights may arise. So the effects resulting here

45

are essentially dependent upon the **individual's previous imprints.** The subjective changes may even extend as far as transforming conditions of the body and/or states of consciousness. This can provide support for processes of disease and healing. Strong emotional responses and the resulting physical reactions that viewers have to films like *Gone with the Wind* or *The Thorn Birds* are an example of this phenomenon.

When the subjectively acting symbol sometimes proves to be very effective, this is in no way a magical result in the sense of energy work! Magic definitely does not function on the basis of an individual's previous imprints and pure belief. Objective energy work, in the sense of changing the structure of an individual life process (magic) by producing effective tendencies inside and outside a human being that favor certain occurrences and qualities of experience and weaken others, basically does not occur when we use subjectively effective symbols. The same applies to working with powers received from light beings such as gods, Bodhisattvas, and angels (Reiki, spiritual healing).

How Do We Use a Symbol that Works Subjectively?

However, subjectively effective symbols can be used to put us into states of consciousness, moods, and physical conditions that will support objective energy work. In this regard, there are many transitions between the two areas. Moreover, depending on our training progress, a subjectively working symbol can become an objectively working symbol! One example of how this happens is through an initiation.

Every symbol whose meaning is not understood by the person who uses it on the basis of appropriate spiritual instruction (learning combined with experience and initiation) is actually just a subjectively working instrument. As a result, the preferable approach is to contemplate or mentally visualize it and consciously connect it with certain states of the body and mind, experiences and perceptions, in the inner and outer worlds. Of course, such symbols can also move the life energies of the body and transform them within certain boundaries. The functions of the nervous system, the meridians known to us from acupuncture, and chakras (non-material energy organs connected to the physical body that organize and represent different life themes), react to the human emotional

46

Views on Symbols

Jean Gebser, the modern Swiss philosopher, believes that every genuine symbol is an effective element of origin and a preforming basic pattern for the state of Being, for all that exists and has developed, which means the entire reality (paraphrased from: *The Ever-Present Origin*, page 244).

C.G. Jung has written the following on the topic of the symbol: "... that it [the symbol] has no content of truth when considered from the standpoint of realism, but it is psychologically true, and it was and is the bridge to the very greatest accomplishments of the human being" (paraphrased from: *Symbols of Transformation*, page 390).

And furthermore...
"Symbols are formed energies, forces, which means determined ideas whose spiritual value is just as great as their affective value" (paraphrased from: *Psychological Types*, page 333).

The mind then rests upon its own depths
and broods upon the darkness of its womb.
What intention and reason never calls forth
Offers itself as it blossoms sweetly on its own
And from the divinely inspired conception by the forces
The archetypal forms of things arise.
(Humboldt, *57ᵗʰ Sonnet*)

life, memories, associations, states of consciousness and their meaningful integration into the overall personality. However, in contrast to objectively working symbols, this effect basically does not extend beyond our personal energy field (aura).

Neurolinguistic Programming (NLP), mental training, and Silva Mind Control, as well as autogenous training, are well-known systems that use the subjectively working symbols in the manner explained above.

Symbols and Mantras that Can Effect Objective Changes

Examples of this are the Reiki symbols and mantras, but also runes or magical amulets and the sacred mandalas (yantras) that have come to us from the Indian *Vastu*, the "Mother of Feng Shui," with whose help the energetic qualities and the living atmosphere of rooms can be changed. Mantras like *Om namah Shivaya* and *Om mani padme hum* are also included in this category.

In order to use these tools in the sense of objective energy work, they must basically be transmitted to us by someone who is already applying them within a certain objective framework and has the ability to impart the system of his/her energy work in a spiritual manner. Another approach is inner attunement to the appropriate system, as well as learning the proper use of the symbols.

Esoteric Buddhism (the spiritual path from which Reiki originally came), for example, takes this latter approach. This is accomplished by doing precise rituals and reciting initiation mantras—often repeated more than 100,000 times—during a period of time that is astrologically favorable for the practitioner, connected with a sequence of visualizations of mandalas and calling upon the appropriate deities in states of deep meditation. Usui used some of these possibilities for self-initiation during his 21-day retreat on Mt. Kurama, a century-old, famous power place close to Kyoto. He fasted there in seclusion near a picturesque waterfall. With support from the power of the sacred place, as well as the extraordinarily favorable astrological constellations in the transits of his birth horoscope, he attained access to the healing force of Reiki and the power of the mantras, symbols, and initiation rituals connected with it in a mystical experience of enlightenment. This astrological situation had more extraordinarily positive aspects for an experience of spiritual enlightenment than anything I had ever seen in my astrological practice and related research. Nevertheless, this beneficial time would have been useless had Dr. Usui not been well-prepared on the basis of his decades of spiritual studies and had he not known precisely when to do which type of practices at what place and for how long.

If the first, rather uncomplicated and generally less strenuous path from person to person is selected instead of the elaborate procedure of the second path, this is called *initiation*[14]. It can, depending upon the characteristics of the appropriate tradition, be translated into practical terms in different ways within the scope of a ritual.

Examples of this are: Reiki initiations, Taoist initiations (Qi Gong and magic), the transmission of *Barraka* within the Sufi tradition, *Shaktipat* in Hinduism, Tantric initiations, Kriyâ Yoga, shamanic initiations into a specific medicine power, and initiations within a magical lodge into a certain degree (for example: Adeptus minor) or a particular spiritual power of a deity.

How Can Subjectively Working Signs Become Objectively Effective Symbols?

In principle, if they are thematically suitable, symbols of the first category that are not too general can be made into tools with precisely defined functions within the scope of the second category through appropriate practices and much personal commitment (devotion), as well as spiritual support from the angels, for example, if they have not already attained this status. To do this, it is usually necessary for us to enter into a state of illumination, at least temporarily, in order to do the work necessary to accomplish this or consciously enter into such a state and be able to dwell there. The function of a mantra or a symbol before its transference into the second category is not necessarily clear in the objective sense. Above all, this is true with regard to artificially created symbols that basically have an arbitrarily and subjectively selected form of manifestation. The same sign, the same word, or the same sentence can be related to very

---

[14] In contrast to self-initiation.

different functions, deities, and energies in various esoteric traditions. Sometimes they may be very powerful, but in other cases they can also have exceptionally gentle effects. The more strongly a symbol's appearance reminds us of structures that can be observed in the physical world, the more narrowly it is basically defined in the range of its possible effects.

How Dr. Mikao Usui Revived the Symbols and Mantras from a Lost Tradition of Healing for Himself

Dr. Usui had to create his own access to a lost tradition and proceeded as described above when faced with the problem that the symbols and mantras he found in the Sanskrit writings did not function in a practical way for him. His three weeks of meditation and fasting on the sacred mountain of Kurama connected him with the spiritual tradition behind the writings, symbols, and mantras. He then achieved the abilities to become a Reiki channel, to initiate others into this spiritual tradition, and was able to create and use the tools of this tradition. He virtually had to go on a mystical journey to the divine source of Reiki to be accepted there personally as the messenger and water-bearer for the divine powers.

Where Do the Objectively Working Symbols Get Their Powers from?

Objectively working symbols draw their powers from light beings such as deities, transcendent Buddhas, and angels—they are actually just loaned to the people who use them. This is how such spiritual powers can have an effect on our moods, feelings, memories, associations, physical conditions, and states of consciousness. They can obviously also effect changes in our energy system. The possibilities of influence inherent to objectively effective symbols may, under certain circumstances and depending on their characteristics, extend far beyond our personal energy field. They can directly influence relationship structures, the probability of occurrences, the state of materials, the functions of electrical devices, the charge of batteries, the surface tension of water, the amount of biophotons radiating from a person's hand, and much more. An example of this is the distant-healing technique of the Reiki System.

Among other things, we can draw the conclusion that the symbols and mantras used by Dr. Usui in his system are *absolutely not Reiki,* but first became applicable for the initiated through the traditional initiations within the scope of the Usui System of Natural Healing. Otherwise, they are just signs and words like any others and are often used as part of the everyday language in Japan within other contexts. They are employed to decorate temples and tombs, whereby their content of meaning is not directly connected with the functions familiar to the Reiki practice.

When the symbols and their mantras are transmitted correctly within the scope of Reiki initiations, each of us can rely on their power and their effect within this system. Symbols and mantras that have been looked up in books—like this one—or learned from friends without the corresponding initiation are simply characters from the realm of the esoteric—but not precise, powerful tools of energy work.

Additional Symbols and Mantras

New symbols and mantras, which the respective Reiki schools often consider to be part of the traditional Usui Reiki, are constantly appearing throughout the world. The following should be taken into account in this respect:

There are three degrees in the traditional Western Reiki System according to Dr. Mikao Usui.

The *First Degree* practices contact treatment. It does not include an initiation that empowers a person to actively use the Reiki symbols or mantras or specific instructions on how to use the symbols.

In the *Second Degree,* three symbols and their corresponding mantras are transmitted energetically. These can now be applied by the initiate for power intensification, mental healing, and distant treatment, as well as for techniques of the Reiki energy work that result from their spectrum of effectiveness. At the least, training in the use of these sacred tools includes distant healing, mental treatment, and power intensification.

Depending on the school, there may just be a pure initiation into the Third Degree, plus teaching of the Master Symbol and its mantra, in the *Third* or *Master Degree.* Or a complete training may be transmitted in the form of initiation rituals into the First, Second, and Third Degrees (possibly one as individual levels).

According to all of the authentic material at our disposal[15], Usui did not teach additional degrees and symbols. The symbols and mantras he used can clearly be traced back to spiritual schools that are widespread in Japan such as Esoteric Buddhism and *Shintô*.

If additional symbols are now incorporated into the Usui System of Natural Healing as tools for the energy work, this can be done in two ways:

A. Symbols and mantras are used that belong to **another** form of energy work, which means that they basically also work with a **different energy.** In this case, Reiki is applied **together** with the other method of spiritual energy work. Of course, the additional symbols then do not work in accordance with the rules in force for Reiki but according to those of the tradition from which they come.

In this case, the simple name of "Reiki" or "traditional Reiki" is misleading because we are not dealing with the spiritual life energy according to which, in this case, the new symbols function—and especially not with Dr. Usui's System of Natural Healing. The rules that are now in play differ from those known to Reiki. But this in no way implies that the respective form of energy work should be seen ineffective or of lesser quality from the start! When we link the various systems of spiritual energy work, this also presents many wonderful possibilities that one system—as much as it may offer—cannot provide on its own. Ultimately, it is important to serve people with a method and not to preserve a method!

B. Additional symbols and mantras are integrated into the power flow of the Reiki system in the same or in a very similar way, just like Dr. Usui made the traditional four symbols and mantras part of the spiritual healing tradition that he founded at that time. Of course,

---

[15] During the era of Usui and Hayashi, the three degrees explained above were divided into six levels. However, the content was essentially the same. Sometimes the Power-Intensification Symbol was transmitted to experienced Reiki students of the 1st Degree. More information about the history of the Usui System of Natural Healing can be found in books like *The Spirit of Reiki* by Lübeck/Petter/Rand, Lotus Press.

this is possible because Dr. Usui was a human being and each of us can theoretically also accomplish what he achieved. The only problem is that this is not as easy as we would like to think it is...

To do this, we require the permission of the guardian deity of Reiki, *Dainichi Nyorai*, who will be discussed very extensively later in this book. We also need a strong personal resonance with this light being, as well as an appropriately profound understanding of the spiritual wisdom teachings connected with this being. Then, we must also—at least temporarily—consciously or unconsciously enter into the state of enlightenment that is necessary, together with the corresponding expertise regarding the task to be accomplished. However, perfection in latter is not an absolute requirement in all cases when there is a very committed cooperation by the angels, Bodhisattvas, and spiritual guides.

Just as the traditional four symbols and mantras strengthen Reiki and allow it to manifest more powerfully in material reality or direct the flow of spiritual life energy into certain vibratory levels or energetic fields of a living being, additional symbols and mantras can have a similar effect. For example, Rainbow Reiki includes four such tools that are connected with the spiritual elements of earth, water, fire, and air. They can be used to direct the spiritual life energy to the areas of a living being's energy systems, to specifically send Reiki to the blockages or structures of certain chakras, or to provide Reiki to the part of a person that is associated with relationships. It is quite obvious that these additional tools should not be called "traditional Reiki according to Dr. Usui."

The next chapter will provide more precise information on how the symbols of the Reiki healing system function, how to receive more power from them, and how to work with them in a more flexible way.

CHAPTER 2

Rei Ki Gong

The work with the symbols and their mantras assumes a central position in the Usui System of Natural Healing. Anyone initiated into the symbols and mantras can do Reiki energy work with them. However, how effective the respective technique is depends upon how these tools are used. In order to help the readers get the highest degree of spiritual healing energy from each symbol, this chapter reveals the finer points and tricks of Rei Ki Gong—which is admittedly an artificial word combining Japanese and Chinese terms. But it fits well with the meaning: There is Qi Gong (work with the life energies in general) and Rei Ki Gong (work with the spiritual life energy). This chapter explains in detail what can be done with the symbols, as well as the practices with them that are practically unknown here in the Western world. They are based on the ancient Taoist and Shinto teachings. The experiences that are possible with these techniques are very profound, so they are worth trying out. Practice one technique per day and always wait at least 24 hours before trying out the next technique. Once you are familiar with the effect, you can obviously continue on as you like in the way that works best for you. When doing a new form of energy work, it is always useful to first become thoroughly familiar with the various effects before intensively practicing with them. This also helps prevent grounding problems and spontaneously occurring, more intensive healing reactions.

The Most Frequent Mistakes When Using the Symbols and Mantras

In the course of my teaching work, I have observed a series of mistakes that very frequently occur regarding the application of mantras and symbols. Interestingly enough, I've noticed time and again on my travels throughout the world for the sake of Reiki that these problems seem to be equally widespread in almost all of the various countries. This section discusses and clarifies these application mistakes for the benefit of everyone who uses the symbols.

Applying the Symbols and Their Mantras Too Quickly and Inattentively

Life energy follows our attentiveness. The more hastily, less concentrated, and quickly we draw the symbols and speak the mantras, the less life energy—no matter what type—can be summoned. It is important to draw the symbols *slowly*, as in Tai Chi Chuan or Qi Gong exercises, and speak the mantras *attentively* and *with emphasis*.

It is correct that the 2nd Degree basically offers the possibility of doing mental energy work. However, this type of application must be preceded by carefully integrating what we have learned. In the practice, this means drawing the symbols slowly and consciously with the palm chakra and saying the associated mantra in a loud and emphasized way, whenever this is possible, in order to bring the mind and body using the tools into the closest possible resonance through this consciousness work relating to the symbols and mantras. It is also a good idea to draw the symbols on paper every few weeks and compare them with the originals, such as those in this book. Mistakes that are hardly noticeable can easily occur when "drawing in the air."

Later, after this practice phase, the symbols can obviously be drawn mentally[16] with the intention of appearing at a certain place. The mantras can also be recited silently. However, in my own practice, I use every opportunity that arises to apply the symbols and mantras directly and in a „hands-on" way to further perfect my own Reiki abilities.

---

[16] If the Reiki symbols are drawn with the hands, the secondary chakras in the palms and/or finger pads do the work of forming the symbol. If the symbol is formed mentally (spiritually), the power of the hand chakras to create it must take effect through the aura. This makes its effect indirect in contrast to the direct, form-giving movement of the hands. Of course, drawing it through the aura has a similar effect to when this is done through the hand chakras if the mind has adopted a clear, precise image of the symbols used and proceeds very consciously in setting up the symbols.

The symbols and mantras will definitely also function to a certain degree, which is adequate for most applications, when they are just used mentally. But there is an enormous increase in the effects when we use them as explained above and continue to practice them. Just like every art, the Reiki skills can also be continually improved through the appropriate practices. Reiki is so wonderful—the more familiar I am with it, the greater my deep respect for the lifework of Dr. Mikao Usui becomes.

Indiscriminate Applications of the Symbols and Mantras

The symbols and mantras all have unique meanings and functions. The better we understand these special qualities, the more successful the results will be in the application. It has been my experience that the less we understand their characteristics and respect them, the less powerful they will become over time.

Many Reiki friends who do not know this come to the conclusion that the energy-work tools passed down to us by Dr. Usui are no longer up-to-date or somehow "watered down" or blocked because of other influences when treatments with them do not produce satisfactory results. That this is not true can be easily demonstrated. The mantras and symbols must simply be used in the proper way. Some of these aspects have already been explained in the previous section. It is also important to increasingly have a better understanding and appropriately apply each symbol with its unique qualities both in the theoretical and the practical sense. In this process, a major problem can be the indiscriminate application of all the symbols and mantras familiar to the Reiki practitioner during the treatment positions. This is comparable to the handyman who uses all of his tools, from the hammer drill to the spirit-level, when repairing the plug of an electrical device because he knows that they are all good, powerful, and expensive—but unfortunately not suitable for every purpose. If used improperly, they may even cause damage. Although it is not possible to directly harm someone with Reiki, I believe that it is already a problem when a person does everything possible in terms of healing and actually doesn't know why he/she is doing it and exactly how it works. This rapidly decreases the effectiveness, and the success of the treatment may be far less than the possibilities of the method—which is obviously quite unfortunate for those who seek healing.

As a result, the symbols should be used in a way that is appropriate to their respective meanings for achieving the best results. A widespread error related to this topic is the belief that the symbols are essentially different from each other only in regard to their strength.

For example: The Power-Intensification Symbol strengthens Reiki, the Mental-Healing Symbol heightens it even more, the Distant-Treatment Symbol makes Reiki even stronger, and the Master Symbol increases the effect the most.

This approach is completely wrong!

Every symbol is a type of special tool that contributes its specific and unique powers to the Reiki System.

The respective chapters of this book contain explanations about the special powers of each of the traditional Reiki symbols, which have been extensively, precisely researched and carefully examined in the practice.

Effective Applications for the Symbols and Their Mantras

There are a great many different ways to use the Reiki symbols and their mantras handed down to us by Dr. Usui. The results can also vary significantly. This section explains how to call upon the highest possible spiritual powers by means of these wonderful tools of healing and personal development. It is important for us to have a responsible approach to the powerful divine forces of healing that are evoked in this way—they always work and do so solely in the sense of life, love, and the divine order. Yet, some people have a hard time opening up to their own purpose and saying "yes!" to the divine truth. It is often easier to do this in little steps. The unbelievable healing force of the symbols can also be used to harmonize difficulties that appear insurmountable. However, the most useful approach is a calm, prudent one because it gives the respective person time to become accustomed to new things in the correct way and really let go of what is no longer useful.

The Right Way to Draw a Reiki Symbol

Preparation: Breathe slowly and consciously several times into your hara, which can be found about two fingerwidths beneath your navel on the center line of your body and about two fingerwidths toward the inside. Leave a little pause each time between the inhalation and exhalation and feel the life energy that collects in your hara as you do this.

Now imagine[17] that a powerful stream of golden light is flowing from your hara over your belly, chest, shoulder, arm, and the hand that is drawing the symbol. Draw the symbol using your palm,[18] this is the biggest chakra in the area of the hand with the golden light in slow, flowing movements. In your mind's eye, the golden light[19] should leave a thick trail of golden metal behind as the strokes form the symbol. The energetic structure of a symbol is essentially formed out of the body's own high-frequency ki from the hand and finger chakras. The loss of the body's own ki is very quickly balanced by the start of the Reiki flow based on the increased activity of these energy centers, as I have been able to determine

[17] In visualization exercises there are frequently problems because the person assumes that everything must appear in the mind's eye exactly like things are seen with the physical eyes. This is not true! All of us blessed with eyesight are constantly visualizing in everyday life by comparing what we see at the moment with what we have seen at some point in the past. Otherwise, we could not recognize it again! When two friends talk about a third person who is not there and say something about his appearance, both of them know what is meant because they remember what he looks like. And this is true even if they don't "see" with their mind's eye. It is completely adequate to be able to describe something that we would like to "see" mentally, coupled with the intention of imagining it in front of our inner eye. It is also obvious that the ability to visualize can be developed much further—even to the quality of intensive daydreams in which the dreamer only sees what appears on his inner "movie screen" despite having his eyes open. Almost everyone has experienced this at some time. So it is only necessary to have this ability ready to use when you want to include it in practices. But it doesn't need to be developed—it has already long been in use. Yet, as mentioned above, just daily visualization is required for the practices in this book. So don't worry about whether you can manage it. You already have everything that you need.

[18] The symbols are frequently drawn with one finger or the fingertips. Although this is acceptable because of the lesser capacity of the finger chakras, the effect is generally much weaker than when a symbol is set up with the palm chakra.

[19] The golden light is purely a stand-in to make the process tangible and controllable for the conscious mind. Reiki is not golden. It has no color at all.

in longer studies by means of aura/chakra-reading. So the body actually does not lose any ki when the symbols are set up, which is also evident in the practice. I have observed that people working with the symbols do not show any type of exhaustion. Instead, there seems to be an extensive vitalization that takes place after a short amount of time.

If the symbols are consciously created from the much stronger ki of the hara, they can fulfill their antenna function, through which Reiki is pulled into this world and directed at a specific task much more effectively, as has been confirmed by the practice. Yet, many more beautiful things can be done by means of the symbol work with the ki of the hara, as shown in the next paragraph…

The Correct Way to Withdraw a Reiki Symbol

When a symbol has had its effect, it doesn't really need to "stand around" anymore. To withdraw the hara-ki[20] with which you have formed it, use the method described below. You may ask why it is necessary to do this. First of all, nothing bad happens when we leave a symbol „standing around." A number of such symbols in a room may be somewhat irritating for people with strong psychic abilities. However, since the symbol will dissolve itself after a while on its own and reunite with the flow of the environmental energies, depending upon the care with which it was set up, the effects should only be temporary.

However, there are strong, pleasant effects that result from a correct withdrawal of the body's own life energy that is saturated with concentrated Reiki. When this high-frequency mixture of life energy is brought back into the hara, it has a lasting effect that is especially beneficial to the organism by improving and strengthening health, as well as developing the spiritual gifts. As a result of this simple technique, which practically happens as a „side effect" when Reiki is used, the hara-ki is transformed

---

[20] In more precise terms, the hara-ki is the archetypal ki of the water elements (according to the Chinese teaching of the Five Elements). It is created from the essential ki of the kidneys and, either when necessary or through conscious effort, is fed into the so-called small energy cycle consisting of the serving and governing vessel, from which all of the other life-energy meridians that are familiar to us from acupuncture receive their power.

more and more into a special spiritual quality. For this process, the very complicated and time-consuming exercises of classic Chinese Qi Gong are otherwise necessary. The transformation of the hara-ki promotes spiritual development of the so-called three hearts, the three *Dan Tiens*. This results in a strengthening of the Shen, the divine spirit in human beings. Over time, this spirit then achieves its full ability to function.

Procedure: With your left hand, if you are right-handed (otherwise with your right hand), draw the structure of the symbols while you imagine inhaling its energy into your hara and gathering it there. Don't worry if this doesn't work while you are inhaling on one breath. Stop your movement while you exhale and then complete the strokes of the symbol with your hand. Then place both hands in the shape of an X with light pressure on your hara and direct your attention to this area. Imagine that the light pressure is creating a type of incline in your energy system through which all of the energy that is currently not needed for anything flows to the hara and collects there as if it were in a cistern. Observe this process for about one to two minutes. Then the practice is over. If you like, give thanks and bow.

The Proper Use of a Reiki Mantra

In order to activate a traditional Reiki symbol, which means letting it do its work, speak the associated mantra three times aloud or consciously within. There are also big differences here as to how the mantra is used. The same principles basically apply as already explained above for the symbols. Through the initiations, even beginners can be sure that the symbols are safely activated when the mantras are used mentally. Yet, when we use the mantras correctly as explained below, the power of the activation can be increased enormously.

Procedure: Say the mantra clearly and, if possible, out loud with emphasis and a full voice. As an alternative, also practice singing the mantras. Invent melodies for them and try out various pitches until you have found the right one for you. After singing the mantra, take another moment to consciously sense the change in the energies in order to develop your spiritual abilities of perception. What has changed inside of you? What has changed in the room? Which area of your body do you feel with special clarity before the application? Which one afterward? Do you feel more lifted up toward heaven or drawn to the earth before or after?

The CR as a General Power-Intensifier

Unfortunately, the Power-Intensification Symbol CR is frequently under-estimated. According to my experience, the CR should basically always be used together with any of the other symbols by applying it after the respective symbol has been employed. The only exceptions occur in certain parts of the initiations into the Reiki degrees.

The CR greatly increases the effect on any of the other Reiki applications, such as the laying on of the hands, the aura or chakra work, mental healing, and distant treatments.

Exact Drawing of the Symbols– Correct Pronunciation of the Mantras

The symbols and mantras have unique meanings. If they are drawn or pronounced correctly, the (metaphorical) key turns in the lock and the door opens. Through the type of energy transmission in the initiations of traditional Reiki according to Usui, a certain breadth of variation is possible in the application of this energy-work tool. However, the safest approach is to follow the rules compiled on the basis of the tricks of the trade to guarantee that everything functions as it should and helps as much as possible. The appropriate chapters of this book contain many examples of how the symbols are correctly drawn according to the rules of Japanese calligraphy, as well as the proper spelling for the original names (mantras) of the symbols. Practitioners should make a habit of writing the symbols at least once a month on paper and comparing them with the models. If the symbols are just drawn in the air, unnoticed errors can easily slip in.

Rei Ki Gong Exercises

The following techniques can help you discover completely new possibilities of spiritual healing work with Reiki. At the same time, they will teach you how to awaken the slumbering power of the symbols and use them in a meaningful way. The symbols and mantras should be used in the following techniques just as they are described above in this chapter in order to achieve the optimal effects.

Correctly Drawing a Symbol, Activating It with the Mantra, and Experiencing the Energy

Gather experiences with the effects of the symbols by using each of the four[21])—Power-Intensification Symbol (CR), Mental-Healing Symbol (SHK), Distant-Treatment Symbol (HS), and the Master Symbol (DKM)—according to the approach explained in the sections on The Right Way to Draw a Reiki Symbol and The Proper Use of Reiki Mantras. Draw it large, with a height of at least one yard, in front of you. Take your time and precisely feel within yourself the special quality of each symbol, both before and after the activation by the mantra. Hold your hands in front of the symbol, and then hold them inside of it. What do you perceive? Keep notes about your new experiences. Be sure to do this exercise even if you have already been working with the Reiki symbols for a long time. It is quite likely that you will experience some interesting surprises.

---

[21] The success of this practice obviously depends upon whether you are initiated into the symbols and mantras of the 2nd and/or 3rd Degree of the traditional Usui Reiki. Although it doesn't hurt, there also is no benefit if you are initiated into the 1st Degree, for example, and attempt to use the symbols from the 2nd and 3rd Degrees. Among other things, this is one of the reasons why Dr. Mikao Usui did his three-week meditation and fasting retreat in order to receive access to the spiritual powers of the Reiki System. If just reading the writings had been enough, he would not have had to subject himself to this great and risky effort.

Withdrawing the Energy of a Symbol and Storing It in the Hara

Take the energy of each of the symbols that you have formed in the previous exercise back into your hara, as explained in the section on The Correct Way to Withdraw a Reiki Symbol. Also note here what you have perceived for each of them.

The technique of building a symbol and withdrawing its spiritual energy into your hara is a wonderful, very effective, and important exercise in its own right. In more precise terms, this is the basic exercise of Rei Ki Gong, upon which all of the other techniques principally build. If you do them every day over a period of several weeks, you will perceive astonishingly positive changes within yourself on all levels of your being.

Taking a CR Symbol into a Chakra

Draw the CR Symbol as explained above in approximately the size of a soup plate about one hand-width over one of your major chakras or that of a practice partner. Activate the symbol by pronouncing its mantra three times. Now carefully use your hands to touch the sides of the symbol, as if it were a material substance. Move it slowly and evenly somewhat into the selected chakra. It is helpful when the person receiving this treatment connects with the chakra through consciously inhaling. Keep the symbol in the energy center for several minutes. Then move it back out again. When you want to end the exercise, absorb its energy back into your hara again. If you would like to have some more exciting experiences right after this, move the CR in sequence through several of the other major chakras. Remember to write down your experiences, at least in key words. At the end of the exercise, always be sure to take the energy of the symbols back into your hara.

This technique powerfully supports inner healing for the energy centers (chakras) of all types, improves their relationships with the rest of the energy systems, and increases their vibration, depending upon how long the symbol stays in the chakra, even into spiritual realms. If this practice is done for a longer period of time (five minutes and more per energy center) and with all six major chakras, this has the best results.

"Snapping" a CR into the Hara

Draw a CR with approximately the size of a saucer about one hand-width above your hara[22] or that of an exercise partner. Activate it by pronouncing its mantra three times. Grasp it at the sides with both hands, as if it existed on the physical plane, and move it into the hara. Guide the symbol back and forth carefully and attentively until you get a feeling if how it interacts with the hara. Now find out where you have to move it in the hara so that it „snaps into place." This will become apparent when the resistance against the movement of the CR in any direction briefly increases and then it once again lets itself be guided without any noticeable resistance in the hara. When you have found the point, leave it there for a few minutes. Then move it out again and take its energy back into your hara, as explained above.

When practiced every day, this exercise will activate and qualitatively improve almost every function of the hara. It is very well suited for providing support to the healing of exhausted adrenal glands

Positioning the CR Over the Client's Body and Making It Resonate

Draw a large CR over a practice partner so that it extends from the crown to the pelvis. Of course, it can also be large enough to cover the entire body. Activate it by pronouncing its mantra three times. Now tap it carefully with the fingers of one hand, like a bell that you would like to ring. Instead, or in addition, you can also tone on the vowel sounds, sing overtones, or recite mantras (for example: *Om Mani Padme Hum*) in order to let the structure of the CR resonate.

How does the CR feel before it begins to resonate? How does it feel afterward? How does it feel when you use the variety of methods mentioned above to make it resonate?

By using the Reiki distant treatment, you can also employ this practice for yourself.

---

[22] The hara is located about two fingerwidths below the navel and somewhat inside the body.

This practice is also very good for clearing, harmonizing, and strengthening the aura. In addition, it intensively improves the ability of the aura to resonate for spiritual influences of all types. As a result, it becomes easier to do things like communicate with angels and other light beings, work clairvoyantly, or go on astral journeys.

Letting the CR Symbol Resonate in Rooms, Power Places, and Gardens

One Feng-Shui application of this technique consists of drawing a CR symbol horizontally in a room so that it fills the entire space. The middle of the symbol should be located somewhere near the center of the room. Activate the CR in the usual way. Then stand at its center, place the palms of your hands together in front of your heart, and begin singing vowels, overtones, or mantras. Do this for about 5 minutes. Then sit down quietly and consciously feel the new energy in the room. What has changed?

This technique can be used with fantastic effects at power places or in group meditations. To do this, have the participants sit or stand in a circle and draw the CR symbol so that it is very large and on the horizontal plane in the circle. Otherwise, this approach is the same as described above. However, other people can continuously alternate going into the center of the circle to get the CR to resonate. It is also possible for several people to work with the energies at the center point simultaneously.

An entire building can also be treated in this way during distant treatments. Also try to have the CR "snap into place" at the center of a building, as with the chakra of a human being. A garden can be treated in a similar way. Here as well, put the center of the CR symbol in the middle of the garden.

"Snapping" the SHK into the Pineal Gland

Draw a SHK symbol approximately the size of a saucer above the crown of your exercise partner. Activate it by pronouncing its mantra three times. Grasp it with both hands at the sides, as if it existed on the physical plane, and move it into the your partner's head until it is about one fingerwidth above the connecting line of the eyebrows, which is at about the middle of the skull. Move the symbol carefully and attentively back and forth a bit until you get a feeling for how it is interacting with the pineal gland. Now find out precisely where you have to move it in the head to that it "snaps into place." You can recognize this by the brief increase in resistance against moving the SHK in any direction. Then it will be possible to move it again without any noticeable resistance in the head. Once you have found the point, leave it there for several minutes. Then move it out and absorb its energy back into your hara, as explained above.

Also vary this technique by additionally using the CR symbol on the same area of the body—directly after the SHK Symbol and its mantra.

With everyday practice, this exercise will activate, harmonize, and clearly improve the functional qualities of the pineal gland and other glands in the brain that work with it.

By using a Reiki distant treatment, you can also apply this exercise to yourself.

This technique is very well suited for supporting the healing of all types of health problems that are related to the endocrine glands throughout the body. In addition, this exercise provides very effective support for spiritual development and some types of mental-emotional disorders respond quite well to it. Experiment with it in the individual cases, and remember that it is necessary to complete any type of intensive energy work by grounding the body through giving a Reiki treatment to the soles of the feet (toes to middle) at the conclusion of the session.

"Snapping" the HS into the Spinal Column

Draw HS Symbol with the palm of your hand above the spinal column of an practice partner so that it is large enough to extend from the coccyx to the back of the head (first cervical vertebra). Activate it by saying the associated mantra three times. Grasp it with both hands on the long sides, as if it existed physically, and move it into your partner's spinal column. Carefully and attentively move the symbol back and forth a few times until you get a feeling for how it interacts with the energetic structure of the spinal column. Now find out exactly where you have to move it in the area of the spine so that it "snaps into place." You will discover this by feeling where the resistance against the movement of the HS increases briefly in every direction and then lets itself be guided back and forth again without any noticeable resistance. Once you have found the point, leave the symbol there for several minutes. Then move it back out again and take the energy of its structure back into your hara, as explained above in the appropriate section.

You can also vary this technique by additionally using the CR Symbol at the same place in the body directly after the HS Symbol and its mantra.

By means of the Reiki distant treatment, you can obviously also do this practice for yourself.

This practice has a healing, strengthening, and harmonizing effect on the spinal column and its surrounding areas.

This technique is well-suited for supporting healing in relation to all types of problems found in the spinal column and back, as well as preventing them. In addition, it generally reduces karmic burdens and other emotional and energetic blockages in the area of the spinal column and back. It strengthens and develops the three main energy channels of the backbone—*Îdâ, Sushumnâ,* and *Pingalâ.* This same principle applies to the four branches of the bladder meridian and the kidneys that run parallel to the spinal column. This approach will increase the individual frequencies of their own energetic structures.

The technique is also well-suited for harmonizing the effects of the Kundalinî force rising.

"Snapping" the DKM into the 7th Chakra

Draw the DKM Symbol with your palm about one hand-width above the crown of a practice partner. Activate it by saying the associated mantra three times. Grasp it with both hands on the long sides, as if existed physically, and move it a bit downward and to one side and then the other. Carefully and attentively guide the symbol back and forth a few times until you have a feeling for how it interacts with the energetic structure of the crown chakra (7th chakra). Now find out exactly where you must move it over the center of the crown and about three fingerwidths above it so that it "snaps into place." You will determine that the resistance against the movement of the DKM in every direction briefly increases and then you can guide it back and forth again without much resistance. Once you have found the point, leave the symbol there for a few minutes. Then move it back out and absorb the energy of its structure back into your hara, as explained above.

You can also vary this technique by additionally using the CR Symbol at the same place in your body directly after the DKM Symbol and its mantra.

By means of the Reiki distant treatment, you can naturally also do this practice for yourself.

With the help of this technique, you can harmonize a material orientation that is too excessive. In addition, it helps us keep a perspective in difficult times and remain true to ourselves and our spiritual path. When used on a daily, long-term basis, it can have a rejuvenating effect. It awakens or increases spiritual powers and supports the meaningful integration of all types of experiences.

Mantra Meditation with the Reiki Symbols and a Breathing Technique

Select one of the four traditional Reiki symbols. Draw it large enough in the air in front of you so that there is room for your entire body. Activate it by pronouncing the associated mantra three times. Step into the symbol. Breathe into your hara and leave a little pause each time between exhaling and inhaling so you can feel the life force. Say the mantra of the symbol 108 times. Afterward, place your hands in the form of an x across your heart area and take a few minutes to feel the spiritual power.

Step out of the symbol and take the spiritual energy of its structure back into your hara, as explained above.

By means of this very intensive practice, the light beings who watch over the selected symbol will become your spiritual teachers. They will show and explain many things to you that are not written in any book. This may sometimes arise in your consciousness during the practice, but it usually only happens after hours or even days. The light beings will only very rarely appear to you. They will not give you any tasks in relation to other people and do not want you to "obey" them. You also will not be required to write a new Bible or save the world. But they will help you to better understand yourself, your path, and the divine. This can support you in solving some of the everyday problems in a spiritual manner.

Don't forget to make notes about your experiences after every practice. It's best to use a special book that only serves this one purpose.

Scanning the Body with the CR Symbol

Draw the CR Symbol with your palm about one hand-width above the 3rd chakra (solar plexus) of a practice partner. Activate it by saying the associated mantra three times. Carefully move your hand with its palm above the center of the symbol. Imagine that it is now sticking to your palm, as if it existed on the physical plane. Now move it over all the areas of the body. Guide the symbol carefully and attentive, paying attention to where you feel distinctly stronger energetic activity in your palm chakra. Then treat this area by remaining above it in the aura for several minutes or until you distinctly feel less power flowing. Then continue to look for other areas that need treatment and do the same process there as well.

When the treatment time is over, absorb the structural energy of the CR Symbol back into your hara.

By means of the Reiki distant healing, you can also do this practice for your own benefit.

Pacing Off the Symbols

Select a symbol with which you would like to practice. Place one hand on the 6th chakra and the other hand on the 2nd chakra. Give yourself Reiki like this for about three minutes. Breathe into your hara as you do this. While leaving the one hand on the 6th chakra, now place the other hand on your 4th chakra, your heart area, also for about three minutes. Now place both hands in the form of an x on your heart, breathe into your hara, and walk like this through the room as if you were painting the symbol on the floor. Repeat its mantra during the entire time that you are pacing off the symbol. It should be repeated at least 108 times while you pace. Stop the mantra recitation when you finish a "stroke" and must go to the beginning of the next stroke. This is necessary for all of the symbols, except for the power-intensification sign (CR). Once you have reached the end of the last stroke, sit or lay down and breathe into your hara for about three minutes while you give yourself Reiki on the 6th and 2nd major chakras, followed by three minutes on the 6th and 4th major chakras. How do you feel about yourself now? How has the room changed? Do you feel more elevated to heaven or drawn to the earth?

Now pace back again through the strokes every step of the way and absorb the energy into your hara, as explained above.

You can use this technique to change the energetic structures of rooms and gardens. However, it primarily serves to more strongly connect you with the power and wisdom of the respective signs and promote deeper states of spiritual self-contemplation.

CHAPTER 3

The Traditional Reiki Initiations

This book extensively explains the traditional symbols and mantras used in the Usui System of Natural Healing in both theory and practice. A very significant aspect is the application of these tools in the initiations, which reveal the variety of Reiki skills to the students. These venerable rituals still seem like miracles to me (Walter) today, even though I have done them for years and have experienced their never-failing, astonishing direct and indirect effects so often on myself and my students.

There are a great many different forms of initiations that can be found throughout the world. I often come across the opinion that it more or less doesn't matter what happens in these rituals as long as they include the desire to awaken the Reiki skills. This attitude is definitely wrong since there certainly is a technical aspect to Reiki. This means that certain functions must be fulfilled to basically transform a person into a Reiki channel and awaken the many different Reiki abilities. In addition, there are a series of measures so that this profound spiritual opening and transformation occurs in a gentle and safe way for every student.

If an initiation would function purely on good will, it would not have been necessary for Usui to do a 21-day retreat with a special meditation technique and fasting at one of the strongest power places in Japan in order to open himself permanently for Reiki. Of course, a great many people have already attempted to have themselves initiated from books or "automatically" through the Internet by clicking the icons. However, I have never encountered anyone who has had his/her Reiki abilities awakened as a result. But it is important to address the following question:

Why Are Initiations Necessary?

Certain abilities of active energy work (healing, for example) and passive energy work (such as clairvoyance) are given to very few people from the start because of an appropriately oriented positive karma that they

71

have attained in past incarnations. But even these great talents must be carefully and patiently developed through training and practice so that they can be reliably put to use in a practical way. Most people who want to acquire such abilities must practice intensively for many, many years to make themselves resonant for these tremendous powers—in addition to the training and practice that are obviously always required. Since the beginning of time, spiritual seekers have faced the great challenge that there are so many wonderful abilities resulting from an intimacy with the divine power that not only make life easier in a natural way but can also be applied in an extremely effective manner in supporting their own path to enlightenment and spiritual awakening. However, when a large part of life must be used for acquiring a few abilities of this kind, there is not much of an opportunity to use them for the actual goal, the process of spiritual realization. In addition, most people hardly have (or had) the time required for such ventures in addition to their everyday duties. And someone must also plow the fields, print and sell the books, bake the bread, and build the houses. There are not enough cozy caves in the mountains of this beautiful world to take in as many billions of hermits as there are people. And who would feed them if they all spent the entire day meditating and dreaming of enlightenment?

In order to progress correctly, we should also have certain spiritual abilities available to us in the short term that actually can only be awakened after long periods of practice and studies in seclusion. This is tricky!

The solution to this Gordian knot is the initiations! In every spiritual tradition that I am aware of, the appropriate abilities are transmitted by the people who are trained and qualified to the students so that it is easier for them to make major progress in their personal development within a relatively short time and—quite incidentally—also be able to helpfully assist their fellow human beings in overcoming typical life problems such as disease, poverty, misfortune, and the like.

Well-known examples of initiations are: *Shaktipat* in Hinduism, the initiations into mantras such as in the system of Transcendental Meditation (TM), and Kriyâ Yoga.

By means of the initiations, certain abilities can basically be awakened in a human being. Yet, training and some experience are always required in order to use them in an effective and meaningful way. Although the initiations may have the effect of stimulating personal development, we still must always tackle the learning experiences, decisions, awareness exercises, experiments in new types of behavior, attempts to overcome the ego, and the like on our own.

Various Types of Initiations

The Reiki initiations are not the only way to awaken spiritual powers in an individual. There are various, basically different types of initiations.

Self-Initiation

Dr. Mikao Usui's 21-day period of meditation and fasting: Special conditions are necessary in order for something like this to function. First, the respective person must have precise knowledge about the area in which he would like to become active with the abilities awakened by the initiation. The correct type of practice must be done, and this should occur for a sufficient amount of time and at a place offering favorable spiritual preconditions. The time period for the initiation must be selected so that the astrological transits support the practitioner's efforts. The inner attitude of the practitioner is a decisive factor. Without a motivation that is humble, coming from the heart, and oriented toward serving in the sense of the Divine Order, even the best external preconditions and strictest practice discipline does not make a spiritual initiation possible since it is ultimately divine grace that does this. The person can prepare for it—but the Creative Force makes the decision!

Initiation Through a Light Being

In rare cases, people are initiated by a spirit while they are sleeping or meditating or in a moment when they hardly expect such an experience. This happens almost always just after long, intensive periods of involvement with a spiritual theme for which there is no human teacher at the time who could initiate and train the respective person. There is a general rule that applies here: If the new ability is not used three times in the service of the Divine Order within one moon cycle—until the moon is back at the same place where it was at the time of the initiation—it will disappear again. Then the initiation no longer exists. Being initiated by angels or similar spiritual beings is normally an extremely impressive experience. It often changes the person's entire outlook on life in a lasting way. The necessary training has either already been conveyed primarily through the appropriate knowledge from books, inspiration, or direct contact with a light being so that this is "just" a matter of having attentive and persistent experiences with the newly acquired talents or it is appropriately transmitted after the initiation. The same principle applies here as above: Those who do not learn and practice will have very little from the gift.

Reactivating an Initiation that Has Been Received in a Past Life

A spiritual ability acquired in a past life is sometimes reawakened on the basis of an effort that is usually unconscious for the most in relation to a spiritual theme. In general, this is accompanied in some way by more or less coherent memories from the respective incarnations. This may also take place within the scope of a regression or meditation.[23] As in the initiation through a light being, the new ability must also be put into practice in the service of the Divine Order three times within the course

---

[23] I (Walter) have had the opportunity to collect many experiences with this type of initiation. New, old abilities have constantly been surfacing within me ever since I consciously decided—around 1988—to (once again) live as a spiritual teacher. Gifts and knowledge received in past incarnations, as well as the experiences of many lives as a High Priest of the Great Goddess in places like Lemuria, pre-Vedic India, Sumeria, Babylon, and Egypt, have gradually arisen through the years within me. Today (2004) more than approximately 85% of the teachings imparted to me come from these sources. During the first years, I was still very uncertain about what was entering my consciousness. Yet, through the confirmation coming from the practical effects that I experienced over and over again, I began to trust increasingly in this great gift. Lemurian Tantra, large portions of Rainbow Reiki, the shamanic White Feather Path, the Three-Ray Meditation, Heavenly Dragon Qi Gong, the Crystal Path, and the training system in spiritual perception (aura/chakra-reading, channeling, astral travel, and clairvoyance) all came back to me in this way and I "only" had to adapt the ancient wisdom to the circumstances of our age.

of one moon cycle, until the moon is back in the same place as it was during the initiation.

In my experience, humility and making a serious effort to follow the spiritual path are both absolute preconditions for self-initiation, initiation through a light being, or reactivation of an initiation from a previous incarnation.

Initiation By a Teacher

This path of initiation is probably the easiest to understand: You attend a seminar or training session, learn something, and receive an initiation so that what you have learned also functions in a satisfactory and lasting way.

Two Different Qualities of Initiations:
Awakening Abilities and Acquisition of Abilities

Initiations can essentially make it possible to access two very different types of abilities:

- ॐ A potential that basically exists within every human being can be awakened. One example of this is initiation into the Usui System of Natural Healing.

- ॐ A potential that does not naturally exist within every human being is practically gifted to a person. An example of this is the gift of working with the healing power of an angel.

The Reiki Initiations

The following section describes the initiation into the 1st Degree of the traditional Usui System of Reiki as an example of what actually occurs in these rituals.

The technical details of the initiation ritual are not covered here. On the one hand, they are not included because this could easily encourage the wrong impression that this is the only correct way to initiate. And that would absolutely not be true! Many paths lead to Rome. Not just any arbitrary path, but many. On the other hand, I am convinced that it is more meaningful to learn the initiations within the scope of the personal encounter in a seminar, by asking questions, and by being able to practice under guidance in order to be really sure of imparting to other people the gift of bringing Reiki into this world.

What Happens During the Initiation into the 1st Degree?

In the initiations into the 1st Degree, a Reiki Master uses the symbols and mantras (sacred words that evoke the spiritual energies and apply them for a specific purpose) that Dr. Usui found in the old scrolls on the methods of the Healing Buddha or developed on the basis of them. Through the initiation that the Reiki Master has received and the symbols and mantras of the 3rd Degree received from his/her Master, he/she is capable of creating a lasting connection to the source of spiritual life energy for any other human being.

The symbols and mantras are used within the scope of traditional rituals that are necessary for activating Reiki abilities and directing the organizing powers into certain chakras that participate in the transmission of the spiritual life energy.

However, these methods cannot function when the person applying them has not received the Master Initiation in the traditional way.

Let's use the analogy of a radio again. It doesn't work without electricity. Because of this, it also was not possible for Dr. Usui to immediately work with Reiki after he had found the scrolls from the ancient treasure of wisdom in Esoteric Buddhism. We can be certain that he tried it. Only after three weeks of fasting and meditating—and through the grace of the Creative Force—did he attain access to the source of spiritual life energy, without which none of the techniques could have been put to use.

Four partial initiations are necessary for acquiring the complete set of skills in the 1st Degree. However, these are summarized into two or even one initiation in many schools of Reiki. In Rainbow Reiki, the four partial initiations are given in order to accustom the students to their new abilities in the gentlest way possible and give them adequate opportunity to consciously enjoy the sometimes profound spiritual experiences.

Every partial initiation fulfills a different important function. Each partial initiation should be separated from the previous one by about 3 hours in order to guarantee optimal integration of the spiritual effects. Partial initiations should not be more than 24 hours apart because otherwise the energetic correlations may be lost and within about 10 days the student's Reiki abilities are very likely to disappear again.

The effect of the Reiki initiations in all degrees only influences the chakras indirectly. On a very deep energetic level, it dissolves the blockages in the area of the karma of a race that keeps people from experiencing a direct, comprehensive contact with the spiritual life energy. This is why, with the exception of attaining the Reiki abilities, which are explained in greater detail below, the spiritual and physical effects of the initiations are different in each individual. Reiki is basically available to every living being. Without the appropriate initiation, the spiritual life energy—in figurative terms—comes in drips and drops. After an initiation, Reiki flows to the initiated person in a powerful, even, and constantly available current that can even grow enormously through regular practice.

Certain chakras are touched by the attunements: They are practically used as gateways. However, the real changes take place on much deeper levels, in the so-called light body[24]. This is a spiritual structure that directs and organizes the non-polar life forces like Reiki. From here, the information is sent to the chakra system to control its processes. The chapter entitled „The Spiritual Energy System of Human Beings" provides more information on this topic.

Which Specific Powers Are Imparted Through the 1st Degree Initiation?

There are essentially five different abilities:

1. The initiated person becomes a channel for Reiki, the spiritual life force. He/She can bring this energy form to earth at any time by laying on his/her hands when they are needed. To do this, he/she does not need to concentrate, complete specific practices, or restrict his/her

---

[24] There is a corresponding training for this in the Rainbow Reiki tradition: The Rainbow Reiki Light-Body Work, which is imparted by qualified teachers throughout the world.

lifestyle. When Reiki is needed, it is enough to lay on the hands or come into contact with the recipient through the aura in order to let the force flow. The recipient always absorbs Reiki. In the narrower sense of the word, it cannot be sent but is just made available.

2. A type of energetic protection is created that prevents the personal energy of the Reiki channel from unconsciously[25] being transmitted in a larger extent to the recipient. This prevents a weakening of the practitioner and keeps the person receiving treatment from being burdened on the energetic level by disharmonious structures of the Reiki-giver. If this protection is not available, it is possible that some energies from the practitioner can penetrate into the recipient's inner energy system, remaining there and causing problems. This is not an inevitable result, but it always occurs to some extent. Depending on the energetic and psychological stability, as well as the strength of the recipient's powers of self-healing, this way of transferring disharmonious energies can have a great variety of consequences.

3. The Reiki channel receives protection that prevents disharmonious energies from the person receiving the treatment to be transmitted to him/her. This allows the practitioner to remain free of empathetic illnesses and seriously disruptive outside energies. However, the ability to feel the other person energetically is maintained. This can also be accompanied by irritations, which is why the hands should be washed after a treatment or an aura-cleansing technique should be used. Even with somewhat normal energetic and psychological stability on the part of the practitioner, there should not be any serious difficulties that occur because of energy perception. It is more like a film that we do not like or a newspaper report that awakens unpleasant associations.

4. The sensitivity for subtle energies is increased. After the 1ˢᵗ Degree seminar, many people notice entirely new perceptions in their hands when they lay them somewhere for a longer period of time or hold

---

[25] Please pay attention to this restriction: A person who is addicted to the helper syndrome and absolutely wants to suffer along with someone else will additionally transmit his/her own life force in addition to the Reiki. Reiki protects us but it respects the free will that the Creative Force gives every human being from the very start.

them in the aura of a living being. Through regular Reiki practice and the appropriate practices, this ability can be perfected to a large degree.

5. All of these abilities will become permanently anchored deep within the energy system of the respective person. They cannot be dissolved by anything because they are ultimately a divine gift that was already present in the human organism before the initiation. It may have been dormant, but it belonged to the person like the arms or legs. Once it has been completely reawakened, it cannot be „put to sleep" again.

Because of this, each person only needs to participate once in his/her life in the initiation into the 1st Reiki Degree. And it is absolutely certain that anyone who has been involved in the initiations of a 1st Degree seminar receives these abilities. There are no unsuccessful initiations as long as they are done by a traditionally trained Master with the symbols, mantras, and rituals that have been handed down. This may sound somewhat presumptuous to some people. After all, we all make mistakes. So why doesn't this also apply to Reiki Masters? And this reasoning is completely right. But it is not the Master who ultimately gives the initiation. He/She only establishes the contact to the source of the spiritual life energy, the Divine Beings *Dainichi Nyorai* and *Dai Marishi Ten,* and serves as a channel for their spiritual power, wisdom, and love. These light beings have considerably more comprehensive possibilities of energy work at their disposal than any human being. A Reiki initiation is something very, very simple for them. They are extremely capable servants of the Creative Force.

What human beings do is imperfect and transitory—this is a typical characteristic of human beings that is important from the spiritual perspective. However, a covenant entered into by the Creative Force is not subject to the laws of the material world and cannot be faulty. This has also been demonstrated in the corresponding experience with the Reiki initiations. No matter whether a Reiki Master is tired, has a toothache or headache, is love-sick, or in a depressed mood—as long as he/she follows the traditional initiation rituals, they will have a completely reliable effect.

I am completely aware that it may be difficult for some people to believe this. I was also doubtful for many years until I finally submitted to the same positive experiences that were constantly repeated.

79

The Individual Steps of the Traditional Reiki Initiation into the 1st Degree

The following are the basic steps of the traditional Reiki initiations into the 1st Degree. Each of these functions can be done correctly in very different ways in terms of the "technical aspects of the energy work." So there are no generally binding standard solutions.

- ✪ Invoking the spiritual lineage.

- ✪ Preparing the aura of the student to be initiated to receive—producing a yin-oriented state.

- ✪ Awakening the Reiki ability and stabilizing this measure.

- ✪ Integrating important major and secondary chakras into the current of the Reiki force.

- ✪ Energetic sealing of sensitive secondary chakras for the lasting stabilization of the Reiki abilities.

- ✪ The conclusion—normalizing the state of the individual's aura, as well as the aura of the entire group of initiates at the end of the initiation; asking for the blessing of the spiritual lineage, thanking it, and taking leave.

In conclusion, I would like to discuss two questions that are frequently asked on the topic of "initiations":

Is It Important to Have Both Hands Initiated into the 2nd Degree?

Some people believe that the three 2nd Degree symbols and their mantras should be given to both hands during the initiation into the 2nd Reiki Degree so that the symbols can be drawn with each of them and the yin-yang relationship remains balanced within the individual. Is this true?

First, here is the good news: An initiation of both hands never hurts anyone. But it also isn't necessary. During the initiation into the 2nd Degree, the mechanically more skilled hand is initiated with the symbols and mantras because this makes it easier to practice drawing the signs with pen and paper. The mechanically more skilled hand has a much better developed kinesthetic sense. This is the sense that informs the brain about the body movements. So far so good.

But once the student of the 2nd Reiki Degree has gotten the symbols and mantras "down" and can draw them from memory without any mistakes, it is usually unnecessary to keep drawing the sign by hand. Later on, the symbols and mantras of the 2nd Degree are primarily used mentally by advanced Reiki students, except when it is a matter of refreshing and practicing the knowledge. The 2nd Degree is a mental technique of energy work.

Since only the appropriate "tool box" of symbols and mantras is made available to the Reiki students through initiation into the 2nd Degree, there is also no shift of the yin-yang relationship in the body. During my training practice with hundreds of 2nd Degree students, I have never observed any unnatural "masculinization," "spiritualization," or any other clear signs of a yang imbalance—most people are right-handed and receive the symbols in this hand—as a result of the 2nd Degree initiations. Since many of my students are also frequently present in my seminars as guests through the years, as well as writing and calling me when they have news about their developmental process, my experiences have a long-term background. But, as I mentioned above, it also never hurts anyone to do this.

Foot Initiations

The Reiki Master, body therapist, and practicing naturopath Gerda Drescher (Switzerland) worked for a number of years to develop a method through which special energetic attunements (foot openings) are done within the context of long-term therapeutic measures for concretely improving the grounding of her clients. According to my research, Gerda was the first Master to work with foot initiations. She has used this method from the start with much therapeutic success and passes it on to her advanced students. In addition to this initiation technique, they are also comprehensively trained in the related physical and psychotherapeutic accompanying measures. She does not represent the viewpoint that:

✪ Foot initiations are a component of the traditional Usui System.

✪ Everyone who is initiated into Reiki automatically needs foot initiations because the body's energy field would otherwise be disharmonious or Reiki would not function properly.

✪ Foot initiations are a "must" in the Age of Aquarius.

✪ Grounding can only be achieved through foot initiations.

✪ Foot initiations are suitable for everyone.

Quote: "Their [referring to the foot initiations] effects have far-reaching consequences. In addition to an increased connection to Mother Earth, this integration of the lower pole also leads to the confrontation with the physical nature, the unconscious, unresolved aspects, and our own shadow. They [the foot openings] are therefore in no way suitable for filling a gap in the market and the wallet or polishing our own ego. Instead, they require a process-oriented approach, as well as responsible therapeutic know-how in accompanying the client! There is nothing that I can say about the effect of other foot openings that someone claims to have received directly from a chosen Master or personally through meditation from Usui, the archangels, the Holy Spirit, or even the Creative Force.

Although my foot openings were developed with intuition, this was still done completely unspectacularly in an empirical way, and this is what makes them especially valuable ... Rei-Ki-Balancing® is an invitation to connect more strongly through our own physical body with Mother Earth (Gaia) and challenges us to let our feet take us on the uncomfortable path of spirituality to wholeness as a process of individuation... Since I know that my work is correct and valuable, I have developed clear training structures and guidelines. It is possible to control the adherence to them through the revoking of a license. The basic training lasts at least 2 to 3 years (depending on previous knowledge) and also includes intensive and deep bodywork, among other things."

According to the information that I have received from Gerda Dre-scher, foot initiations are a very formidable and effective method for healing grounding problems in connection with the therapeutic guidance that she has developed.

PART II –

THE
EAST ASIAN SPIRITUAL BACKGROUND
OF THE TRADITIONAL USUI SYSTEM
OF NATURAL HEALING WITH REIKI

CHAPTER 4

Esoteric Buddhism

Esoteric Buddhism has a long history. The special traits of it are the secret teachings (Jap.: *mikkyô*), whose origins are in part much older than Buddhism itself. The secret teachings consist largely of magical rituals with mantras, mudrâs, and symbols. Their effects are manifested through the power of many light beings such as Buddhas, Bodhisattvas, gods, goddesses, and wisdom kings. Dr. Usui created his system of natural healing called Reiki on based on the secret teachings of Esoteric Buddhism, the Japanese magic *Shugendô*, and shamanism, as well as the path of the gods Shintô and the magical Taoism of China. In Japan, many individual spiritual traditions have merged with each other over the course of the centuries since they outstandingly complement each other. Reiki itself is a brilliant example of this, and the symbols are the evidence. The CR Symbol comes from *Shugendô* and *Shintô*, the SHK and DKM Symbol are from Esoteric Buddhism, and the HS Symbol is based on the wisdom of both magical Taoism and Esoteric Buddhism.

The Roots of Esoteric Buddhism

The origins of Esoteric Buddhism extend much further back in time than most people realize. India was actually not the birthplace of all the ancient philosophies and paths of healing. The Vedic texts may come to mind since they are said to be the oldest in the world and originated in India. India was the final stage of their long development The *Vedas* were first written down between 1200-600 B.C.[26] However, their content came from the very advanced civilization of Mesopotamia, if not even earlier. So these are also wisdom teachings that are at least 6,000 years old. The preserved texts include chronicles of kings, letters, procedures, poetry,

---

[26] There is a more detailed discussion of this topic in the chapter on the *Siddham*.

and, above all, magic spells. The secret teachings of Esoteric Buddhism are essentially based upon the *Vedas*. This knowledge with its magical rituals was brought to India in part by the nomadic tribes of the Aryans. Another part of it, especially the magic practices, are remainders of the great spiritual wisdom from the matriarchal cultures that were wiped out or assimilated by the Indo-Germanic Aryans. Its religion is Brahmanism, which then developed into Hinduism.[27]

Before his enlightenment, the historical Buddha Shâkyamuni learned rituals, magic, and meditation from the Brahmanic and shamanic masters. These practices were also still in use after the enlightenment of Buddha and only passed on to chosen students. This is the foundation for the secret teachings of Esoteric Buddhism. About 500 years after Buddha, people also began to write down his teachings. Each individual section of these sacred texts is called a sûtra. All of the texts together form the *Tripitaka*.

The historical Buddha held three major sermons, each of which represents the basis for one of the Buddhist schools. In his third sermon, he taught Esoteric Buddhism, which he called the Diamond Vehicle (Skr.: *Vajrayana*).[28] Although the roots of the secret teachings are older than Buddhism itself, the esoteric texts were the last to be written down. In

---

[27] Please compare this with the comments in the chapter on Spiritual Cosmology. In addition, there are two good reading recommendations: *Tantra: The Cult of the Feminine*, Andre van Lysebeth, Red Wheel Weiser and *The Once & Future Goddess*, Elinor W. Gadon, Harper San Francisco.

[28] In his first sermon, Buddha taught Hinayana or Theravada Buddhism, in which the individual's enlightenment through meditation is the focus. In his second sermon, he taught Mahâyâna Buddhism. This includes the teachings and practices of the first sermon. Moreover, it also includes the Bodhisattva vow. This means that a person vows to attain Buddhahood for the benefit of all sentient beings. From the perspective of Buddhism, this vow alone and the actions that result from it lead us more quickly to enlightenment. The disciples of the individual schools frequently do not accept the others and claim that only their path is the true one. Yet, by comparing the sutras, it is apparent that the foundations of Hinayana are present in Mahâyâna. In addition, Mahâyâna cannot be clearly separated from Vajrayana since the secret teachings are used in both. I consider it probable that the separation of the individual schools is a later invention. Additional names of Esoteric Buddhism are also *Tantrayana* and *Mantrayana*.

some circles, this has led to the assumption that Esoteric Buddhism was only added much later to Buddhism. This is obviously incorrect because the point in time of the written records is not at all related to its creation. The secret teachings consist largely of instructions for rituals. These were initially called *Vidhi* and later given the name of *Tantra*.

Around Buddha's lifetime, changes occurred in India on all levels. New teachings such as Buddhism and Jainism[29] arose, which also led to a movement away from the rigid order of Brahmanism. The historical Buddha was supportive of the people and called upon his students to be involved with the liberation of the mind instead of just wanting to look after their own well-being with magical rituals. However, he in no way excluded the applications of magic; instead, he gave them an altruistic dimension. He wanted to make it clear to his students that magic is only meaningful when it is used for the highest good of all beings involved. In addition, there is a difference between just applying magical techniques and being willing to develop ourselves so that magic can happen in a natural way and we attain wisdom, love, and consciousness. This ability is developed through what Buddha called the liberation of the mind. In addition, the applications of magical practices were commonplace for Buddha, and this was always done precisely when it was truly necessary.

In the sûtras, magical or even esoteric practices are called *paritta*. Using these, for example, it is possible for a person to be protected against the bites of poisonous snakes and other animals, as well as from various types of calamities. The Buddha personally taught many of these methods, and others were assumed from older shamanic traditions in the course of the dissemination of Buddhism. This applies particularly to the shamanism of the nomadic tribes from North India.

In the First Century, a movement developed in Buddhism that especially allowed two teachings of the Buddha to blossom. This was the reciting of mantras and dhâranîs, as well as the teachings of the Bodhisattvas. A Bodhisattva can be a light being or even a human being. Anyone who promises to attain enlightenment for the benefit of all sentient beings

---

[29] Jainism developed in India at the time of the Buddha and is a similar spiritual tradition in a certain sense. However, it seems that the founders of both traditions never encountered each other during their lifetimes.

and constantly endeavors to lead others and himself/herself to happiness becomes a Bodhisattva. This means that laypeople—like the historical Buddha Shâkyamuni—and monks and nuns can strive for enlightenment. This is logical because Buddha also was not a monk and wasn't even born as one. In order to successfully walk the path of the Bodhisattva, there are especially strong means in Esoteric Buddhism. These are the secret teachings, which include the Reiki symbols, mantras, mudrâs, and appropriate initiations.

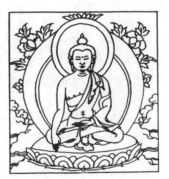

ILL. 1 – SHÂKYAMUNI, THE HISTORICAL BUDDHA

Esoteric Buddhism in China

The main texts that came from India to China were the sutras from the Womb World of the Great Sun Buddha *(Dainichi kyô)* and text groups that are summarized in the Sûtra of the Diamond World of the Great Sun Buddha *(Kongô chô kyô)*.

The Great Sun Buddha *Dainichi Nyorai* is the main figure in both of them. Reiki comes directly from him, which is why he is also closely associated with the Master Symbol (DKM). Other light beings such as Buddhas, Bodhisattvas, guardians, goddesses, and gods are depicted as rays in the mandalas with certain tasks.

In the practices of the secret teachings, the graphic symbols of the light beings were used as the focus during the meditation and in rituals on the path to enlightenment. The meditations have a three-part structure in which mantras are used in connection with special symbols during the meditation. The techniques, which are also known as the Three Secrets (Jap.: *sanmitsu*) of Body, Speech, and Mind, help the adepts perceive their own nature—Buddha consciousness. This generally occurs through the union with Dainichi Nyorai or one of his rays.

The first Tantric texts came to China some time around the Third Century. In the year 230, the Indian monk known as *Chu Lü-yen* translated *Mo-teng-ch'ieh ching*, a text containing various dhâranîs, instructions on astrology, and a fire ritual called *homa*. In the Fourth Century, various Tantric texts were introduced by Central Asian monks. One of the best-known of them was *Dharmaraksa*, who also translated the Lotus Sûtra and the Sûtra of Perfect Wisdom in 25,000 lines. *Fo-t'u-teng* and *Srimitra* are well-known for their magical powers and their deep knowledge of the mantras. *T'an-wu-lan* translated works that described how to heal diseases with mantras and how rain can be stopped with rituals. Such texts continued to increase during the Fifth to the Seventh Centuries. The emphasis on magic continued unchanged while the Buddhist teaching and its rituals started to be systematized. Until the Seventh Century, there were translations into Chinese and commentaries with descriptions of light beings in the mandalas and their functions in rituals, as well as perfected techniques of the secret teachings. Among their goals in particular was the healing of diseases within the scope of developing the mind for an accelerated attainment of enlightenment. Ritualistic energy transmissions and the cooperation with light beings in meditations were used for this purpose.

Toward the end of the Seventh Century, the so-called pure Esoteric Buddhism was finally introduced to China. The Indian master *Subhâkarasimha* (Shan-wu-wei, 637-735) and his Chinese student *I-hsing* (683-727) brought the Sûtra of the Diamond World of the Great Sun Buddha *(Dainichi kyô)* to China. Vajrabodhi (671-741) and his student *Amoghavajra* (705-774) introduced the Sûtra of the Womb World *(Kongôchôkyo)*. From then on, Esoteric Buddhism in China experienced a major upswing. It did not take long for these teachings to arrive in Japan.

Subhâkarasimha and I-hsing

Subhâkarasimha, who came from a royal family in Northeast India, was apparently a very talented child. At the age of ten years, he already assumed the high command over his father's army and ascended to the royal throne at the age of 13 years. Although he had won the power struggle with his siblings, he decided to give the throne to his brothers and went into a monastery. As a monk, he traveled through the entire country and learned magic from many great masters. He ultimately settled at the Buddhist University in Nalanda and studied the practice of the Three Secrets under *Dharmagupta*. Later, he went on pilgrimages to power places and taught the people how to find the Buddha within themselves. As a result, *Dharmagupta* ordered him to go to China. When he reached the Chinese capital of Ch'ang-an in 716, he was already 80 years old.

The Chinese emperor *Hsüan-tsung* (712-756) received him at the palace and gave him the title of "Teacher of the Land" *(kuo-shih)*. As the story goes, *Subhâkarasimha* convinced the emperor to become a Buddhist since the latter was very impressed by the magic of the Indian monk. Emperor *Hsüan-tsung* had shown interest in Taoist magic even before that time.

In Chang-an, *Subhâkarasimha* prepared the first translation of the *Hsu-kung-tsang ch'iu-wen-ch'ih fa,* a text in which a mantra and a ritual are described that greatly help improve memory. In Japanese, this method

91

is called *Gumonji hô*. (Morning-Star meditation). This is the meditation that Dr. Usui did 1,300 years later on Mount Kurama, which resulted in his becoming a Reiki channel. In 724, *Subhâkarasimha* accompanied the emperor to Loyang, where he continued to do his work. His translation of the *Dainichi kyô* (725) was the ultimate spark for the propagation of Esoteric Buddhism in China. The Chinese monk *Wu-hsing* had already taken the original text of the sutras in Sanskrit to China 30 years earlier.

The *Dainichi kyô* describes the philosophical background of the great Sun Buddha *Dainichi Nyorai*. In the first section, it emphasizes that the perception of one's own mind—the primordial nature—is the basis of enlightenment. This is followed by an analysis of the various levels of spiritual awakening. The following six sections discuss the Womb World mandala (Jap.: *Taizôkai*) and magical practices that lead to the individual's recognition of the enlightened mind inherent within every human being.

Subhâkarasimha's student *I-hsing* is one of the most noteworthy figures in the history of Chinese Buddhism. As a young man, he studied the Chinese classics and became famous for his profound knowledge of Taoism. When he lost his parents at the age of 21 years, he became a student of the Zen master *P'u-chi*, who was well-known throughout the entire country back then. With time, his interest in Esoteric Buddhism intensified. He not only studied the teachings of the *Tien-t'ai* School, but also mastered mathematics and astronomy to such a degree that he was commissioned by Emperor *Hsüan-tsung* to revise the calendar in 721. I-hsing began his studies of Esoteric Buddhism under *Vajrabodhi*, who came to Ch'ang-an in 719. *Vajrabodhi* initiated him into the teachings and practices of the Diamond World. In 724, he accompanied *Subhâkarasimha* to Loyang and helped him prepare the translation of the *Dainichi kyô*. Then he wrote an extensive commentary on this sûtra, based on the lectures of *Subhâkarasimha*.

Vajrabodhi and Amoghavajra

As a little boy, *Vajrabodhi* took refuge in Buddhism at Nalanda. In the following years, he read a great deal of Buddhist literature and acquired an extensive knowledge about Hinayana and Mahâyâna Buddhism. He was initiated in South India into the Esoteric Buddhism of the *Vajra-Sekhara* line at the age of 31 years. During his travels through India, he heard of the growing popularity of Esoteric Buddhism in China and decided to also go there to teach. With the help of the South Indian king, he took a ship from Sri Lanka to China and arrived in Ch'ang-an in 719 and Loyang in 720. Very soon after he arrived, he began building platforms *(kaidan)*—power places with mandalas—for initiations into the secret teachings. It did not take long for him to come to the attention of Emperor *Hsüan-tsung*, who called *Vajrabodhi* to him so he could experience his magical powers. The Buddhist healed the presumably incurable disease of the Emperor's twenty-fifth daughter and successfully used rain magic a number of times. During his 21 years of teaching in China, he introduced the rituals of the Diamond World of *Kongôchô kyô*. The sûtra primarily involves the description of the Diamond World mandala and its meditative practices of the five transcendent Buddhas.

Vajrabodhi's best student was *Amoghavajra*, who did more for Esoteric Buddhism than all of the previously described figures. *Amoghavajra* was born in 705 in Central Asia. His father was a Brahman from North India and his mother came from Samarkand. An uncle took him along to China, where he met *Vajrabodhi* in 719 and became his student. After just a few years, he became a master of the secret teachings of the Womb World and received all of the initiations.

After the death of his master, *Amoghavajra* returned to India and Sri Lanka in the year 743 to collect additional material on Esoteric Buddhism. In Sri Lanka he was initiated by the Tantric master Samantabhadra into further aspects and given the appropriate wisdom teachings. He returned to Ch'ang-an in 746 and brought more than 500 sutras and commentaries with him. By his death in 774, he had translated more than 100 of them into Chinese. This has made him the most outstanding translator in the history of Chinese Buddhism.

Amoghavajra endeavored to spread Esoteric Buddhism by building initiation platforms (*kaidan*) in temples within and outside of the capital city. All three emperors during his lifetime promoted him because of his great spiritual healing and rain magic skills, which were expected from the monks of Esoteric Buddhism during that period. When General *Lu-shan* provoked a rebellion in the year 755, Amoghavajra was called upon to carry out a ritual for the protection of the state. As *Amoghavajra* lay dying, *T'ai-tsung* stopped all of the court activities for three full days.

Hui-kuo–Uniter of
the Two Schools of Esoteric Buddhism

Amoghavajra had many outstanding students. One of his youngest students by the name of *Hui-kuo* (746-805) eventually had a great influence on Esoteric Buddhism in East Asia. Since *Hui-kuo* had studied both schools of Esoteric Buddhism on the basis of the Diamond World and the Womb World with the great masters, he was later able to unite the two major lines of Esoteric Buddhism into one school. Although the earlier masters of Esoteric Buddhism were aware of both lines, they tended to just specialize in one of them. *Hui-kuo* appears to be the first to value both as equal and meaningfully complementary to each other. He was convinced that the Diamond World and the Womb World, in which the Great Sun Buddha *Dainichi Nyorai* appears once as the Great God and once as the Great Goddess, inseparably belong together just like man and woman. In the following generations, it became the custom to initiate the monks into both lineages.

Moreover, *Hui-kuo* was the first monk of Esoteric Buddhism to contribute toward spreading the teaching outside of China. When he had already reached a ripe old age, the monk *Kûkai* (774-835) who had traveled from Japan became his best student. The only person to whom *Hui-kuo* passed on the teaching and initiations of Esoteric Buddhism in its entirety was *Kûkai*. This made *Kûkai* the eight patriarch and bearer of the lineage. It is said that *Hui-kuo* had waited a long time for him. *Kûkai* is the founder of the *Shingon* School of Esoteric Buddhism in Japan. *Saichô* (767-822), the founder of the Japanese *Tendai* School, also studied Esoteric Buddhism in China. Very little is known about his teacher *Shun-hsiao* and the transmission imparted to him. After *Saichô* and *Kûkai* returned from China, *Saichô* become one of *Kûkai's* students for a number of years. Only after the visit to China by the two monks *Ennin* (794-864) and *Enchin* (814-891), both of whom had studied Esoteric Buddhism in *Hui-kuo's* lineage, was it fully and completely integrated into the *Tendai* School founded by Saichô.

The merging of both schools obviously implies, as already mentioned above, that *Hui-kuo* must have learned from more than one teacher. Although *Hui-kuo* is the seventh of eight *Shingon* patriarchs[30], his predecessors came from the above-mentioned two schools. *Nâgârjuna*, the first human patriarch (before him were *Dainichi Nyorai* and *Kongôsatta*), developed Esoteric Buddhism in the Third Century by adopting some of the practices and teachings from Brahmanism, the precursor to Hinduism. When *Nâgârjuna* became a Buddhist, he was already a renowned and famous Brahmanic master. He passed on his teaching to *Nagabodhi*, the second patriarch, who in turn imparted them to *Vajrabodhi*. *Vajrabodhi* brought the Esoteric Buddhism of *Kongôchô kyô* to *Tang*-China and propagated it together with his Chinese student *Pu'kung*.

Later, in the year 716, the Buddhist Master *Subhâkarasimha* brought the *Dainichi kyô* to the *Tang* capital city of *Chang'an*. His successor *I-hsing* wrote down the complete teaching of his master and added it to the *Dainichi kyô* as a commentary. *Hui-kuo* then had the good fortune of learning both paths, uniting them, and passing them on to *Kûkai*, the eight patriarch, who soon brought them to Japan.

In addition to these eight patriarchs *Nâgârjuna, Nagabodhi, Vajrabodhi, Pu'kung, Subhâkarasimha, I-hsing, Hui-kuo,* and *Kûkai,* there is still a second list of eight important teachers. This tradition says that *Nâgârjuna* received the *Shingon* teaching directly from the Diamond Mind *Kongôsatta* (Skr.: *Vajrasattva*), a ray of *Dainichi Nyorai*, as he succeeded in using the help of a ritual to open a mysterious iron stupa that human hands had never opened. So here are the patriarchs: *Dainichi Nyorai – Kongosatta – Nâgârjuna – Nagabodhi – Vajrabodhi – Pu'kung – Hui-kuo – Kûkai*. It appears that those who wrote down the history placed more value upon the number 8 than the actual number of patriarchs. In any case, the second series of patriarchs is comparable to the transmission of Reiki. Namely, Reiki was passed on from *Dainichi Nyorai* to *Kannon* and from

[30] Patriarchs are the leaders or lineage-bearers of a spiritual tradition. In Shingon Buddhism and Reiki, they can be traced back to the Great Sun Buddha *Dainichi Nyorai*. There are often additional light beings between the first patriarch and *Dainichi Nyorai*. In Reiki, these are the Goddess of Light and Victory Dai *Marishi Ten* and the Goddess of Great Compassion, *Kannon Bosatsu*. So one line always begins with a light being whose power is transmitted to a human under special circumstances such as Dr. Usui's experience of enlightenment on Mount Kurama. Such a person is then the first patriarch. He can transmit the teachings on an energetic level with initiations and on a professional level through trainings.

Kannon to Dr. Usui. Like *Kûkai*, Dr. Usui gave the complete teaching to not just one person but a number of people. In both cases, this had the advantage of spreading the teaching but also the disadvantage that some people believed they were better than others and some of these called themselves the only legitimate successor of the patriarch.

This shows us that, beginning with the historical Buddha, time and again there have been people who have received a direct transmission of the teaching for which they are striving from a *Bodhisattva* such as *Kannon* or *Kongôsatta* in an experience of enlightenment. In keeping with my observations, it appears that every human being who practices enough and opens up to the forces of light and love is capable of this. And the latter qualities seem to be even more important than just the technical practice. A very important factor is the mental attitude with which we practice—the meaning is the essence.

Esoteric Buddhism in Japan

Esoteric Buddhism officially came to Japan with the Japanese traveling monks Kûkai and Saichô. With these two monks, a great flowering of Esoteric Buddhism began and a large wave of esoteric writings and materials was introduced in Japan. But in more precise terms, sutras like the Sûtra of the Great Sun Buddha *Dainichi kyô*, esoteric meditations such as the Morning-Star meditation *Gumonji hô*, and Siddham symbols such as the SHK Symbol already reached Japan at a much earlier date.[31]

Esoteric Buddhism came to Japan in its original form because the Japanese traveling monks learned from the Indian pilgrim monks and Chinese monks in China. Once in Japan, Esoteric Buddhism was then merged with the Japanese magic *Shugendô*, the Japanese shamanism *Shintô*, and Taoist magic.[32] The various Reiki symbols with their origins in all of the

---

[31] Cf. the chapter on the SHK Symbol.

[32] Some practices of magical Taoism, which in turn adopted the most important spells from Wu shamanism, were also already combined with Esoteric Buddhism in China. Both spiritual traditions complement each other wonderfully.

above-mentioned spiritual traditions show that this fusion is the basis for the Usui System of Reiki.

After their return from China, the monks Kûkai and Saichô founded the esoteric schools of *Shingon* and *Tendai*. Both schools are directly related to Reiki and the symbols, whereby the *Shingon* School has contributed more to the development of Reiki.

Shingon Buddhism is a school of Esoteric Buddhism that was brought to Japan by the Japanese monk Kûkai in the Ninth Century. The roots of this school have a very long history. This form of Buddhism has been given the name of secret teachings (*mikkyô*) in Japan. There are many teachings, philosophies, light entities, rituals, and meditations skillfully combined with each other in a broad spectrum in *mikkyô*. It reminds me (Mark) of Rainbow Reiki, which also skillfully integrated only the best methods of the Reiki System. In addition, there are also astonishing parallels here in terms of the philosophy and in relation to the techniques of spiritual energy work, which had already existed long before Frank Arjava Petter and others researched the origins of Usui Reiki.

The teachings of *Shingon* School are based upon the two sutras *Dainichi kyô* (大日経) and *Kongô chô kyô* (金剛頂経). They contain the first systematic depiction of the secret teachings and their practice. Esoteric Buddhism took root in the countries of India to Central Asia, Ceylon, China, Korea, Japan, Mongolia, Nepal, Indonesia, and Tibet. In Japan, Esoteric Buddhism has maintained its original form for the most part despite numerous advanced developments.

Esoteric Buddhism places a special emphasis on rituals, which include the reciting of sacred words and phrases with magical effects. These magical formulas are called "mantra" (short) or "dhâranî" (long) in Sanskrit, the classic Indian language. In Japanese, they are called the "true words" (*shingon*). This is also where the name *Shingon* School comes from. The script that is used in Sanskrit is called *Siddham*[33]. The SHK Symbol belongs to this *Siddham* script. The signs of this script can be used both as magical symbols and as the alphabet for Sanskrit.

Many ancient ritual writings provide information about the way in which the rituals were performed in Esoteric Buddhism. These are not just

---

[33] Cf. the chapter on the SHK Symbol.

limited to the *Vedas*. However, the parallels between the individual texts are so apparent and incredibly numerous that they must have influenced each other. In Brahmanism, many ritual writings were also created within the context of the *Vedas*, which also sometimes still bear the same names as in Esoteric Buddhism—*viddhi* and *kalpa*. In later times, they were then called *tantra* and *giki* in Japan.

During the *Heian* period (794-1185), the importation of Chinese cultural assets to Japan such as architecture, astrology, philosophy, Taoism, etc., had reached its zenith. In the opinion of most historical works in Western languages, it is generally assumed that at the same time, meaning the beginning of the Ninth Century, Esoteric Buddhism with its two new schools of *Tendai* and *Shingon* were introduced and established in Japan. However, the reality was also different in this point. For one, this can be seen by the fact that there are text sections in the sutras of the *Mahâyâna* that are very similar to those of the *Vajrayâna* of Esoteric Buddhism. It is not even possible to find a precise line of separation between the two on the basis of the text material since the one actually builds upon the other.

Although there are some sutras such as the *Dainichi kyô* that are solely related to Esoteric Buddhism, these were not only familiar but also read and systematically studied in Japan and other countries many years before the official introduction of Esoteric Buddhism.

Furthermore, there were also already individual Buddhist and shamanic ascetics, who lived in the mountains in order to achieve and further develop their magical powers, at that time. However, spiritual training in the mountains has only been officially recognized as an important component of Buddhism since *Kûkai* and *Saicho*.

Kûkai, who is also known posthumously by the name of *Kôbô Daishi*, learned Esoteric Buddhism up to its completion in China from the great Master *Hui-kuo* and became his successor. Kûkai called this teaching *Shingon* (which means mantra, True Word) in Japan. Kûkai found this term to be especially suitable since it appeared in the sutras *Dainichi kyô* and *Kongôchô kyô* and is one of the most important tools.

As *Kûkai* spread Esoteric Buddhism in Japan, it served the protection of the state on the one hand, as had previously also been the case with some of the earlier Buddhist schools. Specific rituals were carried out for this purpose. On the other hand, *Kûkai* also made sure that Esoteric Buddhism could spread among the people. The magical practices characteristic of Esoteric Buddhism[34] such as rain magic, healing, and prevention of misfortune were used for this purpose.

Since the mountains were connected with Buddhism in earlier times, there were also monks who practiced in the mountains. This new *Mountain Buddhism* (Jap.: *sanrin bukkyô*), which followed the shifting of the capital city to *Heian,* the present-day Kyoto, and found a visible expression with the establishment of the two significant monasteries on the mountains *Hiei san* and *Kôya san*, was intended to also have an influence on the people. Magic and fortune-telling had always been widespread among the people. Esoteric Buddhism also provided a very effective system of magical practices and secret rituals with the help of *mudrâs, mantras,* and symbols. These practices were used by ordained monks, free monks (*shido sô*), lay brothers (*ubasoku*), wandering saints (*hijiri*), miracle monks (*genja*), and mountain ascetics (*yamabushi*). By means of their pilgrimages from mountain to mountain, they brought Esoteric Buddhism to the people in the entire country.

With the exception of the influences on Buddhism in India, China, and Korea, the Esoteric Buddhism spread in this manner had long ceased to be pure Buddhism since it became merged with the native gods (*Kami*) from Shintoism and its folkloric and Taoist beliefs. This had a strong influence on the Reiki System of Natural Healing founded by Dr. Usui, even if it was about 1,000 years later. This is why research on the Reiki symbols is so complex. The profound and extensive wisdom of all these influences is one of the major characteristics of the Reiki symbols. And this is why it is impossible to say that the symbols can only be traced back to one single spiritual tradition. This makes Reiki, as we know it from Dr. Usui, also so Japanese because it is in the nature of the Japanese to skillfully combine their own cultural assets with those from other countries—and then even improve them. Yet, the practical application of the life energy of Reiki is much older than any culture of modern history. After all, the character for Reiki is the oldest Chinese character for a female shaman practicing her art in the Wu tradition. Japan is a country that has created

---

[34] And shamanism!

outstanding preconditions for bringing this wonderful healing energy back to humanity.

In principle, time and again over the course of the centuries the most useful energy work in everyday life from the various traditions has been incorporated and merged into a whole. This is why this teaching has also become such a great success. Whenever it encountered practical demands in competition with other systems, it won because it was able to better solve the problems with the help of its energy-work techniques. There is historical evidence for this statement.

The Monk Kûkai (774-835)

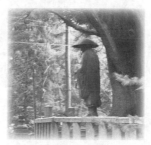

ILL. 2 – THE MONK KÛKAI

Kûkai was not the first person to bring Esoteric Buddhism to Japan. However, he was the one who spread it in a systematic form in Japan. *Kûkai* is probably the most famous Japanese monk of all times in Japan. I (Mark) have never met anyone in Japan who did not know about *Kûkai*. There are places in almost all of Japan that are related to *Kûkai*. These may be places where Kûkai meditated or created other things. But these may also be foods or events that date back to *Kûkai* or are associated with him in some context. Many stories about him have historical evidence to support them. Many others are part of the legends since it is very difficult to prove them. Yet, if even just one-thousandth of what is said about *Kûkai* is actually true, this alone would be a great miracle. To convey an impression of exactly who he was and why *Kûkai* is so important for Reiki and the symbols, the following section describes *Kûkai's* life in the form of brief scenes.

Scenes from Kûkai's life

Kûkai's Youth

Kûkai was born on June 15, 774 on the island of Shikoku in the city of Zentsûji, which is in the province of Sanuki, as the son of a civil servant. His parents *Saeki Yoshimichi* and *Tamayori* gave him the name of *Mao* 真魚 (which means: True Fish). Even in his youth, he surprised his family by making Buddhist sculptures, which he had never seen, out of clay.

101

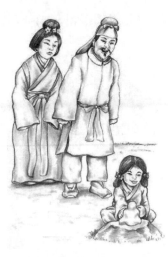

ILL. 3 – KÛKAI AS A LITTLE BOY FORMING A BUDDHA OUT OF CLAY

When he was seven years old, he once climbed a steep mountain. When he arrived at the top, he said: "If my life has any value, I will be rescued no matter what I do." He had hardly spoken these words when he fell into the depths. Just before he hit the bottom, a goddess appeared and caught him. After this incident, he realized the mission of his life. He promised Buddha that he would invest his entire life in helping many beings.

His family had almost no relationship to Buddhism. These occurrences made his parents very sad because they were afraid that their son would one day become a monk. So they decided to keep their son away from Buddhism and have him educated in such a way that he would become a government official in the capital city. They wanted him to visit the university in the capital city. However, students were only allowed to enter if their parents had the status of high-level civil servants, which was not the case here, or when they passed very difficult examinations of nine levels. This is why his parents first sent him to a state school. Here he learned Confucianism, medicine, and politics.

At exactly this time, the capital city was switched from Nara to Nagaoka. *Mao* was very interested to know how the new capital city looked. But he was less pleased that normal citizens from his surrounding area were torn away from their families to do forced labor in building the capital city.

His father promised him that he would travel there with him after *Mao* had finished school so he could attend the university there. In those days, such a journey was strenuous and tedious. The inland sea also had to be crossed by ship, which was always associated with risks. *Mao* promised himself that the career of a civil servant would allow him to help the suffering people. He completed school with outstanding grades. His parents demanded that he become a respected civil servant to raise the status of his family. They were not interested in doing something good for others.

So he traveled to Nagaoka at the age of 15 years in 788 to prepare for his course of studies there. For three years he studied from early morning to late at night. Even when he went somewhere, he always had his books with him. Once he was so absorbed in his book while walking that he ran into a tree and everyone laughed at him. In the year 791, he ultimately passed the entrance examination to the university. He decided to study the subject of *Myôgyôdô*, which meant specializing in Confucianism, history, and classical Chinese. However, it was his goal to climb the ladder of success.

Kûkai's Years of Ascetic Practices

As soon as *Mao* arrived at the university, the endless studying continued. Every ten days, there were inhumanly difficult examinations that were mainly based on mindless memorization.

When the capital city of Nagaoka was barely completed, the decision was made to move it to another place—Heian (the present-day Kyoto). This once again led to forced labor and suffering among the people. Because of intensive rainfall, the harvest was largely destroyed so that there was also a lack of food and the people had to suffer even more. Although *Mao* was forced to study so much, he still had an unbelievable compassion for the people and thought a great deal about how this situation could be improved.

He spent the night before an examination outside under a tree so he could study there. He was very concerned because he still had to learn more than half of the material. Anyone who did not learn everything by heart not only failed but also had poor chances at climbing the ladder of success.

103

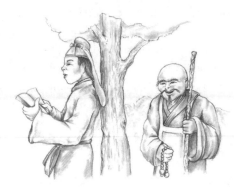

ILL. 4 – KÛKAI'S ENCOUNTER WITH A WONDROUS MONK

While he was studying under the tree, a wondrous monk appeared from out of nowhere. His name has been forgotten, but he had a bare shaved head and a long beard and long eyebrows. He wore a robe, a pilgrimage staff, and a prayer chain. The old monk asked: "What are you doing?"

"I am learning the oldest Chinese collection of poetry by heart," *Mao* responded.

"Oh, then you are probably a student at the university. The course of studies is certainly very interesting, isn't it?"

"No, just the opposite. Constantly cramming is completely boring."

"Precisely. And what you are studying is what people already learned a long time ago. But it has absolutely no use in the present."

"But if I don't graduate from the university, then I cannot become a civil servant. As a civil servant, I would like to have a big career and then influence the government in such a way that the people have an easier life."

"Oooh, now that is interesting. So you believe that you can redeem the people in the world as a civil servant. You don't look like a young man from a family of high standing. No matter how much effort you make, no matter whether or not you become a civil servant, this path will never give you the opportunity to do something good for humanity."

This made *Mao* very angry: "So what should I do if this is not possible?"

"Mmmmh. Try reciting the following mantra once: *Nô bô akyasha kyarabaya on arikya mari bori sowaka.*"

Mao began to recite this sentence in a loud voice. While he did this, the old monk initiated him and explained: "This is a Buddhist *mantra*. If you truly want to lead the people in the world to happiness, recite it a million times."

"Whaaat! A million times! That is a lot."

"Precisely. And this is an ascetic practice from Esoteric Buddhism. It is called *Kokûzô Gumonji hô*." These were the last words of the old monk. Then he left. *Mao* remained standing in silence and didn't know what to say. But then he recited the mantra a number of times and discovered the following: "This is very strange. Until a little while ago I still had the feeling that my heart is very heavy. But now I somehow feel relieved and so clear ... Buddhism ... Perhaps this is the path that I have sought for so long and desired in my heart for all these years?"

He decided to leave the university. His family was horrified. They thought it was extremely stupid that he let himself be talked into such craziness by an old crippled monk. But he had made his decision. He left his family and went to the mountains so that he could meditate there.

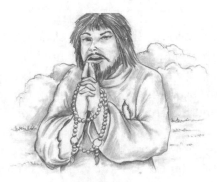

ILL. 5 – THE TIME OF ASCETICISM

Every day from morning to evening, he did the meditation with the mantra. When his clothing was completely in rags and his hair and beard had grown to the point where no one would recognize him anymore, he had repeated the mantra one million times. Then he had a vision. The planet Venus appeared to him.

105

In his joy, he climbed up a cliff at the ocean so that he could see the sunrise. Here he recognized how beautiful the world was and that it would have been a pure waste of time to remain in the capital city to have a career there. Then, as he watched the rising sun, the sky, and the ocean, he recognized himself and gave himself a new name. He called himself: *Kûkai*, which means "sky and ocean[35]." At this moment, big waves hit the cliff.

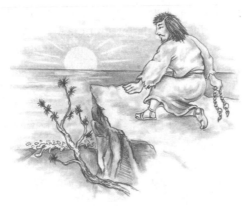

ILL. 6 – SKY AND OCEAN

From here, *Kûkai* traveled to Shikoku, the island where he was born, in order to continue meditating in the mountains there. *Kûkai* climbed the Tairyû Mountain in the province of Awa. From there, he went to Cape Muroto in the province of Tosa. At Cape Muroto, he discovered a cave in which he continued the previously completed meditation for a long time. Whether summer or winter, Kûkai meditated under waterfalls and encountered many challenges. After he had walked around Shikoku, which is still the basis for the best-known Japanese pilgrimage, "The 88 Temples of Shikoku," he climbed Kôyasan, a mountain on the island of Honshû in the prefecture Wakayama.

Looking into the wide valley, he expressed a wish: "One day I would like to establish a Buddhist center here on this mountain..." Then, as

[35] Perhaps this is a coincidence: The *sky* represents the masculine divine principle and the *ocean* is an extremely well-known spiritual symbol for the divine feminine principle. Both are united in the name *Kûkai* like the two central mandalas of Esoteric Buddhism.

he fell asleep under a tree, a goddess with a crown appeared to him. She spoke these words to him: "*Kûkai*, if you would like to experience the ultimate truth of Buddhism, you must learn the secret teachings of Esoteric Buddhism. Go immediately to the *Kumedera* temple. You will find something very important in the central pillar of the east pagoda." *Kûkai* wanted to say something in response and woke up. But then the goddess was gone.

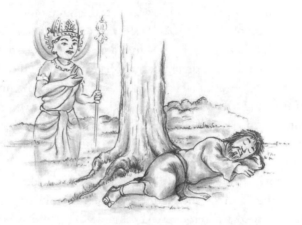

ILL. 7 – INSTRUCTION FROM THE GODDESS

So *Kûkai* traveled to *Kumedera* in 796 and asked about what was concealed in the east pagoda. Not even the head monk was aware of anything there. So they both went in to take a look. *Kûkai* discovered a dusty box that had a sûtra container in it. When he opened it, he found a sûtra that had been unknown in Japan up to that time: *Dainichi kyô* (The Sûtra of the Great Sun Buddha). The monk of the temple was very surprised since he had known nothing about this sûtra in his pagoda.

Kûkai attempted to read the *Dainichi kyô*. Despite his good education, he could only understand very few words. No matter how often *Kûkai* tried to read the sûtra, there were always areas that he could not understand. To be able to understand its contents, he traveled from temple to temple so he could study the sutras there.

In December of 797, he wrote the famous text *Sangô shiiki*. This text deals with his previous background and his decision to now study

Buddhism from the ground up. He wrote it like an autobiography in the form of a novel at the age of 24 years.

The Search for the Secret Teachings

Next, *Kûkai* went to the *Daianji* temple. It was the most famous monastery school in Japan in those days. It was not usually possible to simply walk in to become a monk. But since *Kûkai* was especially stubborn, the monks informed the abbot, whose name was *Gonzô* at that time, of his presence. According to a legend, *Gonzô* was the same monk who taught *Kûkai* the mantra of the *Kokûzô*. "Well, well. So you would like to also learn the secret teachings *mikkyô*. Why do you want to learn them?"

"Buddha told me in a dream that this is what I should do."

"That is very beautiful. However, I also do not know much about the secret teachings. If you want to learn them correctly, you must go to *Tang*-China. But to do this, you must first learn Chinese. You are lucky. Some monks are here from China right now. They can teach you Chinese. So you can stay and become a monk."

This is how *Kûkai* came to fully and completely dedicate himself to the study of the Chinese language. It was not difficult for him since he had already learned written classical Chinese during his youth. Before long, he was also able to interpret Chinese.

Gonzô told him that he had been selected to be a traveling monk and would already be leaving for China in the following year. However, when the ships left in April of 803, Kûkai was not on board. He had not been selected, and such a delegation was only sent to China every 20 years. So he was completely depressed and disappointed.

But then something unexpected happened. While crossing the inland sea, a storm arose and the ships shattered on the rocks. It is said that many people died, but most of the monks were able to rescue themselves and soon returned. As a result, a new delegation was prepared for the following year. To *Kûkai's* greatest joy, he was permitted to go along this time.

In May of 804, two ships set out to sea. *Kûkai* was on one of them. A passenger on the other was the monk *Saichô*, who was already well-known at that time and later founded the *Tendai* School of Esoteric Buddhism in Japan. This time, there were no problems in crossing the inland sea. However, as they sailed into the China Sea a tremendous storm arose. The sailors asked *Kûkai* to pray to Buddha. *Kûkai* went on board and asked *Dainichi Nyorai* for protection and guidance. It did not take very long for the storm to calm down and the clouds to disappear at the level of the sun. But this was not the end of it. The disappearance of the clouds was accompanied by a new wind that forced the two ships in different directions and separated them from each other.

After an odyssey on the high seas that lasted weeks, the ship with *Kûkai* landed on the Chinese coast at Ch'ih-an-chen in the province of Fukien. Unfortunately, the people did not believe that they were actually a Japanese delegation since they did not have the necessary certificate with them. It was namely on the other ship, which had been driven to the north. So they were seen as pirates to whom access to the mainland was prohibited. Then *Kûkai* had an idea. He wrote a petition in the style that he had learned when he was in school. Because of this letter and *Kûkai's* polished style, the people realized that they could not be pirates but must actually be delegates from Japan. So they started on a two-month journey by foot from the coast to the capital city of Chang'an.

In Chang'an, he met the Japanese monk *Yôchû*, who had already lived in China for 30 years. This monk returned to Japan on the ship that had brought *Kûkai*. Later, after *Kûkai's* return, *Yôchû* helped him spread Esoteric Buddhism throughout Japan. *Kûkai* soon also met two monks who were famous in India and China, *Hannya Sanzô* and *Munishiri Sanzô*, from whom he learned the *Siddham* script and more. But since it was not enough for *Kûkai* to achieve mastery in the Siddham script, *Hannya Sanzô* then sent him to the temple of the Blue Dragon (清竜寺), where he was allowed to meet *Hui-kuo*, the seventh patriarch of Esoteric Buddhism.

Hui-kuo was very happy as he received *Kûkai*:

"*Kûkai*, you are finally here. Where have you been so long! I have already been waiting for you for a long time. We do not have much time, and will therefore start with the preparations for the initiations tomorrow. Until today, Buddhism had more of a theoretical nature. It has been like a science that has been mainly focused on intensively studying the sutras. It is very difficult to attain enlightenment in this manner.

However, Esoteric Buddhism follows the teaching of *Dainichi Nyorai* and, with the help of meditation and spiritual energy transmission, can heal diseases, relieve catastrophes, assist many people in finding more happiness and freedom, and achieve full enlightenment in this present life."

Kûkai was obviously very glad to hear this because it was precisely what he had desired for so long.

Kûkai was first initiated into the Womb World mandala and then into the Diamond World mandala. During both initiations into the mandalas, there is a ritual in which the adept approaches the mandala on a table blindfolded and lets a flower fall down on it.

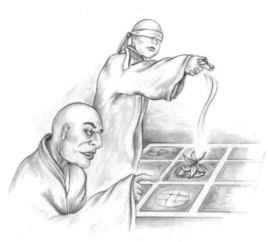

ILL. 8 – ORACLE RITUAL

During both initiations, the flower fell on *Dainichi Nyorai*, which confirmed to *Hui-kuo* that *Kûkai* had been chosen. Even though *Hui-kuo* was already very old, he had never had such a talented student. Because of the rapid progress, it was possible for *Kûkai* to soon receive the highest master initiation. In addition, *Kûkai* received a sacred name of the secret teachings: *Henjô kongô*. *Henjô* is another name for *Dainichi Nyorai* and *kongô* means that someone firmly bears enlightenment in his heart.

Then *Hui-kuo* had the ritual implements, mandalas, sutras, and the ritual rules *giki* of Esoteric Buddhism made for *Kûkai*. These are tools that students require to make the path easier for them.

One night, *Kûkai* was suddenly called to *Hui-kuo*. The latter said: "*Kûkai*, it is good that I have imparted all of my knowledge to you. Go back to Japan as quickly as possible and take the ritual implements, mandalas, and texts with you."

Kûkai was extremely surprised and replied: "But I wanted to stay much longer in Tang-China to further research the secret teachings!"

"Even if you remain in Tang-China, there is nothing more for you to learn here. It is much better if you go to Japan to spread the teaching of Esoteric Buddhism there and lead the people to happiness."

"I understand."

"*Kûkai*, a long time ago we made the promise to spread Esoteric Buddhism. I am now going on a distant journey. I will be reincarnated in the Land of the East and you, *Kûkai*, will be my teacher," were his last words. Then *Hui-kuo* passed away.

A funeral stele was built for the seventh Shingon patriarch *Hui-kuo*, for which *Kûkai* was allowed to write the inscription. *Kûkai's* script was so sublime that even the emperor appreciated it. So he was invited to the emperor and permitted to write for him there. Whenever *Kûkai* picked up a writing brush, he prayed to *Dainichi Nyorai* and let his power flow through him. The emperor was so pleased that he bestowed the name of *Gohitsu wajô* (五筆和尚, Highest Buddhist Priest of the Five Writing brushes) on him.

The New Buddhism

In March of 806, Kûkai left the city of Chang'an. In addition to the Buddhist ritual implements and sutras, he also took many texts on Confucianism, Taoism, literature, and astronomy with him. Shortly before he left on his journey home, *Kûkai* did an esoteric ritual in which he threw a thunderbolt with three tips (Skr.: *vajra*) into the sea in the direction of Japan. This was meant to be a type of guide and help him spread Esoteric Buddhism in Japan.

While on the high seas, the ship with *Kûkai* was caught in a huge storm. So that he would not be thrown from board but still be able to pray, *Kûkai* took a rope and tied himself firmly to the mast. Then *Kûkai* prayed to *Dainichi Nyorai* and *Fudô Myôô*. He asked to safely cross the sea so that he could spread the culture of Tang-China and the secret teachings of Esoteric Buddhism in Japan for the benefit of all beings. Suddenly, the figure of *Fudô Myôô* appeared in the sky. *Fudô Myôô* raised his sword and

111

used it to cut through the wind, clouds, and waves. The ship then sailed calmly through the storm in something like a safe tunnel to Japan.

Once he arrived in Japan, *Kûkai* initially had no possibility of introducing his form of Buddhism, which was new in many ways for Japan, to the court of the Tennô. Since he had been sent away for a period of 20 years but had returned much earlier, he was not permitted to travel to the capital. For two years, he was assigned to stay at the *Kanzeonji* temple in Dazaifu on the island of Kyushu. To give a sign of his presence, he sent all of the goods that he had brought with him from Tang-China to the capital city and wrote a report that listed all of the articles (*Go shôrai mokuroku*).

In the meantime, *Saichô* the monk, who had drifted toward the north on the trip home from China, had already returned before *Kûkai* and was active at the court of Tennô as a renowned monk in the capital city. Since he had only been sent to China for a short time and had already enjoyed a high status beforehand, it was not a problem for him to found the *Tendai* School and promote his perspective of the Esoteric Buddhist teachings, as they were transmitted to him on the Tientai mountain in China.

In the year 807, *Kûkai* finally received permission from the new *Saga Tennô*[36] to go to the capital city and become a monk in the *Takaosanji* Temple (present-day name of *Jingoji*).

Since *Saga Tennô* and *Kûkai* were both ardent calligraphers, it was possible for *Kûkai* to get closer to the Tennô in this way. *Saga Tennô, Kûkai,* and *Tachibana no Hayanari* are known as Japan's most famous calligraphers under the name of *sanpitsu*, the "Three Writing brushes."

When a revolt occurred with the intent of toppling the *Saga Tennô*, *Kûkai* used this event to introduce his form of Buddhism to the Tennô. *Kûkai* convinced the Tennô that it was necessary to support the people in maintaining the peace, which was also very advantageous for the state and the court of the Tennô. Starting in 810, *Kûkai* received permission to carry out rituals for the protection of the state.

To express his thanks, Tennô gave *Kûkai* the temple *Otokuni dera*. This temple was known for the spirits of the dead that appeared there and

---

[36] The Japanese word *Tennô*, which means something like "emperor," always is written behind the proper name. It can be used for both the masculine and the feminine gender.

caused unrest. Yet, *Kûkai* succeeded in leading all of these unredeemed beings to the Light. This was the start of spreading the *Shingon* School of Esoteric Buddhism in Japan.

One day, *Saichô* visited *Kûkai*. The latter requested *Kûkai's* permission to become his student in order to learn the secret teachings of Esoteric Buddhism from him. This act obviously attracted attention since it was extremely unusual in Japan for an older person to become the student of someone who is younger. However, this was also a sign of how strong *Kûkai's* charisma must have been.

From then on, numerous Japanese monks began to study under *Kûkai* and received many initiations into the secret teachings. When *Kûkai* explained to his students that every human being is capable of becoming fully enlightened in this present life, his students were extremely surprised. This was not written in any of the sutras that were available in Japan up to that time. If this was true, then *Kûkai* must have already achieved this enlightenment. *Kûkai* explained to them that this story is found in the *Dainichi kyô*: "...*Gautama Shâkyamuni* was a human being just like we are. As a human being, he succeeded in becoming the Buddha, which means that he attained full enlightenment. Buddha taught that every human being who realizes the three Secrets (*sanmitsu*) of Body, Speech, and Mind can become a Buddha..."

Because they still did not believe him, the monks challenged *Kûkai* to give them a sign that he was the Buddha. *Kûkai* did not personally believe that miraculous acts were necessary, but hardly anyone would have listened to him without them. In order to make it easier for his students to truly trust in the new teaching, *Kûkai* prayed to the Great Sun Buddha *Dainichi Nyorai* and recited his two mantras *om abira unken* and *om bazara datoban*. Kûkai was suddenly filled with golden light and his body changed into that of *Dainichi Nyorais*. The light was so strong that the monks could hardly keep their eyes open. In order to spread his teaching throughout the entire country, *Kûkai* sent the monks who he had trained in his name in four directions to be active in various regions.

However, *Kûkai* was not only involved in the well-being of the court of the Tennô and the monks. Even in his youth, the merciless behavior of the government officials toward the people had shaken him. With Esoteric Buddhism and his knowledge, he now also had the possibility of doing much good for the simple people. In the year 811, *Kûkai* returned to his homeland to help the people there in building a dam as protection against flooding. For many years, the people had tried to build dams but every effort had been in vain. *Kûkai* explained to the citizens that this work would be beneficial not only to themselves but to many other people as well. And he also showed how each of the participants in this work could become a Buddha by means of a special ritual. At the same time, *Kûkai* explained to them the advanced building techniques that he had learned during his stay in Tang-China. The work was easy for everyone to do and it was possible to successfully complete it after just 45 days.

Saichô's student *Taihan* had received an order from his teacher to study under *Kûkai* and constantly stay in the temple with him. One day, *Saichô* ordered him to get an explanation of the *Rishukyô* sutras from *Kûkai*. However, *Kûkai* rejected this request because he recognized that *Saichô* wanted to learn the secret teachings of Esoteric Buddhism without the meditative practices through just studying the texts. But this is not the path to true liberation. Only through the practice, through which we experienced body, speech, and mind in its essence, is it possible to understand the secret teachings.[37] Once *Saichô* had visibly developed his personality through the meditative practices, *Kûkai* was willing to send him the texts when the time was right. *Saichô* was obviously less than pleased by this response. When he had his student *Taihan* called back because of this, the latter preferred to stay with *Kûkai* in order to devote himself completely to *Shingon* Buddhism. This made *Saichô* so angry that he officially turned away from *Kûkai* on the grounds that the younger man supposedly did not understand Buddhism.

Since *Kûkai* had become very successful throughout the country in the meantime, the Tennô gave him land in the mountains to found a monastery so that *Kûkai* could continue deepening the secret teachings for the state and the people. This land was in an area where *Kûkai* had

---

[37] But this does not mean that there are not meditative practices in the Tendai School. Zazen is practiced on a regular basis in the Tendai School. In addition, there are many rituals. On the Hieizan Mountain, there is also the 1000-day meditation *Sennichi kaihô* during which people walk 64 km (about 38 miles) every day in meditative contemplation in order to merge with *Fudô Myôô*. I have spent several days participating in this meditation there. It is quite intense, but also highly recommended.

devoted himself to ascetic practices during his youth—the mountain *Kôyasan* in the present-day prefecture of Wakayama.

With a group of monks, *Kûkai* set out on the journey to Kôyasan. Deep in the mountains, they got lost and didn't know what to do next. Moreover, a snowstorm soon began. The monks complained that they would probably freeze in the flurry of snow that night. *Kûkai* calmed them by saying that he was certain *Dainichi Nyorai* would protect all of them. He encouraged them to recite the mantra of the Bodhisattva who overcomes space and is the bearer of great treasures *Kokûzô Bosatsu*: *Nô bô akyasha kyarabaya on arikya mari bori sowaka.*" They had hardly begun with the mantra when two dogs suddenly appeared in the middle of the forest. Dogs like this were only known at that time on the island of Shikoku, where Kûkai was born.

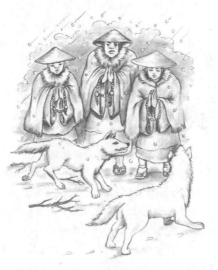

ILL. 9 – DOGS SHOW THE WAY

They barked very loudly and gave signs of wanting to show the monks the way. The monks followed the dogs through the forest for a number of hours. They finally came to a mountain from where it was possible to look down into a valley. *Kûkai* suddenly realized that they had come to exactly the spot where 20 years earlier he had expressed the wish of one day building a Buddhist center. They had reached their goal—with the help of the dogs. But where were the dogs? They had disappeared. Not even their tracks could be seen in the deep snow. *Kûkai* explained that they were Bodhisattvas in the form of dogs.

Very near by, they discovered something shiny in the crown of a fir tree. It was the three-tipped thunderbolt that *Kûkai* had thrown into the sea before his journey back to Japan. This fir tree still stands there today. The thunderbolt is kept in the treasure-house on Kôyasan. Any visitor can admire it.

Until the spring of 818, the monks carried out rituals to consecrate this place, which resulted in the creation of a power place that still has a strong aura for its visitors from all over to world to this very day.

The teaching hall was completed after five years of construction. The completion of the treasure pagoda took many more years. *Kûkai* soon also received the commission from Tennô to build the east temple *Tôji* in the capital city of Heian (present-day Kyoto) in order to pass on the secret teachings there. So *Kûkai* often had the opportunity to travel through the country and help the people on the way.

In addition, he took the time to specifically travel through the land in order to give assistance to the people there. Whenever he was asked for help, he always made an effort to go where he was needed. This is why there are also so many historical places today that remind us of *Kûkai*.

In 828, *Kûkai* founded the first public school next to the *Tôji* temple, where anyone was permitted to study irregardless of class or financial situation. The poor people in particular even received their meals there, and a system was also introduced that resembles the modern scholarship. At this school, which was called *Shugei shuin*, an entire series of subjects was taught that people do not necessarily expect from a Buddhist monk. These subjects included Confucianism, Buddhism, Taoism, law, engineering, medicine, astronomy, and music.

In addition to the Buddhist treatise, *Kûkai* also wrote many literary works and even authored Japan's first sign lexicon for Chinese characters, the *Tenreiban shômyôji*.

In the year 835, *Kûkai* returned to Kôyasan. He knew that this would be his last journey to Kôyasan. On March 15th, he informed his students that on March 21st at the hour of the Tiger (early morning at 4:00 a.m.)

he would go into the light realm while in deep meditative absorption[39]. In addition, he said that there would be no reason for mourning and uproar because the Kôyasan would remain and he himself would stay in a building by the name of *Okunoin* and grant eternal protection and guidance...

Twenty years after his death, *Kûkai* was honored by the Japanese Tennô for his outstanding services with the posthumous name of *Kôbô Daishi*.

The Pilgrimage of Shikoku

Kûkai has kept his promise of protection and guidance to this day. I (Mark) am personally acquainted with many people who can confirm this. If the reader ever wants to enjoy an extremely wondrous experience and perhaps is even interested in also encountering *Kûkai*, I can warmly recommend the pilgrimage of the 88 temples on the island of Shikoku. Just contact me about it.

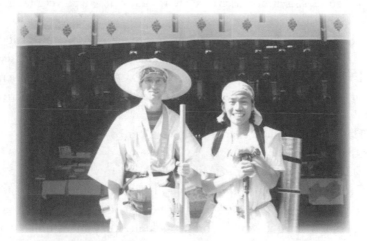

ILL. 10 – MARK HOSAK ON THE PILGRIMAGE OF SHIKOKU

[39] Perhaps it is no coincidence that Dr. Usui selected the same time period—even if this was many years later—for his 21-day meditation on Mount Kurama and had his experience of enlightenment in the early morning around 4 to 5 a.m.

Kûkai was born on the island of Shikoku. For many years, he also meditated and founded numerous temples there, as well as doing miracles. Shikoku is the smallest of the four major islands of Japan. This is a place where it is possible to experience virgin nature that is rarely found anywhere else. *Kûkai's* 88 sacred places are found partly in the Japanese primeval forests, partly at the ocean, and partly on the mountains or in the cities and villages. The pilgrimage consists of walking from one temple to the other while concentrating fully on the various practices of the secret teachings during this time. The presence of light beings and power places can be clearly felt. This obviously also is true for laypeople.

At the end of my second pilgrimage, a monk and ritual master explained to me the secret teachings on the Kôyasan mountain. He told me that the roots of Reiki can be found in the secret teachings and symbols of Esoteric Buddhism, which the monk *Kûkai* brought to Japan more than 1,200 years ago. He said that the Reiki power itself comes from the Great Sun Buddha *Dainichi Nyorai*. A method for experiencing the deep mystical knowledge of Reiki and the secret teachings is the pilgrimage of the 88 temples itself because there are so many active power places and light beings there.

The first time I went there myself in order to do my university research, I had already heard a great deal about the miracles on this island. But it was difficult for me to believe in them. Only my own experiences of everyday life taught me the truth. Each day I was allowed to experience many small and sometimes even major miracles.

Here are a few brief examples that happened to me in the very first days that I was there:

On the way to the *Dainichi* Temple (No. 4), which is dedicated to the Great Sun Buddha *Dainichi Nyorai*, I asked a woman in her garden where the path was. She explained to me that it is better to first go to temple No. 5 since it would soon be dark and that one is much closer. But I absolutely wanted to visit the temples in the right order. So she finally explained the path to me. As I continued, the dog that had been in the woman's garden came along with me. He always walked a little ahead of me and looked back to see if I was also really following him. I had the impression that he was smiling. The dog knew exactly where the path was and accompanied me in the twilight until I saw the gate of the temple from the distance. I joyfully went to the temple but the dog was no longer there. I just thought that he had probably disappeared into the bushes somewhere.

On the path to the next temple, this dog suddenly appeared again. He absolutely wanted me to go in a different direction than I had planned. The dog barked loudly and ran back and forth, showing me that I should follow him. Until then, I had only come across the idea that a dog could show me the way in films. But the dog did not stop until I gave up and followed him. Just like before, he walked ahead of me the whole time and kept looking back at me to see if I was also actually following him. Then I discovered a guidepost at the edge of the path in the darkness and realized that the dog had shown me the right way. But when I wanted to look at him, he was gone without a trace. I was completely perplexed. I had just taken my eyes off of him for a brief moment. How could he have disappeared so quickly? This incident was on my mind until the next temple, where I spent the night.

I could not yet understand the exact meaning of this experience at that time. I had also not yet become more closely acquainted with the life of the monk *Kûkai*. And so I also did not know that my experience was directly related to *Kûkai* and the secret teachings.

Many months after the pilgrimage—winter had come and there are no heaters in Japan—I was wrapped up in my futon as I read the life story of *Kûkai*. When I came to the part in the book where *Kûkai* and some other monks were shown the right path in the mountains by the dogs, I remembered my experience with the dog during the pilgrimage. I immediately knew that there was a correlation here. When *Kûkai* explained that they were Bodhisattvas in the shape of dogs, I felt a deep joy. At the same time, a warm energy spread throughout my heart and I was no longer cold... Although it was already the middle of the night, I hurried to the woman in the next room, who came from Taiwan. I even disrupted her meditation that she had been working on for months. Because she was knowledgeable about many sutras, she was surprised that I had had such experiences that are usually only granted to high monks. As a result, she was convinced that I probably must have been a monk in a previous life. I explained to her that any person can enjoy such experiences and that I would help her do so, which soon happened on the Kôyasan as well...

The next summer, I went back to Shikoku to do the pilgrimage once again. This time, I was accompanied by a friend from Germany who made the trip especially for this purpose. On the way to temple No. 4 I told him the story of the dog. Suddenly, he interrupted me and asked: "Do you mean this dog?" I couldn't believe my eyes. He stood directly in front of us and smiled again...

On the pilgrim's hut, the character *dôgyô ninin* (同行二人) is written in Chinese. This means that even when we go on the pilgrimage alone, we are still not alone. *Kûkai* always walks on our right side. His symbol is the pilgrimage staff, a true companion on all paths. It means that we must carefully put down the pilgrimage staff before every break in order to also give *Kûkai* a break.

As I climbed up a set of stone stairs in the Japanese primeval forest, I came to a bronze statue of the monk *Kûkai*. It was already getting dark and I didn't quite know where I should spend the night. I thought to myself that if *Kûkai* is always present, I should also be able to make contact with him. And so I created the contact with the Reiki symbols. I had barely greeted him when the bronze statue was transformed into the true-to-life figure of *Kûkai*. A radiantly warm light came from him that also filled me completely. I asked: "*Kûkai*, what should I do now? Where should I go?" He responded: "Take the path of your heart." I had not reckoned with such an answer. So I asked: "What is the path of my heart?" Once more I heard his voice: "You will experience it if you continue to go on the pilgrimage with me!" Then he suddenly dissolved in the golden light, which soon disappeared as well. And so I stood in the darkness in front of the bronze statue again. I felt the same warmth in my heart as I had at certain times before. Yet, I still did not know where I should go. My mind told me that I should go to the left. Then I remembered the voice of *Kûkai* "Take the path of your heart." So I decided to go to the right and soon reached an ancient temple that was deserted by humans but protected by light beings. I was able to spend the night here.

Today I know that the path of the heart is not just the decision of whether to go left or right, but much more. The book that you are now holding in your hands is a part of it...

CHAPTER 5

Taoism and the Traditional Reiki Symbols

The Chinese teaching of Taoism is very significant for the creation of the traditional Reiki symbols—especially for the HS Symbol and partially also for the DKM Symbol—because these two symbols are a special form of Taoist talismans. The following brief introduction to Taoism is intended to clarify the background within the context of the Reiki symbols.

There are three well-known teachings in China: Buddhism, Taoism, and Confucianism. Of these, only the latter two actually came from China. Although the word "religion" is generally used in the West, the term "teaching" is more common in China. There are two main words for Taoism in China: *Daojiao* and *Daojia*, both of which begin with the syllable *Tao* or *Dao*. *Tao* can mean either the path or the teaching. Both of the terms are related to the main currents of Taoism. *Daojiao* is the magical form, and *Daojia* is the more philosophical approach. Since it more closely replicates the Chinese sound, the modern English pronunciation sometimes also uses Daoism instead of Taoism.

Philosophical Taoism

Daojia comes from the Chinese work *Daode jing* by *Laotse* and *Chuang-tse*, who are seen as the founders of Taoism. The goal is mystical union with the *Tao* through meditation and imitation of the Taoist nature in thought and action. At the same time, the *Tao* has a metaphysical meaning and is not influenced by moral rules about the "path of the people" like Confucianism. According to the *Daode jing*, the *Tao* is the original principle that is the basis of everything—a reality that comes from the universe and flows back into everything again. Enlightenment (the third character in the DKM Symbol; Chin.: *ming*, Jap.: *myô* 明) as the goal of the meditation in the Taoist sense is the return (Chin.: *fu*) of the beings to the *Tao*. Total emptiness must first be achieved for this purpose so that the eternal stillness can be maintained in order to ultimately be able to perceive the return of the ten thousand moving things to their origin. Once there, everything is still and in its natural original state. The natural primordial state is something that Dr. Usui frequently addressed by challenging his students: "Human being—the crown of Creation—return to your natural primordial state." This is also emphasized by the bridge explained in the chapter on the HS Symbol. The HS Symbol, as the source of Reiki energy from which everything comes and also returns to once again, is the bridge to the DKM Symbol (*Daikômyô* 大光明) in the sense of Taoist enlightenment.

In *The Book of Changes* (*I Ching*) "The Return" (Chin.: *fu*) is explained with *yin* and *yang*. When one of these has reached its climax, it returns back to the other until this in turn has reached its culmination. And so it continues on. The hexagram *Fu* shows precisely this movement. Beneath a solid *yang* line, there are five broken *yin* lines. The third character (*myô* 明) describes exactly this process. Seen from the perspective of the sign, the moon (*yin*) is to the left and the sun (*yang*) is to the right.

Magical Taoism

Magical Taoism, *Daojiao*, has as its main goal the attainment of immortality. It uses meditations, magic, alchemy, physical and breathing exercises, as well as Tantric techniques, for this purpose. Depending upon the school, the various practices are emphasized more or less. The schools, which only became merged with Taoism between 220-120 B.C., go back in part to much older traditions such as Wu shamanism. This is also the era in which the energy work with light beings began in Taoism. The sorcerers of that time initiated this development. According to early reports from the Third Century B.C., they were called the "Lords of the Formulas" and were masters in Chinese astrology, spiritual healing, clairvoyance, geomancy, and sexual practices. For the purpose of healing and rituals, they used symbols in the form of talismans and cooperated closely with light beings, as is now customary in Rainbow Reiki. These sorcerers developed into the Taoist priests who carried out rituals with talismans and magic formulas for healing and other purposes. They frequently lived in monasteries under strict ascetic rules.

In the Second Century A.D., Taoism became especially popular because it was possible to heal diseases in many people with the help of talismans and rituals. The Taoist Master *Ko Hung* (284-364) soon summarized the various methods for attaining a long life in his encyclopedia, *Pao p'u tzu*. The esoteric aspect, which deals with making talismans and using magic spells, is the basis for Dr. Usui's creation of the HS Symbol.[40]

Taoism probably came to Japan at the latest in the Seventh Century. The Japanese historical work *Nihonshoki* begins with the characters *yin* and *yang* and tells of the arrival of Taoist masters. The height of Taoist practices such as divination and exorcism occurred in Japan during the Heian period (794-1185) with the development of the path of *yin* and *yang* (Jap.: *onmyôdô* 陰陽道). This mainly involved the making of amulets and magical practices. An office was even created at the Tennô's court for this purpose.

Among the best-known Taoist rituals in Japan is the *Taizan fukun* of the god *Taishan*, who decides upon the length of a human life. The basis of the secret rituals called "cutting the nine sign" *Kuji kiri*[41] also comes from Taoism, but was optimized in Japan through skillfully combining it with Esoteric Buddhism and the Japanese Shugendô and Shintô forms of magic.

The correlation between Taoism and Esoteric Buddhism was certainly familiar to the monk *Kûkai*[42] since he had learned both in China and also taught them in Japan at the first public university in that country.

It is not really clear whether the Taoist ideas of making talismans and magic had already entered into Esoteric Buddhism in China or not until it reached Japan. But we do know that Taoism continually influenced Buddhism in China through the course of history. Shintô and Shugendô, as well as many old offices in Japan were so directly influenced by Taoism that they were permeated by its ideas, as Professor Fukunaga Mitsuji has demonstrated in his book on Taoism and Japanese culture.[43] Long before

---

[40] Cf. with the chapter on the HS Symbol.

[41] Cf. with the corresponding chapter.

[42] Kûkai is the eighth patriarch of the *Shingon* School of Esoteric Buddhism, which can be traced directly back to *Dainichi Nyorai*. Cf. the chapter on Esoteric Buddhism.

[43] Cf. with the chapter on Shintoism and Sugendo, as well as Fukunaga, Mitsuiji: *Dokyo to nihon no bunka*. Jinbun Shoin. Kyoto, 1982.

his experience on Mount Kurama, Dr. Usui had access to these combined teachings. Without them, there would neither be the Reiki symbols nor Reiki as an art of spiritual healing in its current form.

Many centuries later, there was a phase in Japanese history during the *Edo* period (1600-1868) when Taoism was systematically suppressed. It lasted until the beginning of the *Meiji* period (1868-1912). During this time, a belief arose that Shintoism, which was strongly influenced by Taoism, was a pure Japanese, native religion.[44] This was first claimed by the 国学 *kokugaku*[45] disciple *Hirata Atsutane* (1776-1843), who had studied all of the Taoist texts from China and came to the conclusion that Taoism did not come from China to Japan, but was originally brought from Japan to China. Furthermore, the word Taoism (Jap.: *dôkyô* 道教) was soon removed from the Japanese texts. This is also one of the reasons why there is relatively little material on Taoism to be found in Japan today. However, if we compare the Japanese with the Chinese texts, as well as consider the offices at the Japanese court of the Tennô and many aspects of Shintoist art with China, the contribution of the Taoist influence cannot be denied.

Be that as it may, the magical practices of Taoism have influenced Shintô and Esoteric Buddhism so strongly through the centuries that the magical practices have been preserved despite the new name they were given. Whether or not Dr. Usui was informed about the details of these developments is unknown. In any case, the magical elements of Taoism contributed to the development of the healing art of Reiki, which is useful throughout the world.

---

[44] However, there are many good reasons to presume that Shintoism actually developed from the teachings of Wu Shamanism and native shamanism imported to Japan from China. There are simply too many obvious parallels between the two systems.

[45] A scientific school during the Edo period that developed into a national movement on the basis of philological-literary studies. Through the research of the old Japanese literature and reformation of the state thinking, Shintô increasingly took the center stage of state thought as the path of truth. "Un-Japanese" elements such as Buddhism or Confucianism were rejected.

CHAPTER 6

Shamanism and Shintô

Shamanism

Japanese shamanism has a long history, the origins of which go back to cultures that have hardly been researched and explored even in Japan itself. For example, an entire series of pyramids of gigantic dimensions have been discovered on the Japanese mainland and off the coast. According to all of the current facts, these have no relation to the earliest known culture of the *Jômon* (10,000 B.C.-400 B.C.). Scientists date the two pyramids in Northern Japan in the Prefecture of Tôhoku as being older than 8,000 years. At the foot of the big pyramid, there is a city of stone overgrown with trees than are more than 1,000 years old. Its buildings have nothing in common with those of the *Jômon* culture. It is interesting to note that shamans have been especially common in such areas since ancient times. Some of their traditions are still practiced to this day.

In Japan, as also in Korea, the female shamans play a leading role in shamanism. They are called *miko* (巫 or 巫女) in Japanese—a term that is exclusively used for women. It also depicts the lowest third of the first character for Reiki (靈氣)[46]. In short, the female shamans pray to the gods so that they will send blessed water (rain) to the earth.[47]

[46] In the Chinese character for Reiki, which is identical with the Japanese, the symbolically depicted female shamans are clearly associated with the ancient tradition of the Wu shamans. In Wu shamanism, which also had a substantial position for many centuries at the court of the Chinese emperor, the veneration of the sacred mountains (the Wu knew of their spiritual powers and medicinal herbs, and the gods who liked to come down there) played an important role, as well as the very important magic dance for rain, which is also depicted in an abstract form in the symbol for Reiki. The central source of a Wu female shaman's spiritual power is the unification of the divine powers of heaven and earth in her heart. In Chinese, the *Rei* is called *Ling*. Some of the oldest meanings of this word and its characters are: magical reality; magic power; life

➤

125

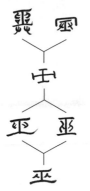

The character 巫 is composed of the components for work 工 and two people 人 together. In combination, this indicates a method with which the gods are invoked. An additional meaning is concealed in the original sign. The two people are sitting there on their knees and holding their hands as if they were offering something to the gods, perhaps a spiritual sacrifice and as if they were giving Reiki.

ILL. 11 – KANJI ORIGIN FOR FEMALE SHAMAN

➢

energy of the principle of darkness Yin (the Great Goddess) or the deities in general. The character *Ling* also describes the mask of a Wu female shaman, with whose help she establishes contact to the spiritual force of a light being in order to use it for acts of magic. This resonance can extend to the complete invocation of the deity. The symbol *Ling* is considered by far to be the oldest symbol denoting the Wu shamans. It is synonymous with their characteristics and their central spiritual power. The main quality of the Wu is that they can come into a personal close relationship with light beings and ancestral spirits (ascended masters). The ancient book *Ch'u-yü* says on this topic: "… Only when someone from the people was gifted with great spiritual power and held fast to his clan, as well as being capable of strict spiritual purity and discipline, … then a light spirit or a deity would come down to him. This was called *Hsi* in a man and *Wu* in a women." The Sacred Marriage (*Hieros Gamos*) played a central role in the initiation of the Wu into her spiritual powers and in special magical rituals. The chapter on "Spiritual Cosmology" contains more information on the Sacred Marriage. The deity from whom the Wu receive their spiritual power is *T'ai-I*, the All-One. The corresponding deity in Esoteric Buddhism is Dainichi Nyorai. Moreover, the Wu maintain close relationships with the Five Totem Animals, with which we are familiar from Chinese Feng Shui. These are light beings that personify the five elements and organize their flow of power into the world. It is rather certain that the Wu brought their cult to Japan and established the central portions of Japanese shamanism and the cult of the sacred mountains and their gods there. The Wu tradition later merged for the most part with Taoism and invigorated it with much practical and very effective energy work. There are strong parallels between the Wu and the early Indian forms of spiritual energy work that was practiced by masters living in the outdoors, from whom Gautama Buddha learned. Spiritual energy work with the Five Holy Animals is also taught in Rainbow Reiki.

[47] More details on this in the chapter on the Reiki characters.

There are also male shamans. They are called *Geki* (覡). The character is composed of the terms "female shaman" and "seeing." The shaman is therefore the one who seeks the gods through the female shaman by seeing her and learning from her. This indicates that the original shamanism in Japan must have had a matriarchal nature, as was true for the Wu shamans in ancient China.

There are two basic types of female shamans. The first group is called *Kannagi* and belongs to the court of the *Tennôs* and the Shintô shrines. This is where the female shamans play the role of a helper in the rituals; however, in most cases they have lost their original function and technique, as well as their magical powers. In particular, this role includes tasks like selling ritual objects (candles, incense, sake, amulets, etc.) to the believers. They wear red-white clothing and are active in almost every shrine and at every shrine festival to this day. In earlier times, they were the daughters or other family members of the Shintô priests. Any young girl of a shrine community can assume this function today. Most of them have no special training and do their "job" for pocket money as long as they are still virgins.

The second group involves much more. They are called *Kuchiyose* and enjoy a long-term, intensive training with many initiations and practical exercises, including ascetic practices in the deepest forests of Japan. After the training, they may remain in their home village and carry out powerful rituals of all types for the inhabitants there. Or they travel from village to village and attune themselves to the feelings and needs of the inhabitants there. They also perform healing and light-filled rituals and then take this energy with them to the next village. In a ritual manner, they then convey the feeling of the previous village, giving the villages the possibility of achieving a better understanding of each other on a deep spiritual level. This dissolves possible conflicts with love and through the help of the gods to everyone's satisfaction.

In their rituals, they use techniques such as ecstatic dancing, dream work, astral travel, channeling, fortune-telling, healing with the power of the light beings, and making herbal remedies that are additionally charged with aspects of the light beings' power and much more. In difficult circumstances of death, special rituals for the liberation of the soul are performed. Even today, they are often asked to seek personal advice from guardian angels and the deceased.[48] "The Mountain of Fear" (Jap.: *Osoresan* 恐山)

in Northern Japan's Prefecture Tôhoku is especially well-known for this purpose. This mountain is an old volcano with a fantastic crater lake and a bizarre landscape of stone and sulfur crystals. In many places, there is hot, sulfurous gas or water streaming out of the ground. There are many small and large pagodas of natural stones piled up between them. The hot springs are known beyond that region particularly for their curative effects and many people like to visit them. It is said that the souls of all deceased pass through here on their way to the light worlds. This is why is it also especially easy to make contact with them there.

Kami–The Spirits, Gods, and Light Beings of Japan

As in many ancient spiritual traditions of the world, people in Japan also assume that not only the beings of the world have souls but also everything else: springs, rocks, trees, etc., because they are all made of the creative force. The light beings, which maintain the connections between the individual, apparently lifeless parts or "unconscious" beings (animals) of the material world and the creative force are generally called *Kami* in Japan. The spirits and gods of Japan (Jap.: *Kami*) may be at home in stones, rocks, entire mountains, individual trees, forests, or even animals. Or, for example, they may be the tree itself. The power places where they live are generally decorated with various symbols such as thick ropes, red gates (Jap.: *torii*), or strips of paper folded into lightning bolts.

In many cases, shrines with one or more altars are located there. In addition to the *Kami* of nature, there are also the heavenly *Kami*, such as the Sun Goddess *Amaterasu* or her brother, the Storm God *Susanoo*, who are worshiped in very large palace-like shrines. All of the *Kami* have special abilities and strengths. Depending upon which goal is to be achieved with the shamanic work, the *Kami* are invited to the rituals as needed.

---

[48] These activities are also practically identical with those of Chinese Wu shamanism.

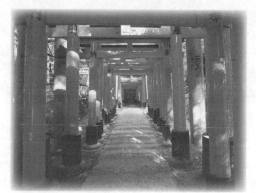

ILL. 12 – SACRED GATES IN THE FUSHIMI INARI SHRINE, KYOTO

Shamanic Work with the Kami

The so-called "invoking" of the *Kami* can be interpreted in a number of different ways. With the help of shamanic practices, it is possible on the one hand to invite a *Kami* into one's own body (invocation). This means that the *Kami* can communicate with other beings through the medium. In the same way, it is possible to learn something from them or to receive special abilities for a shorter or longer amount of time. On the other hand, the *Kami* can be invited to rituals and festivals in order to participate in them. In both cases, a fair exchange always takes place. For their help and support of the shamans and/or laypeople, the *Kami* receive various return services such as festivals in their honor where they are symbolically carried through the city in altars or entire shrine complexes are built where anyone can come to do something good for the *Kami*, to contact them, or to thank them.

When visiting the *Kami* in shrines, I (Mark) have repeatedly been struck by how very playful they are. Before people enter a shrine through the gate, they must first throw little stones onto the ridge of the gate. If other stones fall down as a result, these must also be thrown back up again. This is fun, but it can also be extremely strenuous and some people then stay outside. Fortunately, stones do not have to be thrown onto every gate. That would become extremely intense, as can easily be seen in the illustration.

129

Incidentally, the *Kami* are not just found in the outdoors or in shrines in Japan but also in the house altars or even in the car, wallet, and other things that require protection. They really strive to do their work well...

The Rule of the Female Shamans

About 1900 years ago, there was a shaman queen in Japan by the name of *Himiko* (also known as *Pimiko*). Her name means "Sublime Child of the Sun." During this period, Japan did not yet have its own script. Written records about this kingdom existed only in the neighboring China, which was more technically advanced at that time. In the Chinese text *Wo-jen-chuan* (The History and Topography of Japan in the Third Century) from the *Wei-chi* (History of the Wei Dynasty), compiled by Chen Shou (233-297 A.D.), Japan was called the "Land of the *Wa*," which later became one of the common names for Japan in general. Queen *Himiko* ruled the land from 180-248 A.D., after she had united large portions of ancient Japan. The center of her kingdom was the city of Yamatai. Queen *Himiko* ascended to the throne at the age of 14 years as a young shaman. She led a shamanic life by performing numerous rituals with offerings for the gods and spirits, accomplishing a great deal for her people with her magical powers. However, few people ever saw her because she very much valued reclusiveness. Her servants—who were also female shamans—conveyed her words to the people. This occurred less through speeches than by traveling from village to village in the above-described manner of loving diplomacy. When *Himiko* died, a large cairn was built for her. She was followed by a longer series of more shaman-queens and empresses.

This form of government by a female shaman was probably not a rarity in and around Japan. If we compare this with the Ryukyu Islands (today: Okinawa), which at that time did not yet belong to Japan, shamanic queens also ruled their people in a similar manner there up into the 19th Century.

Centuries later, the *Nihongi* described how *Himiko* descended directly from the sun goddess *Amaterasu* or may have even been her; this is called avatar, which means the embodiment of a deity in a human being that occurs not through karma but through free divine will. An avatar fulfills the Bodhisattva vow during his or her lifetime.

This is also the origin of the idea that the Tennôs of Japans were not of divine descent but actually were gods themselves. However, the last Tennô (Shôwa Tennô) was forced to revise this in his radio speech on capitulation in the Second World War on August 15, 1945.

I believe that the rituals and practices related to these ideas are even more interesting than the political discussion. In the original shamanism of Japan, there is namely a form of rituals in which the adepts call the gods or spirits into themselves or merge with them so much that they can no longer be differentiated from them (invocation).

From Shamanism to the Japanese Shintô Religion

Influenced by the lively contact with the mainland and the rigid Confucian ethics, men were later allowed to become Tennôs after many generations in which the women ruled. However, with the introduction to Buddhism in the years 538 or 552, a shift occurred in the history of Japanese shamanism. The question soon arose whether just the original spirits and gods or the newly introduced Buddha should be prayed to in the future. There were even combative confrontations in which the adherents of Buddhism emerged as the victors. In precise terms, instead of religious interests this was related to—as is probably the case for most aggressive religious conflicts—the hunger for power of individual people, which was actually neither in the interest of shamanism nor Buddhism. Since then, it became necessary to clearly separate native shamanism from the imported religions by giving it the name of *Shintô* (神道)—Path of the Gods. In English, Shintoism is also used as a synonym of Shintô.

In addition to Buddhism, the Taoist way of thinking also came to Japan. Taoism in its magical form has a great deal in common with Shintô so that a renewed mixture of both spiritual traditions occurred. After all, this had already happened once in China with Wu shamanism. Soon there were quarrels again, this time about whether Buddhism should be recognized as the sole state religion. Furthermore, the adherents of Buddhism claimed that their religion was the only effective one and attempted to repress Shintoism and Taoism as the path of the devil, which they fortunately never succeeded in doing.

Up into the Sixth and Seventh Century, shamanism still played an influential role at the Japanese court of the Tennô. Because of the strong influence from China and the adoption of many cultural assets that ranged from technical achievements to religion to the form of government, shamanism was ousted from the court of the Tennô and ultimately labeled a folk religion. Under the influence of the magical practices of Taoism and Esoteric Buddhism, it soon developed into *Shugendô*[49].

Shintoism and its rituals, which focused on the Tennô family, were preserved. In the Tenth Century, the rituals that were important for the court of the Tennô were summarized in texts such as the *Engi Shiki* (927). This gave Shintoism the status of a religion that was complete in itself and definable with a system of myths, rituals, priestly lineages, and shrines. Incidentally, this text extensively explains the effects of the CR symbol for the first time.

The Connection Between Shintoism and Buddhism

Since the introduction of Buddhism and its official recognition in the year 594, the nameless shamanism was given the name of *Shintô*. Despite repeated political-religious difficulties, both religions coexist with each other up to this day in Japan. An unavoidable reconciliation of both religions soon occurred as Buddhist temples were built next to or on the grounds of Shintoist shrines and shrines found their way into temples. At the beginning of the Eighth Century, Buddhist monks recited their sutras in front of the Shintô shrines to tell the *Kami* about the new teaching. Sutras and sacred objects were exchanged between the temples and shrines to introduce the light beings of both religions to each other and make them happy. For example, after abundant offerings were made to the shrine of the war god *Hachiman*, he donated large sums to finish building what is still the biggest Buddhist temple of Japan, which is called *Tôdaiji*. As a result, *Hachiman* had the title of Bodhisattva bestowed upon him some years later.

---

[49] See the next chapter for more information.

At latest in the early *Heian* Period (794-1185), as the monk *Kûkai* made Esoteric Buddhism popular in Japan and simultaneously taught Taoism at the first public university of Japan, which he opened, there were mutual reconciliations and the deep blending of Buddhism and Shintô.

It was recognized that the Indian Buddha, the Taoist gods of China, and the Japanese *Kami* were solely various names for the same light beings. So, for example the *Sun Goddess Amaterasu* can be equated with the Great Sun Buddha *Dainichi Nyorai*. Accordingly, the *Kami* were also associated with the *Siddham* symbols of Esoteric Buddhism, and Buddhas were called incarnations or appearances of the *Kami* and vice versa. This was especially promoted by the character of the rituals in Esoteric Buddhism and in the magical-shamanic Shintô. There is namely an important common factor. In the ritual work with the light beings, both spiritual traditions focus on inviting the light beings into one's own body in order to merge with them, among other things. This facilitates lasting learning from the light beings, as well as the development of the highest spiritual powers. With these powers, it has been possible to create something like a healing art by the name of Reiki–the Usui System of Natural Healing ...

Ryôbu Shintô

The combination of Shintô and Esoteric Buddhism is called *Ryôbu Shintô*. *Ryôbu* is related to the two large mandalas of the two worlds (Womb World and Diamond World)[50] in the Esoteric Buddhism of the *Shingon* school. The two mandalas are graphic depictions of the universe and its phenomena. The correlation with Shintô is extensively described in the Japanese book *Tenchi Reiki Ki* (Records of the Spiritual Life Energy from Heaven and Earth). It is not certain whether this book comprising of 18 scrolls originates from this time. Some people believe that it was written by *Kûkai*. Others say that it was probably first created in the *Kamakura* Period (1185-1333). Independent of this, it provides a comprehensive explanation of the various Shintô-Buddhist rituals and symbols.

[50] These two mandalas and their diverse spiritual relationships are nothing other than an abstract depiction of the Sacred Marriage (*Hieros Gamos*), which is innocuous to the layperson. It is the sexual unification of the Great Goddess with the Great God, through which the material world is created anew time and again.

Another development is *Watarai-Shintô*, which was created by *Watarai Ieyuki* (1256-1351). In his five books on Shintô (*Shintô Gobusho*), he extensively explains the symbols, rituals, purification (spiritual purifying techniques), and ritual architecture (a type of Feng Shui) in Shintô and Buddhism, in addition to the mythology. At this point, it becomes clear that the Reiki Symbols were compiled from many different spiritual traditions that were basically connected by ancient shamanism and *Dainichi Nyorai* in many forms of manifestation. For more than 1,300 years, the combination of various spiritual traditions has been a completely normal process. Accordingly, there is hardly a person in Japan who feels that he or she belongs to just one of them. Statistically seen, about 80% of the Japanese today are Shintoist and another 80% are Buddhists. Since a population of 160% is not possible, this is a sign of the openness and devotion to various traditions next to each other and with each other. Although there was an attempt during the second half of the 19th Century to once again separate Buddhism and Shintô from each other, even now the worship of the Shintôist *Kami* in little shrines is located next to the Buddha in Buddhist temples and the worship of Buddhist light beings is present in Shintôist shrines. I have noticed that the clear sublime presence of the light beings is particularly tangible especially in the temples and shrines where both are combined with each other.

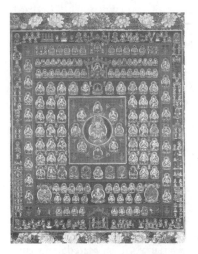 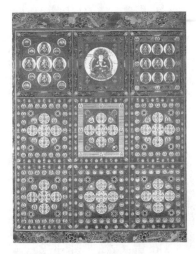

ILL. 13 – WOMB WORLD AND DIAMOND WORLD MANDALA

CHAPTER 7

Shugendô—Japanese Magic

My (Mark's) special interest in researching the origins of the Reiki Symbols lies in the time before Dr. Usui. Within the scope of my many years of involvement with this wonderful energetic method of healing, I came across the correlations with *Shugendô*, the Path of the Magician, early on. There are namely mountain ascetics in Japan called *Yamabushi* who do many interesting and unusual things that are probably connected both directly, as well as indirectly, with the Usui System of Reiki and the Reiki symbols. Here, as well as in Shintô and Esoteric Buddhism,[51] it is important to explore both the native and the imported elements that have lastingly influenced *Shugendô* in order to have a deeper understanding of it.

Shugendô reflects a special characteristic of Japanese culture that I would like to briefly explain. When something new is introduced in Japan, the old is not thrown away but continues to live in the new. After a while, the old and new are then so skillfully combined, and frequently even improved, that they merge in such a way that they can hardly be separated. The result is then something typically Japanese.

In simple terms, *Shugendô* is a form of Japanese magic in which the useful magical elements of many cultures have flowed together and been integrated through the centuries—possibly even the millennia—into the practices of everyday life. With the great variety of origins for the individual Reiki symbols and their applications, Reiki itself shows a strong similarity to this characteristic of the *Shugendô* itself through the skilled and probably unique combination of Buddhism, Taoism, Shintô, and *Shugendô*.

I consider it to be very probable that Dr. Usui also studied with the *Yamabushi* before his meditation on Mount Kurama because they frequently climbed Mount Kurama for ascetic purposes at that time and still do today. Another reason is because many of the methods and applications of the symbols, such as the CR symbol, are tremendously similar in the

---

[51] Cf. the corresponding chapter.

Usui System of Reiki and *Shugendô* and date back to the *Engi Shiki*, an old ritual text from the 10th Century.

The Development and Background of Shugendô

Its development was promoted to a considerable degree by the nature-worshipping pre-Shintoist path, which experienced a unique expression of concepts and practices under the influx and influence of Esoteric Buddhism and Taoism.

The term *Shugendô* first arose during the Middle Ages and was considered to be something like a folkloristic form of Buddhism in Japanese history. When read from the back to the front, an analysis of the characters 修験道 (*Shugendô*) reveals that this is about "the path" (*dô*) that is taken by "performing magical practices in the mountains"(*shu*) for acquiring "supernatural powers and their miraculous effects" (*gen*).

The character *shu* means: "ruling, regulating," as well as "performing, practicing, and exercising." *Shu* also occurs in many terms of Buddhism and always means "cultivating, training, and practicing" there as well.

The detailed meaning of the character *gen* is: "sign, apparent proof, and the performance of miracles." *Gen* also appears in the Buddhist sutras *Shô mudô kyô* and *Darani shû kyô* with the meaning of "proof of the miraculous power." The character combination of *shugen*, which frequently appears in the literature within this context, is an abbreviation of *shujugen*, which means the "acquiring of miraculous powers through practicing magical formulas."

Even early literary sources such as the *Shoku Nihongi* from the year 797 describe miraculous powers such as those of a Buddha, a spiritually realized human being. The Eighth Century is still quite early for Japan since there was no script in Japan until the introduction of Buddhism in the Sixth Century and its own script systems only developed over time.

The book *Shô mudô kyô* states the following about *Fudô Myôô*, a wrathful manifestation of *Dainichi Nyorai*:

"If there are people in the masses who want to perform such rituals (*hô*) and go to the silent and lonely mountains and forests seeking a pure place to practice and concentrate on their practices and read the sutras, then they will encounter *Fudô Myôô* and achieve the goal of their practices... If the *Fudô Myôô* sutras and dhâranîs are correctly intoned in this way, then they will achieve the great perfection... Anyone who wants to try out the effects of the ritual can make a mountain move, cause water to flow against the current, and do everything according to his own will."

The same topic is discussed in the book *Darani shû kyô*:

"Anyone who recites the magic formulas (*ju*) will quickly attain magical powers of all sorts... If there should be someone who practices this ritual, these magical formulas, brings offerings to the *Bonten* (light beings/angels), and therefore hopes to achieve miraculous powers (*gen*)..."

It is difficult to determine when the term *Shugendô* developed. In the book *Nihon Ryôiki* from the year 822, *Shugendô* was described as follows in the biographical information about *En no Gyôja*, the founder of *Shugendô*:

"...Practicing the ritual (*hô*) of the magical formula (*ju*) of the Peacock King, achieving extraordinarily miraculous powers (*i genriki*)..."

This reveals that *shugen* means something like "practicing magical formulas and achieving miraculous powers."

The term "magical formulas" means *mantras*. However, since the origin of both terms is different, I will be separated them from each other at this point:

The Sanskrit word *mantra* is *shingon* in Japanese and means "true word."[52] This is also the source of the name of the Japanese *Shingon* School of Esoteric Buddhism founded by the monk Kûkai. In Japanese, the word *ju* means "spell" and was already used long before—and obviously also after—the introduction of Buddhism. The Japanese do not keep these terms strictly apart. Yet, it is quite meaningful here to precisely define the terms used in order to achieve clarity about their origins and the correlations with the Reiki symbols.

The mountains are very well suited for practicing the rituals of Esoteric Buddhism, performing difficult practices (*kugyô*), and therefore accumulating good karma. The peaks of the mountains are places between earth and heaven—not completely here and not completely there—that are especially appropriate for magical rituals. People who practiced mi-

[52] see next page

raculous powers in the mountains were called miracle-working monks or miracle ascetics (*genja*) during the *Heian* Period (794-1185). Those who were especially gifted in exercising the miraculous powers were called *ugen no hito*.

Kûkai, after he had been initiated by a miracle-working monk, also went into the mountains to devote himself there to his Morning Star meditation[53]. This is the same meditation that Dr. Usui performed on Mount Kurama. At that time, *Kûkai* did not know what effects these practices would have on his life. He simply devoted himself to the course of his spiritual development and progressed on his life path with the practices in this manner. Later on, he was then able to accomplish great miracles to help many people. The accomplishment of miracles was namely the main reason that he was able to convince the Japanese Tennô of the effectiveness

[52] The meaning of the word *mantra* in the ancient Indian sacred language of Sanskrit has five parts and is based on the qualities of a Buddha (a spiritually realized human being): 1. truth; 2. reality; 3. what describes things as they are; 4. not deceitful, false, or underhanded; 5. not contradictory. When the word *mantra* was translated into Japanese, the translators selected the term "truth" (true word) from its five detailed meanings. The Buddhist saint Nâgârjuna defined mantras as "esoteric (meaning that their meaning is concealed beneath the surface) words. Kûkai (*Kôbô Daishi*) said the following about the effect of mantras: "A mantra surpasses rational comprehension. It extinguishes ignorance when we meditate on it and recite it. One single mantra contains a thousand (in the sense of "countless many") truths. Saying mantras can help the practitioner to become spiritually realized in the here-and-now. Practice the mantra time and again until perfect stillness has been realized within you. Then also continue to practice it until you have penetrated through to original source of being." A mantra can be the name of a deity, a Buddha, Bodhisattva, or avatar—or a sequence of words or syllables charged with the sacred force that express the specific powers of a divine being. Mantras can also be intensified, deepened, and expanded in their effects through specific spiritual postures (mudrâs) and visualizations (sacred symbols/characters, mandalas, or deities). A personal mantra, into which the student has been initiated by his spiritual teacher, contains the heart of the teachings that the guru would like to transmit to the student to supporting his process of spiritual awaking. Mantras call in, represent, organize, and project the flow of spiritual powers.

[53] The Morning Star is the planet Venus, which has been equated with the Goddess in most of the great cultures of world history. For more on the significance of the Great Goddess for the spiritual awakening and the practical use of sacred forces, please compare the corresponding explanations in the chapter on Spiritual Cosmology.

of Esoteric Buddhism and its superiority over all the other religions that were being practiced at this time.

Mountains as Power Places

Within the scope of his research, Dr. Usui studied various methods of healing such as Shintô, Taoism, Esoteric Buddhism, and Shugendô. He finally went to Mount Kurama to mediate there with a specific goal in mind. On the 21st day of his meditation, he achieved this goal in a vision and became a Reiki channel and Reiki Master.

Life in seclusion for a certain amount of time has the advantage that the abilities achieved can later be used for the benefit of all in worldly life. So the goal of life in the mountains is not fleeing from the civilized world but acquiring abilities for a better life in civilization. In this sense, esotericism should also not be used to flee from the material world and everyday life but instead create a "here and now" that is especially beautiful for all participants in the sense of the divine order. And this is precisely what Dr. Usui did. He studied and researched holistic methods of healing as his basis. By means of the appropriate practices, he then attained the healing power of Reiki in the mountains. Once he returned to civilization, he brought more happiness, health, love, meaning, and prosperity into the world through his abilities and perceptions.

The most important aspect in *Shugendô* is working at the power places in the mountains (*sangaku shinkô*). The origins of this work extend all the way back to Japan's prehistoric period. This phenomenon is not just limited to Japan. There are similar forms of energy work with power places and light beings throughout the entire world. Because of their tremendous similarities, they probably all date back to the same, prehistoric culture.

The mountains were sometimes identified with the gods, as in India, Tibet, Europe, and China. In other places, they were seen as the abode of gods and worshipped as such. In Japan there are mountains from which some of the Japanese gods were said to have descended to earth. All such power places became the goal of pilgrimages and sites of shamanic rituals and meditations. These were also frequently the places where the seemingly incurable diseases of the people who sought healing vanished into thin air.

The magical places between the spiritual world and the material world, and the easily resulting closeness of the people to the gods makes rituals and energy work especially effective. For example, climbing a mountain symbolizes the transition from the human world to the divine world in Indonesia on the Borobodur. In India, staying in the mountains was the fourth stage of an ascetic's pilgrimage. In the spiritual sense, meditation in the mountains was considered to have special merit. Mountains, as well as rivers, served the purpose of purifying on various mental and spiritual levels. In terms of cosmology, mountains[54] such as the famous *Meru*, are considered to be a bridge between earth and heaven. The temples of Esoteric Buddhism in particular, such as the Kurama Temple and the temple cities of Kôya and Hiei established by Kûkai and Saichô, were built on sacred mountains. In my own life, I have discovered that spiritual experiences occur here especially through the high energetic vibration and presence of so many light beings.

In the Japanese power-place work in the mountains, ritual tools such as mirrors and jewels (Shintoist origin) or clay vessels with sutras and dhâranîs (long mantras of Buddhist origin) are buried. Similar practices also exist in Rainbow Reiki, in which special healing-stone mandalas are buried in the earth to spiritually energize such places and connect them with other power places and Ley Lines.[55]

Connections with Shamanism

During the course of the centuries, a fusion occurred between *Shugendô* and the magical practices of Esoteric Buddhism, Taoism, and Shintô. An important precondition for this was the mutual factor of doing energy

[54] Cosmological mountains such as Meru are based on the ancient Indian concept that a mountain stands at the center of the universe or another world, forming the meeting place and abode of the light beings. There are differences in the structure of such a mountain-world system, depending upon the spiritual tradition. What they all have in common is that they are reminiscent of a three-dimensional mandala and depict a bridge between the world of the humans and that of the gods.

[55] Cf. *Rainbow Reiki* by Walter Lübeck, Lotus Press. Translated by Christine M. Grimm.

work in the mountains. The roots of Shintô and *Shugendô* may be similar in certain respects, yet they each developed in different directions and mixed over and over in later times. This usually happened through the pilgrimages undertaken by ascetics of all spiritual directions as they came into contact with the shamans, the folk beliefs, and the mountain ascetics (*Yamabushi*) in the mountains and villages. As the mountain ascetics began to gather students, they formed the basis for the monasteries that can now be found there.

The shamans played an especially important role in ancient Japan, as they probably did in most of the ancient cultures. Within this context, shamans are understood to be especially qualified people in the service of a community who can come into contact with beings from the subtle world through states of trance or ecstasy. They open up to a community on the heart level so that they can take this mood with them to the next village in order to help the people there better understand their neighbors. They heal with the help of light beings, perform miracles to harmonize problems that cannot be solved in other ways (such as rain-making), and bring spiritual wisdom to the people. In this way, shamans emerge when there are unusual diseases, occurrences, and festivals as mediators between people, human beings and nature, as well as between humans and light beings. Since the *Heian* period (794-1185), it has been proved that shamans used mantras for securing peace, preventing harm, and making it rain, which came from Esoteric Buddhism and Taoism[56]. For example, the *Tendai* monk *Ryôgen* (912-985; posthumously called *Jie Daishi*) developed a magical cult for warding off danger from Esoteric Buddhism and Taoism. A well-known method is the amulet technique where symbols are painted in a ritual manner on a piece of paper, which is then pasted to the entrance of residences.

[56] On the other hand, Taoism, which originated in China, experienced a strong influence on its magical practices by the preceding *Wu* shamanism. In other respects as well, there are a tremendous amount of similarities between the ancient Chinese Wu shamanism and the Japanese shamanism and Shintô. Cf. the chapter on Shamanism.

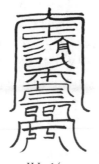

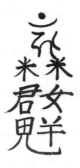

ILL. 14 –
TALISMAN OF THE NORTH STAR

ILL. 15 –
TALISMAN FOR VICTORY
IN THE BATTLE

In addition to the Buddhism at the court of the Tennôs, it has been observed that mountain asceticism was common among the Buddhist monks since the early Eighth Century. The monks in the mountains usually had little connection with monastic life. This is why they were also called *free monks* (Jap.: *shido sô*), meaning that apart from the state clergy they turned to Buddhist practices, magical rites, and cults of folk beliefs. They practiced exorcism of various types, read the sutras, predicted the future, healed diseases, and performed shamanic rituals with the gods. In addition, there was also the mountain asceticism of the laypeople (Jap.: *ubasoku*), who pursued very similar goals without being ordained as monks.

Those who had chosen the path of the Buddha without the approval of the government, who devoted themselves to religious asceticism, and who had selected the mountains as the place for these practices, came into contact with the folk magicians and shamans who practiced there. These often belonged to the circle of the mountain people (Jap.: *yamabito*). The mountain people, who lived in the power places of the mountains every day or even those who practiced there, made up a large portion of the original native peoples and were well-known as shamans for their special powers of healing. As is apparent today, Buddhism was influenced by the mountain people and the mountain people were influenced by Buddhism. Since Taoism was also becoming increasingly popular in Japan at the same time, it was brought to the people on the same path as well. The merging of native magical practices, Buddhism, Taoism, and Shintô led to the development of *Shugendô*.

One of the early shamanic-oriented magicians, a mountain man *yamabito* who was known for his powers and attracted much attention with his prophecies and magic until he was finally slandered and banned, was named *En no Gyôja*. He is also known as the founder of Shugendô, in as far as we can speak of founding instead of a development over many years.

Before the introduction of Esoteric Buddhism, it had been difficult to spread Buddhism among the people since they had already been practicing a very effective magical tradition (Jap.: *Jujutsu* 呪術; literally.: handwork/art of magic) that was adapted to their everyday needs and problems for a long time. Only when the Buddhism in Japan also included the magical practices was it possible for it to take hold among the people in the countryside. Even in the Eighth Century, a high degree of interest in magical practices was observed in the monasteries. However, the practices imported from China were much more interesting for the monasteries than the native practices. Soon after the native magic was officially prohibited in the year 729, the monasteries began teaching *Siddham,* mantras, and mudrâs, which promised effects very similar to those of the native magic. Soon only the free monks like Kûkai had the opportunity of learning the native magic before their ordination. Kûkai was very lucky to be permitted to learn both. During the early years of his monk career, he went on pilgrimages as a free monk through the forests. Here he came into contact with the shamans and mountain ascetics who lived there and was allowed to learn many important things from them. He later became an ordained monk in a monastery and traveled to China to study Esoteric Buddhism there. Thanks to his comprehensive previous experience and great talents, he became one of the eight patriarchs[57] of the *Shingon* School. During his stay in China, he also studied Taoism, technology, the art of engineering, astronomy, and the Indian *Siddham* script. After he returned to Japan and was a distinguished monk, he once again traveled across the country, as in his youth, to help the people. In addition to teaching them how to build dams and bridges, he showed

---

[57] The patriarchs of the *Shingon* School of Esoteric Buddhism are traced back to *Kongôsatta* and *Dainichi Nyorai* in an uninterrupted series. In terms of Reiki, Dr. Usui is the first patriarch of Reiki and was initiated directly by *Kannon* and *Dainichi Nyorai.*

them how to connect Esoteric Buddhism with their native shamanism in order to make their difficult lives easier.

In addition to Kûkai, there were many other monks who brought Buddhism to the people and learned from the local shamans at the same time. Buddhism in Japan had to embrace the shamans and either share or assume their tasks and functions. This is the only way that Buddhism, newly introduced from China, had the possibility of being accepted by the people since state-supported Buddhism was initially just a privilege of the court of the Tennôs and the aristocracy, as well as a pure object of study in the monasteries.

CHAPTER 8

Light Beings

Dainichi Nyorai
大日如来
(Chin.: *Palushena*; Skr.: *Mahâ Vairocana*; Tib.: *Rnam-par-snang-mdsad*)

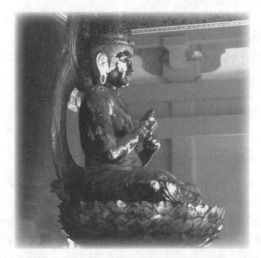

ILL. 16 – THE GREAT SUN BUDDHA DAINICHI NYORAI

Dainichi Nyorai is the Cosmic Buddha of Esoteric Buddhism and is directly related to the DKM symbol[58]. This being is the king and queen of the Buddhas in one, which is why he is the only Buddha to wear a crown. The translation of this name is the "Great Sun Buddha" of the light and the truth. His origin probably dates back to a very ancient sun cult. In Buddhism, the *Dainichi Nyorai* is the Buddha who dwells in the spiritual center of the universe. The light of wisdom radiates from his pores. This light can manifest as the form and aspect of all the other Buddhas and

[58] Cf. chapter on the DKM Symbol.

bears every quality of all of the Buddhas within himself. The historical Buddha Shâkyamuni, who lived about 2500 years ago, is also an emanation of *Dainichi Nyorai*. When *Dainichi Nyorai* appears in a group, he is always placed at the center of all the other Buddhas. Other names for him are *Shana, Roshana, Birushana, Daibirushana, Makabirushana, Henjôshana, Henjô, Henjô Nyorai*, and *Daikômyô Henjô*. His Shinto archetype is the Sun Goddess *Amaterasu Ômikami*.

He is the highest Buddha of Esoteric Buddhism. Through his tremendous power, the light of his teachings is spread throughout the entire world. *Dainichi Nyorai* sits at the center of the Mandala of the Two Worlds. In the Diamond World (*kongôkai*), he embodies the masculine aspect of the sun (Taoist: *yang*). In the Womb World (taizôkai), he embodies the feminine aspect of the moon (Taoist: *yin*).

Dainichi Nyorai grants happiness to this world, heals diseases of body, mind, and soul. He can appear in three forms: as Buddha, he remains himself; as Bodhisattva he embodies the dissemination of the teachings; and as the wisdom king *Myôô*, he attends to the practice of the teaching.

The Origin of the Name Dainichi Nyorai

The name *Dainichi Nyorai* is a translation from Indian Sanskrit and means *Mahâ Vairocana* (Great Shining One). However, in India there is also a light being *Vairocana* (Shining One). They are basically both the same. While the first name is only found in Esoteric Buddhism, the second name is used in both Esoteric Buddhism and Mahâyâna Buddhism.

There are two approaches for translating this name into Japanese or, more accurately, into Chinese[59]. In the early phase, the pronunciation of the Chinese character that is similar to Sanskrit was used. So *Vairocana* became *Birushana* in Japanese and *Mahâ Vairocana* became *Maka Birushana*. These names are found in the sutras of *Mahâyâna* (for example, the Flower Garland Sûtra; Jap.: *Kegon kyô*) and early Esoteric Buddhism (for example, the Sûtra of Becoming a God Through the True Words of the Goddess *Fukû kensaku*; Jap.: *Fukû kensaku jinpen shingon kyô*).

[59] The *sutras*, including the names, were directly translated from Sanskrit into Chinese. There are no translations into Japanese because the *Sutras* were adopted together with the Chinese script in Japan.

By way of contrast, the name *Dainichi* is the translation of the actual meaning of *Mahâ Vairocana* and stands for the "Great Sun." In his honor, the Sanskrit name *Tathagata* (Jap.: *Nyorai*) was added, as it is for many other Buddhas. Another possible, but also very esoteric translation of *Mahâ Vairocana* is *Daikômyô Henjô* (遍照, The Great Radiant Light that Illumines the Entire World).

The term *Dainichi* appears for the first time in the translation of the Sûtra of the Great Light (Jap.: *Dainichi kyô* 大日経) of the two *Shingon* patriarchs Zenmui Sanzô (637-735) and Ichigyô Zenshi (683-725) from the years 724. This sûtra is an especially important text of Esoteric Buddhism. In it, *Dainichi Nyorai* personally describes the lasting spiritual power transmission of *Mahâ Vairocana* for becoming a god. This is also a translation of the original title of this sûtra (Jap.: *Daibirushana jôbutsu jinben kaji kyô* 大毘盧遮那成仏神変加持経). In other words, it is about Reiki initiations. The monk Kûkai[60] found this sûtra before his journey to China under the pagoda of the temple *Kumedera*.

Since the *Dainichi kyô* is not easy to understand, Ichigyô Zenshi wrote a commentary on this sûtra (*Dainichi kyô sho* 大日経疏). Kûkai was the first to bring this commentary to Japan. The text explains the background for the name *Dainichi Nyorai* that has been included here.

The *Siddham* of *Dainichi Nyorai* are the symbols *a* and *vam*. They represent the totality of compassion and wisdom, the path of enlightenment, stability, and creation.

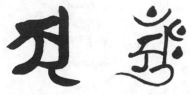

ILL. 17 – THE *SIDDHAM* A AND AHM

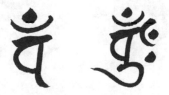

ILL. 18 – THE SIDDHAM VAM AND VAHM

60 Cf. the chapter on the Esoteric Buddhism.

Various aspects of the divinity as expressed in the Siddham trinities. In addition to *Dainichi Nyorai*, *Ashuku Nyorai* (*Siddham hum*), *Fudô Myôô* (*Siddham ham*), and *Kannon* (*Siddham hrih*) are embodied.

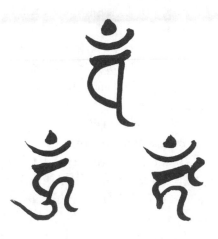

ILL. 19 – SIDDHAM TRINITY: ABOVE IS VAM, LEFT BOTTOM IS HUM, AND RIGHT BOTTOM IS HAM

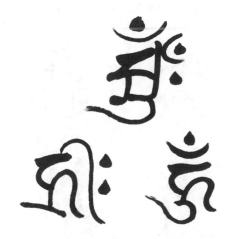

ILL. 20 – SIDDHAM TRINITY: ABOVE IS AHM, LEFT BOTTOM IS HRIH, AND RIGHT BOTTOM IS HUM

Special Emanations of the Dainichi Nyorai

Dainichi Nyorai as the Bodhisattva Diamond Mind (Kongôsatta)

(Chin.: *Wozi Luosa-zin*; Skr.: *Vajrasattva*; Tib.: *Rdo-rje Sems-dpa*)

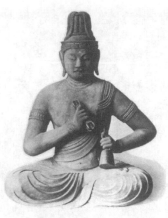

ILL. 21 – DIAMOND MIND KONGÔSATTA

In the Shingon School, the Diamond Mind represents the active aspect of *Dainichi Nyorai*. The secret teachings (*mikkyô*) of Esoteric Buddhism are transmitted through him. According to the legend, he lived in an iron tower in Southern India until *Nâgârjuna*—the first *Shingon* patriarch—opened this tower and passed *Dainichi Nyorai's* teaching of the Mandalas of the Two Worlds on to him. We need to imagine that *Nâgârjuna* himself became the Diamond Mind and could actively work like *Dainichi Nyorai*. His three successors *Nâgabodhi*, *Vajrabodhi*, and *Amoghavajra* brought the secret teachings to China and passed them on to the Chinese monk *Hui-kuo*, who was *Kûkai's* teacher. So *Kûkai* is ultimately also a manifestation of the active power of *Dainichi Nyorai*.

In the secret rituals of Esoteric Buddhism, the Diamond Mind plays the main role as the active force. Without its initiations and the *Siddham* symbols, the rituals have little effect. In his right hand, he holds a five-pointed diamond scepter in front of his chest and a diamond bell in front of his belly with the left hand. His spiritual partner is the goddess *Tara*, also called *Dai Marishi Ten*. The HS symbol has a close connection with Diamond Mind and his *Siddham* syllable of *hûm* (s. page 349). It represents the purifying of the mind in all incarnations on all levels.

149

Fudô Myôô

不動明王

(Chin.: *Budong Fo*; Skr.: *Acalanatha*)

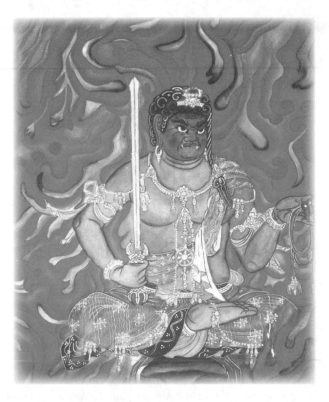

ILL. 22 – THE IMPERTURBABLE WISDOM KING FUDÔ MYÔÔ

In Japan, *Fudô Myôô* is the most important of the five wisdom kings of magic and mystical knowledge. The wisdom kings act as the guardians of the Buddhas and symbolize their power and their victory. They fight the causes of suffering and diseases such as the attachments that are obstacles to happiness, success, and health.

Fudô means "imperturbable" and *Myôô* is the "king of light." So a translation of his entire name would be the "Imperturbable King of Light." Since light represents wisdom here, he is usually called the Wisdom King. His mystical name is *Jôjû Kongô*.

150

Dainichi Nyorai as the Medicine Buddha (Yakushi Nyorai)

薬師如来

(Chin.: *Yaoshi Fo*; Skr.: *Bhaisajyaguru*; Tib.: *Sangs rgyas*)

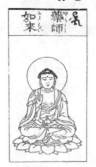

ILL. 23 – THE MEDICINE BUDDHA YAKUSHI NYORAI

When *Dainichi Nyorai* appears as the Medicine Buddha[61], he shows himself in the form of a Bodhisattva with a high crown and without jewelry. He may hold his hands in one of the three mudrâs of teaching, meditation, and wisdom, depending upon through which aspect healing should occur.

Dainichi Nyorai as the Goddess of Loving Eyes (Ichiji Kinrin Nyorai)

(Skr.: *Ekaksara Usnisacakra*)

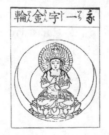

ILL. 24 – LOVING EYES ICHIJI KINRIN NYORAI

Loving Eyes merges the powers and energies of the Mandalas of the Diamond World and the Womb World, combining the energetic forces of the Great Sun Buddha *Dainichi Nyorai* and the Diamond Mind *Kongô-satta* on the energetic level. This is shown through the wisdom mudrâ *Chiken in*.

---

[61] Also see the chapter on the Medicine Buddha.

151

Dainichi Nyorai as the Bodhisattva of the North Star (Myôdô Bosatsu)

(Skr.: *Sudrsti, Dhruva*)

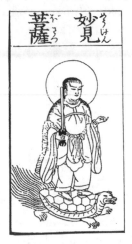

ILL. 25 – BODHISATTVA OF THE NORTH STAR MYÔDÔ BOSATSU

Dainichi Nyorai can appear here in both the feminine and the masculine form. As the Bodhisattva of the North Star, *Dainichi Nyorai* is the source of ambrosia and elixirs such as that of immortality from a type of enchanted garden. At the same time, he is the guardian of horses because he manifests himself as the White Horse and messenger of the Shinto gods. He is always depicted in mandalas within the context of the seven stars of the Great Bear (Big Dipper).

The Five Transcendental Buddhas–
Dainichi Nyorai and the Five Jinas

The transcendental Buddhas are the guardians of spiritual wisdom. At the same time, they are also close emanations of *Dainichi Nyorai* himself. In the mandalas of Esoteric Buddhism, they are associated with the directions and each has their own place. Each individual one represents certain magical powers and effects that can be achieved through initiations, rituals, and meditations.

Dainichi Nyorai – Immaculate Mind and Path to Enlightenment

Ashuku Nyorai – Accumulation of Mind and Awakening of the Heart
(Chin.: *Achu*; Skr.: *Aksobhya*; Tib.: *Mi-bskyod-pa*)

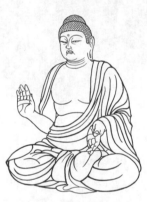

ILL. 26 – ASHUKU NYORAI

Hôshô Nyorai – Devotion and Asceticism
(Chin.: *Baosheng Fo*; Skr.: *Ratnasambhava*; Tib.: *Rin-chen-hbyung*)

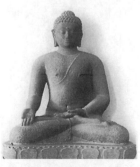

ILL. 27 – HÔSHÔ NYORAI

153

Amida Nyorai – Pure Mind and Spiritual Awakening
(Chin.: *Omituo Fo*; Skr.: *Amitabha*; Tib.: *Oepame*)

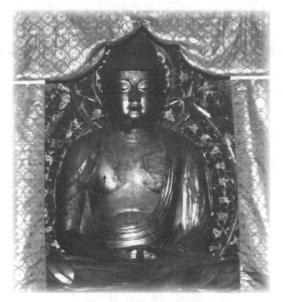

ILL. 28 – AMIDA NYORAI

Fukûjôju Nyorai – Five Senses & Entering into Nirvana
(Skr.: *Amoghasiddhi*; Tib.: *Don-grub*)

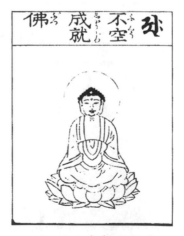

ILL. 29 – FUKÛJÔJU NYORAI

Monju Bosatsu
文殊菩薩

(Chin.: *Wenshu*; Skr.: *Manjusri*; Tib.: *Jam-dpal*)

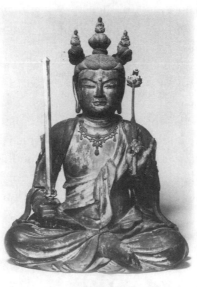

ILL. 30 – MONJU BOSATSU

Monju Bosatsu has very different forms of manifestation and areas of action. He is usually depicted with a sword in the right hand and a lotus
blossom in the left. The sword symbolizes his ability to discriminate between things in relationship to the effect that they have. The lotus stands
for purity and the nature of sentient beings. *Monju Bosatsu* represents the
wisdom that is perceived in the degree to which we apply the knowledge
that we have acquired. This is why he is also a patron for all spiritual
tasks and plans that fulfill a higher purpose. People like to pray to *Monju
Bosatsu* for support in achieving a personal goal whose realization benefits
very many beings.

Monju Bosatsu teaches sentient beings that everything is related to
everything else, that space connects sentient beings even if there are great
distances between them, and that there are no beings in the entire universe
who can exist alone without an exchange with the surrounding world.
His mantra of *Om a ra pa ca na* stands for the world of learning and the

155

world of spiritual wisdom. His symbol is the *Siddham* of *mam*. It represents the emptiness of all existing things. When he is worshipped as the guardian of knowledge, the mantra *Om araha shanô* is employed. Then he rides on a lion with a lotus blossom as a saddle. He carries a sword in the right hand and a scroll in the left. When *Monju Bosatsu* carries a sûtra instead of a sword in the right hand, this represents the wisdom of liberating the mind.

When the Japanese monk *Gyôki* (668-749) went to Mount Wutaishan in China for several years to become immersed in Buddhism there, it became clear that he was an incarnation of *Monju Bosatsu*. Back in Japan, he committed himself to the founding of the *Tôdaiji* temple (which is still the largest wooden building in the world), in which the Great Sun Buddha *Birushana* (*Dainichi Nyorai* of Mahâyâna Buddhism) is worshipped. In the Womb World of the Great Sun Buddha *Dainichi Nyorai*, *Monju Bosatsu* sits at his side in the southwest on a white lotus and points to the wisdom of the Heart Sûtra.

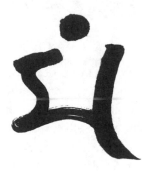

ILL. 31 – SIDDHAM MAM

Kokûzô Bosatsu–He Who Overcomes Space and Brings the Great Treasure
虚空蔵菩薩

(Chin.: *Xukongzang*; Skr.: *Akasagarbha*; Tib.: *Nam.mka'i-snying-po*)

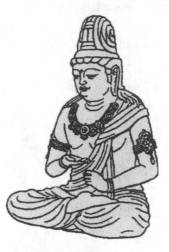

ILL. 32 – KOKÛZÔ BOSATSU

Kokûzô Bosatsu is the Bodhisattva who brings the people the greatest treasures. In his mantra, he is called the "Bringer of the Treasures." His mantra is: *Nô bô akyasha kyarabaya on arikya mari bori sowaka*." When Dr. Usui performed the Morning Star meditation of *Kokûzô Bosatsu* on Mount Kurama, he ultimately received a great treasure on the 21st day—the initiation into Reiki and the symbols. As we can also see in the example of Dr. Usui, these are not material treasures like a car or a sack full of gold but spiritual treasures that are intended to do something good for humanity. In Sanskrit, the word "treasure" also refers to "the space that connects sentient beings."

His *Siddham* symbol is *trah* and it helps in the liberation of the mind so that it can access unlimited knowledge and achieve the ability of also applying it in a creative way. When correctly applied, his *Siddham* symbol *tram* leads to an initiation into a spiritual power such as in the example

157

of Reiki. Dr. Usui probably used the symbol *trah* in the Morning Star meditation and *tram* for the initiation.

The body of *Kokûzô Bosatsu* is golden. He wears a garment and jewelry. The crown on his head displays the five transcendental Buddhas with *Dainichi Nyorai* at the center. His facial expression is decidedly friendly and radiates great joy and peace. He sits in the half-lotus posture on a lotus blossom with his left foot on his right knee. He holds a white lotus blossom with a slight reddish tinge in his left hand. On top of it is a lapis-lazuli blue lotus blossom that radiates golden light. In his right hand, he holds a flaming sword.

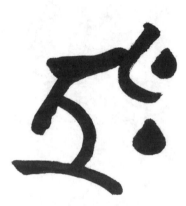

ILL. 33 – SIDDHAM TRAM

Kannon–The Goddess of Great Compassion
観音

(Chin.: *Kuan Yin, Kuan Shi Yin*; Skr.: *Avalokitesvara, Âryâvalokitesvara, Lokesvara*; Tib.: *Spyan-ras-gzigs* or *Tara*)

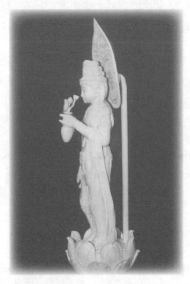

ILL. 34 – KANNON, THE GODDESS OF GREAT COMPASSION

Kannon is the Goddess of Great Compassion. She is a Bodhisattva, which means a being who has sworn to lead all beings to happiness. Despite her primarily feminine traits, she is also seen as a masculine being in some countries. She is especially important for Reiki because she:

✿ Is the spiritual being behind the SHK symbol;

✿ Is in the second place of the empowerment lineage in the Reiki initiations since Reiki—the spiritual life energy of *Dainichi Nyorai*—is transmitted to human beings through her.

Kannon appears in many of the sutras. The most important are the *Hokkekyô, Kegon kyô,* and *Muryôjukyô.* These tell how she can hear the voices of all beings that need help. She does everything in her power to

159

help these beings. There was a time in which she went into the hell realms and freed one being after the other. That was hard work. But the hell realms were barely empty before they filled up again with new people. This made her so sad and angry that she literally exploded. Other light beings soon set out and put her back together again. However, they did not know which part belonged where so she had many arms and heads when she was completed. Since then, there are 33 forms of *Kannon* with a great many abilities. The ones important for Reiki will be explained below. In the end, some tears flowed from her eyes in various colors. As the tears fell to the ground, they turned into *Tara* goddesses of different colors who have been helping *Kannon* since that time.

Kannon does not just work alone. She often appears in the company of other light beings. These include the Paradise Buddha *Amida Nyorai*, whose *Siddham* is also the SHK symbol. When a person dies, *Kannon* glides to the soul of the deceased and lets it step onto a lotus blossom, which then brings it into the Paradise of the *Amida Nyorai*.

There are some pilgrimages in Japan for *Kannon*. They developed as the wandering monks brought the liberation teaching of *Kannon* to the people and established many little miracle-working sacred towers and temples, where her healing powers can still be experienced today. There are obviously also numerous stories in Japanese literature, some of which are included below.

True Stories About Kannon–The Goddess of Great Compassion

The stories in the following refer to all the goddesses of the Kannon pilgrimage temples in Western Japan (Saikoku pilgrimage).

The Goddess Who Sacrifices Herself (Migawari Kannon) of the Nariaiji Temple

A monk once lived on the remote mountain where the *Nariaiji* Temple stands today. The people who lived in the village at the foot of the mountain always brought him food. But one winter there was so much snow that the village residents no longer could climb the mountain. When the monk was almost starving to death, he prayed to the sacred goddess *Kannon* (*Shô Kannon*), whose sculpture stood in his hut, for just enough food for one more day. When he had barely spoken this request, the monk saw a deer in front of his hut that had been killed by a wolf. As the Buddhist monk that he was, he was actually not permitted to eat meat. But since this food appeared as a response to his prayer, he decided to eat it and cooked the thigh in his pot. His strength soon returned as a result of this meal.

When the snow melted, the village inhabitants went up the mountain to see him. They found some wooden splinters in his cooking pot. Furthermore, they noticed that the thigh of his *Kannon* sculpture was damaged. They immediately went to get the monk to show him what had happened. Only then did the monk understand what *Kannon* had done for him. He wept as he immediately repaired the sculpture with the wood from his cooking pot and took greatest pains to make sure that no traces could be seen of the injury.

The *Nariaiji* temple that was later established on the mountain was named after this gracefully perfected sculpture. *Nariai* means "beautiful perfection" and *ji* stands for "temple."

The Goddess Who Sacrifices Herself (Migawari Kannon) of the Anaoji Temple

The wife of a man by the name of *Uji no Miyanari* from *Tamba* wished from the bottom of her heart that her evil husband would become a good man. For this purpose, she had a sculpture of the goddess *Kannon* made. She hired a monk and sculptor from Kyoto by the name of *Kansei*. He lived with them in their home until the sculpture of *Kannon* was completed. *Kansei* also believed in the power of *Kannon* and recited the sûtra *Kannon kyô* every day. When the finishing touches had been made on the sculpture, *Miyanari* and his wife were so delighted that they give *Kansei* many gifts. *Miyanari* even gave him his favorite horse. *Kansei* happily packed his horse and set off on the path back to Kyoto.

But *Miyanari* very quickly regretted his generosity. He followed *Kansei*, laid in wait, and then ambushed and killed him with an arrow through the chest. Then he took his horse and the other gifts and returned home.

When *Miyanari* arrived at home, he was amazed to see that exactly the same arrow that he had shot at *Kansei* was stuck in the chest of the *Kannon* that *Kansei* had carved. Furthermore, blood now dripped out of the sculpture from where the arrow had pierced it. When he turned around in fright, his horse with the load that he had given *Kansei* had disappeared.

He immediately set off on the path to Kyoto to find out what these strange things meant. When he arrived in Kyoto, he found *Kansei* in perfect health and the same was true of his horse. He asked how *Kansei's* return trip had been. When he heard that *Kansei* had arrived home without any incidents, it became clear to him that *Kannon* had sacrificed herself for *Kansei* to save his life. This touched *Miyanari* so very deeply that he became a truly noble pious man from that time on. His wife's wish had been fulfilled in a way that she never would have expected.

The highest monk, *Anaho Gyôkô* of *Anaoji*, explained that this legend is one of many stories that show the power of *Kannon* and that *Kannon* is also present in our modern age whenever one person helps others. Because of other miracles, this *Kannon* is so famous that emperors, monks, and the common people have gone there through the centuries to pray to her. Unfortunately, the sculpture was stolen in the year 1968 after it had been declared an important cultural asset of Japan and has not been found to this very day. This is the first art theft in the modern history of Japan.

The fact that a sculpture can serve as a healing medium can be explained as follows: After its completion, the sculpture is always just a sculpture like any other work of art. Only when the eye-opening ritual of *kaigen kuyô* is performed for the sculpture does it receive its healing power.

The Healing Goddess Kannon of the Rokuharamitsuji Temple

The monk *Kûya* established the *Rokuharamitsuji* Temple in Kyoto and carved a Kannon sculpture, which he initiated himself, in the year 951. At that time, epidemics were raging in Kyoto and he wanted to eliminate them with help of the goddess Kannon. For this purpose, he placed the sculpture in a little altar shrine on a wagon that he pulled through Kyoto. With a special herbal tea, which he brewed himself and infused with the power of the goddess, he was able to heal many people with *Kannon's* help.

The Healing Goddess Kannon of the Tsubosakadera Temple

A man by the name of *Sawaichi* once lived in the vicinity of the *Tsubosakadera* Temple with his beautiful wife *Osato*. One day *Sawaichi* became blind. Afterward, his wife *Osato* began to sneak out of the house late every night. *Sawaichi* noticed this and believed that she secretly went to a lover. He inconspicuously followed her one night. But to his surprise, he discovered that *Osato* went to the *Tsubosakadera* Temple to pray to the Goddess *Kannon* for the restoration of his vision.

He was so ashamed of his own mistrust that he believed his wife deserved a better husband. So *Sawaichi* went to the ocean and threw himself down a cliff. When *Osato* heard of this, she followed her husband into death. But *Kannon* rescued both of them and restored *Sawaichi's* sight.

The current abbot of *Tsubosakadera* says that according to the history of the temple, *Osato* prayed 1000 nights to *Kannon* in order for her husband to be healed. There are many rituals in Esoteric Buddhism that last 1000 days. In addition to special rituals, mantras, mudrâs, and symbols are used. During the Meiji Period (1868-1912), which means during Dr. Usui's lifetime, a theater play (*Jôruri-style*) was created from this touching story that soon became famous throughout the entire country. I assume that Dr. Usui was inspired by such stories in his search for Reiki and wove the appropriate practices into his System of Natural Healing, as we can recognize in the SHK symbol.

The Healing Goddess Kannon of the Kokawadera Temple

The hunter *Ôtomo Kujiko* came to the area of *Kokawa* in 770 to hunt for fun there. One night, he saw a radiant light on the *Kazuragi* mountain. When this light touched him, he developed strong pangs of remorse for the meaningless killing of the animals. He built a little hut in the same place where he had seen the light. One day, *Kujiko* was visited by an ascetic in the form of a child who asked permission to spend the night there. The next morning, the ascetic asked *Kujiko* if he had any kind of wish, and *Kujiko* told him that he had long desired to have an altar of the Goddess. In response, the ascetic carved the sculpture of the 1000-armed *Senju Kannon* within seven days. And then he disappeared.

163

At about the same time, the daughter of the wealthy *Satafu* from *Kawachi*[63] became very ill. Even though the family tried everything they could to heal her, she continued to be so ill that they could only wait for the approaching death. The ascetic suddenly appeared in the form of a child and healed the daughter. In gratitude, *Satafu* showered the childlike ascetic with gifts, but he refused them all. The only thing that he accepted was the *hakama*[64] woven by the daughter herself. After the ascetic finally just said one single sentence, "I live in *Kokawa* in the Province of *Nachi*," he disappeared.

The following year, *Satafu* went with his daughter to *Nachi* in order to look for the village of *Kokawa* where the ascetic lived. But no one had heard of the village of *Kokawa* or the ascetic. Close by, they discovered a little river that they followed since the name *Kokawa* means "little river." They soon reached *Kujiko's* hut. As they peaked inside, they discovered the sculpture of the 1000-armed goddess *Senju Kannon*. From her hands hung the *hakama* that the girl had given the ascetic. They immediately realized that the ascetic who had saved the daughter was a manifestation of the goddess in the form of the childlike ascetic. As a result, *Satafu* became a monk and soon had a temple built on the spot where the hut stood, giving it the name of *Kokawa dera* (Temple on the Little River). Even today, many people still go on a pilgrimage to *Kokawa dera* and are healed there with special rituals in relation to the SHK symbols.

[63] Today this is a section of Osaka in which a very distinct dialect is spoken.
[64] A *hakama* is a Japanese pant skirt.

Other Appearances of Kannon

The Eleven-Headed Kannon
(Jûichimen Kannon 十一面観音)

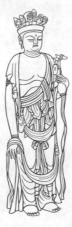

ILL. 35 – THE ELEVEN-HEADED KANNON

This *Kannon* is one of the oldest figures of Esoteric Buddhism. The eleven heads can be traced back to the Indian storm god *Rudra*, who has eleven names. The eleven heads also represent the eleven worldly illusions that keep people from oneness and love. As a result, each face also has a different expression that is intended to help people let go of the illusions (three compassion-inducing, three wrathful, and three grimly smiling faces, plus a face of the Paradise Buddha Amida and a wildly laughing face). Since the Eighth Century, the Great Purification and Protection Ritual with Fire and Water (*Omizutori* お水取り) is performed for this purpose in the *Nigatsudô* hall of the *Tôdaiji* Temple in Nara. Water for purification is drawn from a sacred fountain and large torches are lit for the transmission of protection. Many thousands of visitors stand under the fire rain every year in order to be touched by the glowing sparks, through whose spiritual power transmission (*kaji*) a protection from fire occurs. The temple chronicle *Tôdaiji yôroku* describes how the monk *Jicchû* (726-?) first performed this ritual during the 50s of the 8th Century after he had observed it in the realm of the future Buddha *Maitreya* in honor of the Goddess of Great Compassion *Kannon*.

165

Kannon with the Net and Rope
(Fukû Kensaku Kannon 不空羂索観音)

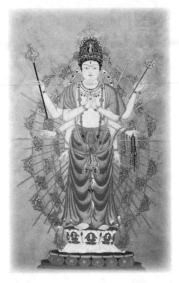

ILL. 36 – KANNON WITH THE NET AND ROPE

This *Kannon* carries, as the name already indicates, a net and a rope. With these tools, she rescues the beings that swim in the sea of ignorance. The net is so fine that no being can slip through the mesh. In addition, she heals sickness, bestows wealth, gives beauty, ensures success in business life, and protects people from natural catastrophes.

She has one, three, or eleven heads; three eyes; six, eight, or ten arms, of which two hands are folded in prayer in *Gasshô* in front of the chest; one hand with a rope or prayer beads; other hands with a frond, pilgrim's staff, or lotus blossom. She wears an especially richly adorned crown with a standing Paradise Buddha *Amida* on her head. With a garment of buckskin, she is also known as the *Kannon* of Hunting and Fishing, *Rokuhi Kannon*.

Sacred Kannon or the Original Kannon
(Shô Kannon 聖観音・正観音)

She is the original *Kannon*, as she is known from the Indian tradition. She frequently also appears in the company of other light beings. She sits on a lotus pedestal and wears a high crown with the Paradise Buddha *Amida*. Her right hand is raised in the mudrâ "Do not fear" and the left points downward in the mudrâ of granting wishes. Sometimes she holds a lotus bud in the left hand that is opened up by her right hand. When she holds her hands together in *Gasshô*, there is often a crystal quartz or jewel between them. This is an early depiction of the *Gasshô* meditation with healing stones.

The Kannon of Purity
(Juntei Kannon 准胝観音)

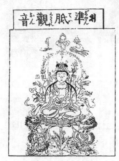

ILL. 37 – THE KANNON OF PURITY

Juntei is called the "Pure Mother of the Buddhas" or the "Mother of All Buddhas" because she rules over the sacred mantra *Butsumo Juntei darani*, through which the 70 million Buddhas of the past have attained enlightenment. As a mother figure, she grants the wish for children. Everything that she touches is purified. She makes peace between people fighting each other, heals diseases, and purifies hearts and fills them with love.

She has one head, three eyes, and eight arms (less frequently two or four). The middle hands are not folded but show the gesture of turning the wheel of the teaching. One hand frequently holds a little axe. She is often accompanied by two companion figures on a lotus pedestal or by two dragons that hold lotus buds.

167

Thousand-Armed Kannon
(Senjû Kannon 千手観音)

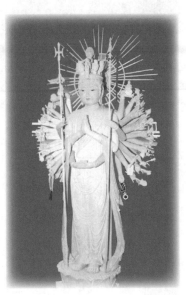

ILL. 38 – THOUSAND-ARMED KANNON

Kannon has, as the name already says, 1000 arms and also eleven or twenty-seven heads (in sculptures less heads can be shown, see above). In most of the hands she holds objects that are symbolic of the individual possibilities and rituals. Among the *Kannon* goddesses, she is the most important for Reiki since her *Siddham* is the SHK symbol.

In the famous long temple hall of *Sanjûsan Gendô* in Kyoto, the longest wooden building in the world, there is a gigantic, centrally seated *Kannon* that is about 11 feet high. In addition, there are 1000 gold-plated standing *Senjû Kannons* that are almost as tall as human beings and show all of the individual facial expressions. It is said that anyone who searches long enough can find his own countenance there.

Esoteric Buddhism has rituals with her for the prevention of disease and protection against fire. The corresponding Shintoist deity is *Seiryû Gongen* in the Daigoji Temple.

Wish-Fulfilling Kannon
(Nyoirin Kannon 如意輪観音)

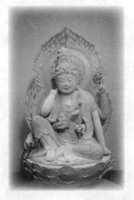

ILL. 39 – WISH-FULFILLING KANNON

She has one head. Initially, she had two arms and then developed six in Esoteric Buddhism for rescuing the suffering being in the six realms of existence with various objects such as the wish-fulfilling gem, the wheel of the teaching, the prayer beads, and a lotus blossom. The wheel of the teaching is sometimes held on the raised index finger of the uppermost left hand. She is usually surrounded by an aura of flames and wears a high crown with a small *Amida*. The right hand is on the chin and the elbow is resting on the raised right knee. One hand is in the gesture of calling upon the Earth Goddess as a witness. She is most clearly recognizable because one knee is raised while the other leg is in a meditation posture; the soles of both feet touch each other here as in the Rainbow Reiki *Gasshô* meditation.

Kannon with a Willow Branch
(Yôryu Kannon 楊柳観音)

She is also called the Medicine *Kannon* because she bows to the will of all beings as flexibly as a willow branch in the wind. Or it may be because this willow branch has the power to cure all diseases. The statue depicts a sacred *Kannon* who either holds a willow branch or carries it in a water vessel in the right hand. She is also depicted with white garments sitting on a rock.

Bishamonten
毘沙門天

(Chin.: Duowen; Taoist name: *Molishou;* Skr.: *Vaisravana;*
Tib.: *Rnam Thos-kyi Bu)*

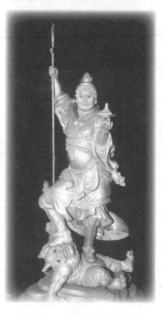

ILL. 40 – BISHAMONTEN

ILL. 41 – SIDDHAM VAI OF BISHAMONTEN

Bishamonten is considered to be one of the light beings of the devas in
Buddhism. As a god of prosperity, he is the guardian of the north. This is
where he possesses great wealth. He is the protector of the goddess *Kannon*.
His mythology can be traced back to the Indian God of the Crocodiles
Kuvera. He is sometimes also called the "Black Warrior." As one of the

four guardian kings (*Shitennô*), he is the main figure and is then called *Tamonten*. In Japan, his wife is *Kichijôten*, the goddess of great happiness, beauty, and merit.

He has been worshipped independent of the other guardian kings as a light being of healing since the 9th Century. He is particularly well-known for his ability to perform distant healing for the *Daigo Tennô* (885-930) on the *Shigi* mountain in the *Chôgosonshiji* Temple.[65] In his honor, the scroll *Shigisan Engi Emaki* was painted in the 12th Century. Since the Heian period (794-1185), *Bishamonten* has been worshipped in the syncretic monastery grounds[66] on Mount Kurama as the light being of prosperity. In the Middle Ages, many warriors also had the nickname of *Bishamonten* because they worshipped him as their patron saint. Furthermore, people believed that he brings with him the ten types of the treasures of happiness in addition to material prosperity. This is also the reason why he was accepted into the ranks of the Seven Gods of Happiness (*Shichifukujin*) in the 17th Century. The little pagoda on the palm of his left hand is the treasure tower of the teaching of the *Dainichi Nyorai*, which he protects on the one hand and from which he gains great treasures on the other hand. He holds a lance or staff of wisdom in the right to direct the wealth into the proper channel. He is usually seen trampling on the demons of the destructive winds called *Biranba*. In the Mandala of the Two Worlds, he sits in the posture of a South Indian yogi. He wears a crown with a bird's head. In his left hand he holds a relic pagoda and the staff of wisdom in his right. His face is usually blue and his armor is covered by a robe with seven jewels. His aura radiates in eight directions with three-pronged *Vajras*. Sometimes he is also pictured with mice that are chewing apart the bowstrings of the enemies.

---

[65] Cf. the chapter on the HS Symbol.
[66] A monastery in which Buddhism, Shintoism, and *Shugendô* are equally represented.

The Great Goddess Dai Marishi Ten

大摩利支天

(Chin.: *Molizhi*; Skr.: *Mârîcî, Vajravarahi*; Tib.: *Hod-zer Chna-ma*)

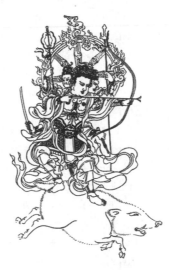

ILL. 42 – THE GREAT GODDESS DAI MARISHI TEN

The name Dai *Marishi Ten* comes from the Sanskrit (*Mârîcî*) and means "radiant light." In the Vedas, Dai *Marishi Ten* was depicted for the first time under the name of *Usas*, Goddess of the Dawn (the metamorphosis from the moon to the sun). In the Brahmanic mythology, Dai *Marishi Ten* is considered one of the spirits of the storm. Since she is portrayed with horses, there is a connection with the sun god *Sûrya*. However, Dai *Marishi Ten* is definitely not identical with him because she rules both the sun and the moon. She is always shown together with a branch of an ashoka tree. This is important since the historical Buddha *Shâkyamuni* transformed from a Bodhisattva to a Buddha under such a tree, which is a symbol for enlightenment. Dai *Marishi Ten* helps the beings come closer to the sun—enlightenment—through the light of the moon. The tree is an important symbol for Buddha, just as the pagoda is for *Dainichi Nyorai*. It is interesting to note that in the case of Dai *Marishi Ten*, both symbols are present. In more precise terms, the inside of the pagoda also contains the tree symbolized by a wooden central pillar under which the relics of the historical Buddha are preserved. This is why Dai *Marishi Ten* is also the bridge between *Shâkyamuni* as a Bodhisattva to his enlightenment as the embodiment of the completely illumined state of *Dainichi Nyorai*. In the symbol language of Reiki, this is the connection between the HS and the DKM symbol since the HS is the bridge to the DKM. This is also the reason why Dai *Marishi Ten* is depicted in very early sculptures together with *Dainichi Nyorai*. She either displays the mudrâ of teaching or wears a pagoda in her crown. With this background, Dai *Marishi Ten* is closely related to the HS symbol, which, as will be described below, is depicted as the pagoda of the state of awakening or realization of Buddha consciousness. As the ruler over the sun (日) and moon (月), she also appears in the third *Kanji* of *myô* 明 in the DKM symbol. With the sun in the right hand, Dai *Marishi Ten* banishes the night, and with the moon in her left hand she brings light into the darkness. This right/left division is the same as in the Chinese yin/yang symbol and the Mandala of the Two Worlds in Esoteric Buddhism:

Yin – left – moon – Mandala of the Womb World – feminine
Yang – right – sun – Mandala of the Diamond World – masculine

In China, she is seen as the Mother of the North Star, which stands for *Dainichi Nyorai*. In Japan, she became the Goddess of War and Victory. She is also a companion of *Taishaku Ten*, the protectress of the Samurai, as well as of the four Buddhist worlds, and the Goddess of Fire. Since she even nourishes from the sun as the fire and is simultaneously the transformation of the light, she can be seen as the mother of the Sun Buddha *Dainichi Nyorai*.

In the Chinese text *Mo-li-chih-t'a-ching*, the earliest Indian translation from the 6th Century, rituals are explained that describe how she can be worshipped and which effect the individual methods have. In Tibet, she is often a companion of the Green *Tara* because both are archetypes for the Great Goddess. In the 8th Century, *Amoghavajra* translated an expanded version into Chinese. This text mentioned that little pictures of this goddess should be worn on the head or as an amulet. At the beginning of the

9th Century, this knowledge was brought to Japan by Kûkai together with the secret teachings (*mikkyô*) within the scope of Esoteric Buddhism.

Dai Marishi Ten cannot be seen by anyone or even captured. Consequently, it is not possible for her to be harmed in any way or experience difficulties. She is the Goddess of Heat Flames. This quality indicates her strength to do things of which no one else is capable. She has six to eight arms and carries a Vajra staff, a needle, a bow and arrow, and rides in standing on a wild boar. This wild boar symbolizes her true character, which—like the heat flames—can never be captured. She circles *Dainichi Nyorai* at such a high speed that she appears to be invisible to the eyes.

Because of these qualities, she is worshipped by the Samurai and especially by the Ninja in Japan. Through her, humans can attain the power to become invisible and not be perceived nor harmed by any opponent. The story of the famous *Kusunoki Masashige*, who concealed a little Dai *Marishi Ten* figure in his armor and put the fear of God into his opponents with the mudrâ *ongyô in*, is especially well known.

Amulets and practices with Dai *Marishi Ten* can ward off disruptive influences and turn away people who impede our development. In addition, they protect against robbery, drowning, and burns.

The mantra of *Dai Marishi Ten* is: *Om marishiei sowaka.*

The *Siddham* symbol is: *ma*

The two mudrâs of *Dai Marishi Ten* are:

Her mandala consists of two combined triangles. She is at the center and is surrounded by four *Dâkinîs*.

CHAPTER 9

The Medicine Buddha Yakushi Nyorai and Reiki

薬師如来

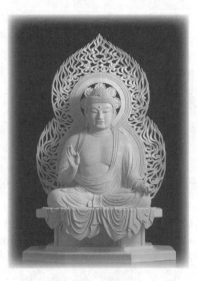

ILL. 43 – THE MEDICINE BUDDHA YAKUSHI NYORAI

I (Mark) became particularly well-acquainted with the Medicine Buddha in Japan during the Buddhist pilgrimage of "The 88 Temples of Shikoku," in which an individual walks about 1500 kilometers on foot from temple to temple. No matter how good the footwear and the stamina, everyone suffers from strong signs of fatigue and severe blisters on the feet sooner or later because of the 40 degree C heat with its 100 percent humidity. My companion and I were no exceptions. In a temple where the Medicine Buddha was worshipped, there was a sign with his mantra. As in every temple, I sent Reiki to the Buddhas as an offering without asking for anything. As a thank-you, I was allowed to have many wondrous experiences. Because of the bad state of my feet, I know that I—as in the year before—would have to call off the pilgrimage because of exhaustion

175

and being worn out unless a special miracle occurred. I was already used to miracles happening here, but not the healing of blisters. So I came up with the idea of reciting the mantra of the Medicine Buddha until we reached the next temple (about 35 km). I told my companion about this plan and invited him to join in reciting the mantra. But he was not the slightest bit interested in it. So I recited the mantra of the Medicine Buddha alone: *Om koro koro sendari matôgi sowaka.*

After about two hours, it occurred to me that my feet and legs were no longer hurting and that I felt much more fit. I was completely enthused. Somewhat later, there was another side effect but its full extent only appeared long afterward: I had already suffered from a toothache for some time, which then went away completely. When I later went to the dentist to have a thorough examination done for this tooth in particular, he could not find anything wrong with it. The dentist just thought that I had probably dreamed up the pain. He did not want to hear about the mantra. On the other hand, my companion's condition became considerably worse so that he was barely able to walk a few days later and had to take trains and cable railways. Unfortunately, not even that could convince him to try out the mantra of the Medicine Buddha... Before my journey home to Germany, my Japanese professor gave me a sculpture of the Medicine Buddha that now crowns my altar.

Like all of the Buddhist light beings, the Medicine Buddha also has a name, *Yakushi Nyorai* 薬師如来, his own *Siddham symbol, mantra,* and *mudrâ.*[67]

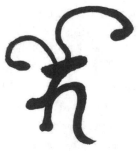

ILL. 44 – SIDDHAM SYMBOL BHAI OF THE MEDICINE BUDDHA

---

[67] The initiations into the symbols and mantras of the Medicine Buddha are included in our seminars and trainings. Contact us for more information.

As the name already suggests, *Yakushi Nyorai* is related to medicine and healing. A literal translation says that he is the "Master of Medicine" and the "Healer of Body and Mind" among the Buddhas. He is appropriately depicted in art with a medicine bowl in the left hand and sometimes also with an arura plant[68] in his right. His color is blue, which represents the harmonization of all diseases here. In addition to healing emotional, mental, and physical diseases, a person can also be reborn with his help in his Pure Land in the East—a Buddhist Paradise. There is also a parallel to the SHK symbol since the *Amida* Buddha who is associated with this symbol also has his own paradise by the name of "Pure Land" in the West.

However, the *Siddham* symbol of *Yakushi Nyorai* is not the SHK symbol but the *Siddham* symbol of *bhai*. This plays an important role for the energy work with *Yakushi Nyorai* in healing. However, *bhai* is not one of the Reiki symbols. From what we know about the work of Dr. Usui and Dr. Hayashi, there is also no indication that *Yakushi Nyorai* ever played a role in the Reiki System of Natural Healing. In addition to *Yakushi Nyorai*, there is an entire series of other healing light beings in Buddhism. The quality of the healing is usually not indicated by their names. So the Goddess of Compassion, *Kannon* with the SHK symbol, has the power of mental healing through the dissolution of habits and ways of thinking that cause suffering. The Imperturbable Wisdom King *Fudô Myôô* cuts off attachments to anger with his sword so that the resulting consequences—most illnesses such as high blood pressure and gallbladder ailments, and accidents—no longer have a basis and disappear as a result. In this way, the great variety of light beings with their numerous aspects can eliminate the causes of suffering and disease. So this is also a form of healing. In the West, we also call this personality development.

---

[68] The arura plant is the bitterest plant that I have ever eaten. According to Traditional Chinese Medicine, the taste quality of bitter in the Five Element theory stands for the heart, the small intestine, and sexuality, as well as for the ability of spiritual awakening and the associated meridians (spiritual energy channels in the body), which are organized by the element of fire. So the arura plant in the hand of *Yakushi Nyorai* is an expression of his competence as a great healer of the heart, as well as the related physical, mental, and spiritual qualities.

The way in which Dr. Usui was initiated into Reiki during his enlightenment on Mount Kurama initially was not related to *Yakushi Nyorai*. Reiki is traced back to the Great Sun Buddha *Dainichi Nyorai*. In the transmission lineage, *Yakushi Nyorai* is not mentioned. In *Dainichi Nyorai's* two Mandalas of the Diamond World and the Womb World, *Yakushi Nyorai* only appears in rare cases and also only in Japan. He is not even mentioned once in the associated sutras. Yet, there are some distinct similarities and connections with Reiki. The *Siddham* symbol *bhai*, just like the SHK symbol, also facilitates the healing of the mind and the rebirth into a paradise. In more precise terms, the healing of the mind is the most important precondition for the healing of physical diseases and simultaneously the basis for rebirth into a Buddhist paradise. A comparison of the function of the two symbols shows some differences, which make it possible to apply Reiki in an even more focused way.

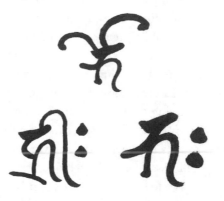

ILL. 45 – SIDDHAM TRINITY, ABOVE BHAI, LEFT BOTTOM HRIH,
AND RIGHT BOTTOM BHAH (FOR SHÂKYAMUNI)

Excellent results can be achieved even with the First Reiki Degree. By using the symbols of the Second Degree, in addition to power-intensification and distant healing we can work in a more focused way with the help of the SHK symbol, i.e. problems can be harmonized successfully with considerably less effort. The inclusion of the symbol *bhai* of *Yakushi Nyorai* further increases the possibilities that are already available. As applies to the Reiki symbols, an initiation by a specially trained teacher is necessary here in order to achieve a high degree of effectiveness and depth of the applications. Although some of the exercises can be done without an initiation, only coincidental results are possible with the symbols in this approach.

In Japan, *Yakushi Nyorai* is worshipped in a very special way because of his healing power, as well as because of his "Pure Land" (Paradise) in the East since Japan itself lies completely in the east of Asia as the "Land of the Rising Sun." The sun and the paradise in the east indicate a connection between *Dainichi Nyorai* and *Yakushi Nyorai*.

When *Yakushi Nyorai* was still a Bodhisattva, he had made twelve different promises that are all related to healing in the narrower and in the broader sense. These include his wish that the world would be enlightened by his blue light. Because of his ability to radiate blue light, he is frequently identified with *Dainichi Nyorai* in Japan, in contrast to all the traditional teachings: *Dainichi Nyorai* also has the ability to radiate light—in this case, golden light—from his body into the world. In the *Shingon* School of Esoteric Buddhism, he is therefore sometimes put in the place of *Dainichi Nyorai* in the Diamond World Mandala. Despite this, *Yakushi Nyorai* is simultaneously worshipped as an independent Buddha.

The Yakushi Nyorai Trinity

The indirect relationship to *Dainichi Nyorai* can also be explained from the point of view of his companions. Like the other Buddhas, *Yakushi Nyorai* also appears in the company of other light beings. In most cases, these are *Nikkô Bosatsu* (日光菩薩) on the right and *Gakkô Bosatsu* (月光菩薩) on the left (or the other way around seen from the perspective of *Yakushi Nyora*). *Nikkô Bosatsu* is the Bodhisattva of the sunlight and *Gakkô Bosatsu* is the Bodhisattva of the moonlight. From the perspective of *Yakushi Nyorai*, the combination of the first *Kanji* of these two names results in the third *Kanji* (*myô* 明) of the DKM symbol. The second *Kanji* of both names—*kô* 光—is also contained in the DKM symbol in the second position. The *Siddham* symbol of the *Nikkô Bosatsu* is also identical with the symbol (and mantra) *a* for *Dainichi Nyorai*.

The best-known example of this trinity is probably the Medicine Buddha Temple by the name of *Yakushiji* in Nara from the year 680. When

179

the *Tenmu Tennô* [69] (631-686) became severely ill, she hoped to become well again through the power of *Yakushi Nyorai* and had this temple build. And she actually regained her health. Because of this case of healing and others, *Yakushi Nyorai* was soon known throughout the entire land at the court, in the monasteries, and also among the people.

ILL. 46 – THE SIDDHAM OF THE MEDICINE BUDDHA TRINITY: LEFT CA, CENTER BHAI, AND RIGHT A

The *Sûtra of the Medicine Buddha* (Jap.: *Yakushi kyô*) was recited on a regular basis in the temples when rituals were performed in honor of *Yakushi Nyorai*. During the rituals of *Yakushi keka,* hunting was stopped, captured animals were freed, and sometimes even wars interrupted as an offering to *Yakushi Nyorai*. The ritual has the effect of quickly healing diseases that normally are incurable without some sort of miracle. On the national level, wars were ritually ended in order to prevent epidemics and natural catastrophes with the power of *Yakushi Nyorai*. To intensify the light-filled healing force of the sun, magical candle rituals were simultaneously performed in the *Tendai* School of Esoteric Buddhism for *Yakushi Nyorai* and *Dainichi Nyorai*.

The Seven Bodies and Forms of Yakushi Nyorai

As a healer, *Yakushi Nyorai* can manifest in seven forms. When painted, they are depicted above or around *Yakushi Nyorai* himself. Each of them has their own mudrâ and also their own *Siddham* symbol. In place of the medicine bowl, they carry a wish-fulfilling gem in the hand. They are often also just portrayed through the appropriate *Siddham* symbols as help in rituals and meditations:

[69] The Japanese title *Tennô* can be added behind the names of both males and females. Its approximate meaning is "emperor/empress."

The Virtuous King of Bliss (Jap.: *Zen Myôshô Kichijô ô Nyorai*)

The Buddha King of Light and Sound of Insight of the Precious Moon Gem (Jap.: *Hôgetsu Chigen Kô on Jizai ô Nyorai*)

The Buddha of the Golden Gem, Who Has Completed the Highest Practices (Jap.: *Konjiki Hôkô Myôkô Jôju Nyorai*)

The Excellent and Affliction-Free Auspicious One (Jap.: *Muyû Saishô Kichijô Nyorai*)

The Buddha of the Thunder-Sound Dharma Sea (Jap.: *Hôkairaion Nyorai*)

The Buddha of the Victorious Wisdom of the Dharma Sea, Who Roams Freely Due to His Spiritual Powers (Jap.: *Hôkaishô Sui Yûgi Jintsû Nyorai*)

Lapis-Lazuli Master of Healing (Jap.: *Yakushi Rurikô Nyorai*)

Lapis Lazuli and the Medicine Buddha Yakushi Nyorai

Like all the light beings of Buddhism, a color is also associated with *Yakushi Nyorai*. His body is radiant blue like the healing stone lapis lazuli. His name always appears in the sutras with the lapis lazuli so that this healing stone has become associated with the Medicine Buddha himself. The color lapis-lazuli blue plays a leading role in many of the healing applications with *Yakushi Nyorai*.

The mine of Badakshan in the Hindukusch Mountains in northeastern Afghanistan, which is quite difficult to reach, is still one of the most significant places where lapis lazuli is found. Already in the Fourth Century B.C., expeditions were sent there on a regular basis since the people were already familiar with the enormous curative effects of this healing stone. This can also be seen in the Buddhist sutras. The healing stone most frequently mentioned in them is the lapis lazuli. Since ancient times, it has been associated with the Great Goddess and helps in persistently following our personal vision without false modesty and lazy compromises. Its healing force is especially effective on the fifth major chakra, whose

181

essential mantra in Esoteric Buddhism is the "*a,*" which realizes the divine power manifested in the heart in the physical world.

In Buddhism, he is a symbol for the pure and the rare. In the very first chapter of the *Lotus Sûtra,* the Buddhas are compared with golden pictures in lapis lazuli, which very much resemble the golden pyrite inclusions in lapis lazuli. This comparison is also one of many indications that major portions of the Buddhist teaching are much older than what is now known as Buddhism. Later, the teacher of the Buddhist teaching is also compared with a mirror made of lapis lazuli that reflects all appearances free of distortions. This is very reminiscent of the healing effects of lapis lazuli itself. According to Gienger[70], lapis lazuli is known as the stone of truth. As already mentioned, it is especially good for the fifth chakra because it so promotes self-expression that unpleasant things can more easily be conveyed in language instead of simply swallowing them. Those who succeed in expressing their own opinion in an open, honest, and clear way, without leaving shambles behind them, and those who strive to always describe things as they are, have created many preconditions for a happy and healthy life. A valuable means for achieving this is a purifying of the mind from the inside out. Especially the Medicine Buddha *Yakushi Nyorai* has the power of promoting this high art in everyone. The recurring colds and stomach problems then disappear. The strengthening of this chakra with the power of *Yakushi Nyorai* is a useful method for this purpose. The process will be explained in the practices below.

The Medicinal Plant
of the Medicine Buddha Yakushi Nyorai

In some of the depictions of *Yakushi Nyorai,* he holds an arura plant (Skr.: *harîtaki,* Lat.: *terminalia chebula, phyalanthus emblica, terminalia belerica*) in his right hand. It is not seen in Japan because this plant does not grow there. While the lapis lazuli, as described above, gives expression to truth, this medicinal plant has the effect of seeing the world without distortions

---

[70] Cf. *Healing Crystals: The A-Z Guide to 430 Gemstones* by Michael Gienger, ISBN 1844090671, published by Earthdancer 2005.

as it really is. The arura plant is well-known in Indian medicine. As the Latin terms show, there are precisely three types. They are known as elixirs for long life. They are particularly effective against diseases of the eye and for improving vision. In the latter case, the plant helps us be able to look things in the eye that we have not wanted or been able to see up to now. In addition, it has proved itself as a healing remedy for skin problems, bleeding, purulence, extreme mucous formation, and pain during urination. Furthermore, it has a stimulating effect on the stomach's fire, also promoting the cleansing organs on the energetic level and sharpening the senses. Arura is a medicinal plant that equally effects the body and the mind. In meditations with *Yakushi Nyorai*, a healing energy for the mind arises from its fruit that also has an effect on the body. Since the arura plant does not grow in Japan, a ritual for the energetic connection to the awakening of its powers of healing has become especially popular there in Esoteric Buddhism.

The Siddham Symbol Bhai of the Medicine Buddha Yakushi Nyorai

Like every Buddhist light being, *Yakushi Nyorai* also has his own *Siddham* symbol, from which the healing power of the Medicine Buddha originates. Through the ritual application of the symbol, healing occurs for the practitioner it through the activation of the 12 powers from within. These include an easy pregnancy and simple birth, the healing of infertility, longevity, spontaneous healing, successful learning, healthy growth, protection during sea journeys against storms, and protection against epidemics and catastrophes. In addition, a special meditation promotes personality development and rebirth in the Paradise of the East becomes possible.

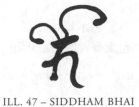

ILL. 47 – SIDDHAM BHAI

183

Practices with the Medicine Buddha

Practice 1:
Mental Healing with the Power of the Medicine Buddha

Establish distant contact with the Medicine Buddha by addressing him as Yakushi Nyorai. Greet him with the words: "Dear Medicine Buddha Yakushi Nyorai, I come to you as a sick person and request healing. I come to you as an ignorant person and request teaching. I come to you as someone who does not know the way and ask for protection and guidance. I come to you as someone who is helpless and ask you for power in order to better serve. As compensation, I send you Reiki. Please use it as you wish for the benefit of all." Then give Reiki to the Medicine Buddha by holding your hands in front of you with the palms facing outward.

*

Now begin the mental healing in the usual way with the SHK-CR name. Ask *Yakushi Nyorai* to send his healing force through you and your hands. During the entire treatment phase, recite the mantra: *Om korokoro sendari matôgi sowaka.* As you do this, imagine how brilliant light flows out of your hands in the color of lapis lazuli and completely fills the body of the recipient. Next, go to the feet and ground the recipient in closing for some minutes.

*

Give thanks and take leave of the distant contact with Yakushi Nyorai in the usual way at the end of the session by saying or thinking: "Dear Yakushi Nyorai, I thank you for the treatment and your help. I would like to request permission to call on you again soon. I wish you the blessing and protection of the Creative Force on your path." Then blow between your hands and rub them together in the usual way when ending a Reiki distant contact.

Practice 2:
Reiki Meditation with Yakushi Nyorai (a)

Establish distant contact with the Medicine Buddha by addressing him as Yakushi Nyorai.

Greet him with the words: "Dear Medicine Buddha Yakushi Nyorai, I come to you as a sick person and request healing. I come to you as an ignorant person and request teaching. I come to you as someone who does not know the way and ask for protection and guidance. I come to you as someone who is helpless and ask you for power in order to better serve. As compensation, I send you Reiki. Please use it as you wish for the benefit of all."

*

Assume the mudrâ of the Medicine Buddha by raising your right hand to the level of the heart with the palm facing outward and placing the left hand on your left leg with the palm facing upward. While you recite his mantra—*Om koro koro sendari matôgi sowaka*—108 times or a multiple of that, imagine how a shining blue lapis-lazuli radiates from you to all beings.

*

Give thanks and then take leave at the end of the session in the usual way when ending a Reiki distant contact.

Practice 3:
Reiki Meditation with Yakushi Nyorai (b)

Establish distant contact with the Medicine Buddha by addressing him as Yakushi Nyorai.

Greet him with the words: "Dear Medicine Buddha Yakushi Nyorai, I come to you as a sick person and request healing. I come to you as an ignorant person and request teaching. I come to you as someone who does not know the way and ask for protection and guidance. I come to you as someone who is helpless and ask you for power in order to serve better. As compensation, I send you Reiki. Please use it as you wish for the benefit of all."

*

Assume the mudrâ of the Medicine Buddha by raising your right hand to the level of the heart with the palm facing outward and placing the left hand on your left leg with the palm facing upward.

Visualize yourself as the Medicine Buddha sitting on a lotus blossom with the disk of the moon. Your body is lapis-lazuli blue and completely empty. You have one face and two arms and are wearing a three-part

185

monk's garment. In the right hand you hold an arura plant as if you wanted to hand it to someone. In the left hand you hold a medicine bowl in your lap.

Stroke by stroke, the blue *Siddham* seed syllable *bhai* is now created in your heart. From the *bhai* now arises clockwise a chain formed by the mantra of the Medicine Buddha *Om koro koro sendari matôgi sowaka*.

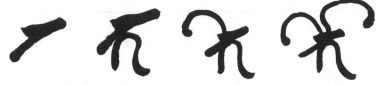

ILL. 48 – SEQUENCE OF STROKES FOR THE SIDDHAM BHAI

While you recite his mantra—*Om koro koro sendari matôgi sowaka*—108 times or a multiple thereof, imagine how shining blue light radiates from your heart to all Buddhas and Bodhisattvas. Once blessed, this light returns to you and fulfills your heart. Now the blue light radiates from your heart to all beings, purifying their mind and healing all diseases.

The blue light ultimately returns to you. Your form dissolves in the light and merges with the *bhai*. Place your hands on your heart and feel what is happening inside of you for at least 5 minutes.

*

Give thanks to Yakushi Nyorai and end the distant contact in the usual way.

Practice 4:
Distant Healing with the Power of Yakushi Nyorai and Reiki

Establish distant Reiki contact with the person you would like to treat.

Establish an additional distant contact with the Medicine Buddha by addressing him as Yakushi Nyorai. Greet him with the words: "Dear Medicine Buddha Yakushi Nyorai, I come to you as a sick person and request healing. I come to you as an ignorant person and request teaching. I come to you as someone who does not know the way and ask for protection and guidance.

I come to you as someone who is helpless and ask you for power in order to better serve. As compensation, I send you Reiki. Please use it as you wish for the benefit of all."

*

Assume the mudrâ of the Medicine Buddha by raising your right hand to the level of the heart with the palm facing outward and placing the left hand on your left leg with the palm facing upward. Request healing on all levels for the person who is to receive treatment.

Visualize yourself as the Medicine Buddha sitting on a lotus blossom with the disk of the moon. Your body is lapis-lazuli blue and completely empty all the way into your fingertips. You have one face and two arms and are wearing a three-part monk's garment. In the right hand you hold an arura plant as if you wanted to hand it to someone. In the left hand you hold a medicine bowl in your lap. Recite the mantra of the Medicine Buddha 108 times: *Om koro koro sendari matôgi sowaka.*

Now hold your hands in *Gasshô* in front of the heart separated by about one hand-width distance and visualize your client between them. The head is on top and the feet are at the bottom.

On the entire body in the front and in the back, imagine drawing one each of the *Siddham* symbol *bhai.* In addition, draw a large CR symbol. Activate each of them by saying the name of the mantra three times.

At all the places that appear to be important to you, draw little CR symbols and activate each of them by saying the name of the mantra three times.

Then recite the mantra of the Medicine Buddha during the entire treatment: *Om koro koro sendari matôgi sowaka.* At the same time, imagine that lapis-lazuli blue light is radiating from your hands into your client and all diseases dissolve like an ice cube in warm water. Give the soles of your client's feet Reiki for three minutes to support grounding.

*

Take leave of your client from the distant contact in the usual way.

Give thanks to the Medicine Buddha and visualize how your form dissolves into light.

Also take leave of the Medicine Buddha from the distant contact in the usual way.

Practice 5:
Chakra Treatment with the Power of the Yakushi Nyorai

Establish distant contact with the Medicine Buddha by addressing him as Yakushi Nyorai.

Greet him with the words: "Dear Medicine Buddha Yakushi Nyorai, I come to you as a sick person and request healing. I come to you as an ignorant person and request teaching. I come to you as someone who does not know the way and ask for protection and guidance. I come to you as someone who is helpless and ask you for power in order to better serve. As compensation, I send you Reiki. Please use it as you wish for the benefit of all."

*

Visualize yourself as the Medicine Buddha sitting on a lotus blossom with the disk of the moon. Your body is lapis-lazuli blue and completely empty all the way into your fingertips. You have one face and two arms and are wearing a three-part monk's garment. In the right hand you hold an arura plant as if you wanted to hand it to someone. In the left hand you hold a medicine bowl in your lap.

Draw a SHK symbol on the chakra to be treated and activate it by saying the name of the mantra three times. Also draw a CR symbol on the crown and activate it by saying the name of the mantra three times. Say your client's first and last names three times.

Now recite the mantra *Om koro koro sendari matôgi sowaka* during the entire treatment. At the same time, imagine that lapis-lazuli blue light is radiating into the chakra of the recipient.

*

Give thanks to the Medicine Buddha and visualize how your form dissolves into the light. Also take leave of the Medicine Buddha from the distant contact in the usual way.

Practice 6:
Making Lapis-Lazuli Healing Oil Infused
with the Power of Yakushi Nyorai

Prepare a container of natural material such as wood or clay and fill it with some oil.

*

Establish distant contact with the Medicine Buddha by addressing him as **Yakushi Nyorai.** *Greet him with the words: "Dear Medicine Buddha* **Yakushi Nyorai,** *I come to you as a sick person and request healing. I come to you as an ignorant person and request teaching. I come to you as someone who does not know the way and ask for protection and guidance. I come to you as someone who is helpless and ask you for power in order to better serve. As compensation, I send you Reiki. Please use it as you wish for the benefit of all."*

*

Visualize the Medicine Buddha and his two companions as the sun and moon in the lapis-lazuli blue night sky in front of you. Send Reiki to the Medicine Buddha by holding your hands with the palms facing in his direction. While you do this, recite the mantra *Om koro koro sendari matôgi sowaka.*

Take the container with the oil in one hand and use the other (initiated) hand to draw the SHK symbol above the oil. Then activate it. Now also draw a CR symbol and activate it as well. Say or think three times: "this oil, this oil, this oil" and hold your hand above it. For intensification, draw some more CR symbols.

Now ask the Medicine Buddha to fill the oil with *Amrita* (divine, healing nectar). Also ask for the blessing of the Great Goddess (moon) and the Great God (sun).

While you recite the mantra *Om koro koro sendari matôgi sowaka*, visualize how a lapis-lazuli blue light radiates from the Medicine Buddha and golden light shines from the sun and moon through your crown chakra into you and is transferred into the oil through your hands.

Remain in this state for at least 10 minutes or until you clearly notice that it is enough.

*

189

*Give thanks and take leave at the end of the session from the distant contact to **Yakushi Nyorai** in the usual way by saying or thinking: "Dear Yakushi Nyorai, I thank you for the treatment and for your help. I would like to request permission to call on you again soon. I wish you the blessing and protection of the Creative Force on your path."*

Then blow between your hands and rub them together.

The oil charged in this way can now be rubbed on your chakras and reflex zones.

CHAPTER 10

Mudrâ

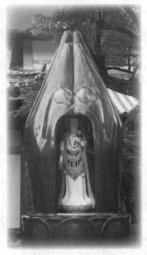

ILL. 49 – REIKI LIGHT BEING MUDRÂ

Mudrâs are symbolic gestures that make it easier for the practitioner to achieve certain states of consciousness such as deep relaxation or contact with specific spiritual beings. Or they are applied to achieve practical results with energy work such as calming an aggressive dog or healing a snakebite. However, without initiation it is very difficult to achieve clear effects by simply making a mudrâ. Just like the symbols and mantras, they are important tools on many shamanic and esoteric paths such as in Esoteric Buddhism, Taoism, Shintô, Hinduism, etc. They also play an especially important role in Reiki. For example, even during the first Reiki initiation, we are asked to place our hands together in front of our heart. This hand position is also a mudrâ and is called *Gasshô* in Japanese. Correspondingly, there are also many different forms of the *Gasshô* meditation and some other techniques with which we can do all kinds of useful and beautiful things.

This mudrâ and others can also be found in the sculptures of many religions. On the basis of the mudrâs in the Buddhist sculptures and Buddhist painting of India, Tibet, China, Korea, and Japan, it is possible to determine which Buddhist light beings are involved, as well as which functions and/or qualities these light beings have. As a result, they serve as visual

191

symbols on the one hand, as well as providing help in the sense of instruction for meditation and other spiritual practices. Just like the Reiki symbols, they are the keys to deep experiences and spiritual wisdom. Like a type of library, they contain an area of philosophical perception in an extremely condensed form that only reveals itself to those who have been trained accordingly. This book imparts some of the knowledge necessary for deciphering the symbols. For example, they are used in rituals such as a Reiki initiation or for increasing concentration or directly accessing the power, wisdom, and love of a light being, and much more. This is done in order to work for the benefit of all sentient beings and to maintain the divine order.

In addition, each individual mudrâ also has deep esoteric meanings. This means that much concealed knowledge is contained in the mudrâs that can hardly be grasped without a good spiritual teacher and the appropriate practice. Thanks to the great wealth of possibilities, there is an entire series of practical mudrâs in Esoteric Buddhism.

In Japan, the mudrâs were systematically used for the first time after the return of the monk Kûkai, the founder of the Japanese *Shingon* School of Esoteric Buddhism, from China. The same also applies to the *Siddham* symbols and mantras, as well as the dhâranîs. They had already existed before this time but only in a limited number and few initiates could understand them or even use them for such powerful rituals as healing and meditations for increasing inner and outer powers within the scope of personality development.

In general, there are two different types of mudrâs:

ॐ Mudrâs without objects in the hands (*mugyô*),

ॐ Mudrâs with objects in the hands (*ugyô*).

In the *Dainichi kyô* (Skr.: *Mahâvairocana Sûtra*), there is a description of 31 mudrâs for the great Buddhas, 57 for the great light beings, and 45 for additional light beings. But there are also many more than these. In order not to exceed the topic covered, this book only introduces the mudrâs that are related to Reiki and the symbols, as well as to its light beings.[71]

---

[71] There are sometimes slight variations in the positions of the hands for some mudrâs. This may have several reasons. Some variations reflect individual aspects in meaning and effect, but others differ from country to country or from school to school. The mudrâs are shown here first in the way that they have been traditionally used and secondly as they are suitable for Reiki.

The Mudrâ of Giving Reiki

Double Semui in

(Skr.: *Abhaya mudrâ*; Chin.: *Shiwuwei Yin*)

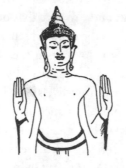

ILL. 50 – THE MUDRÂ OF GIVING REIKI

We hold both hands facing away from us as if we were giving Reiki to someone in front of us. On the one hand, this mudrâ primarily symbolizes protection and peace. A common name for it is also the so-called "do not fear" hand position. It looks like a natural hand position but it has been considered to be a sign of good intentions since ancient times. In India, this mudrâ done with just one hand was originally a gesture of the king when he made exercised his power. Buddha used this mudrâ when he was attacked by an angry elephant, who then immediately became a harmless and loving creature. When sculptures show the index finger pointing slightly forward, this is an indication that the sculpture is from the *Shingon* School of Esoteric Buddhism. In Ghandara, this mudrâ is also interpreted as a gesture of preaching. This can be compared with the *Avatamsaka Sûtra* and the *Brahmâjala Sûtra* in which it is written that the *Dharma*—the teaching of *Dainichi Nyorai*—radiates from all of his pores in the form of light into the entire universe, brightening even the most remote and darkest places there. If these light rays are enlarged, it becomes apparent that in reality there are an infinite number of Buddhas, meaning emanations of *Dainichi Nyorai*. These emanations also include the Buddha nature inherent to every being that can be awakened through spiritual personality development, resulting in enlightenment and spiritual awakening.

Among other things, this double- or single-handed mudrâ is used in Reiki for aura work and during the blessing at the end of each initiation. It expresses that we as Reiki channels have the strength and power of *Dainichi Nyorai*—the king of all Buddhas who manifests as light and can transmit it to the beings in the universe. It is not unusual for my Reiki students and clients to tell me that they see a golden or bright light during the treatment, and I'm sure that other people have also had such experiences. This light is the omnipresent manifestation of *Dainichi Nyorai*. There are also 12 Sun Angel mantras that can make the various archetypal aspects of *Dainichi Nyorai* available to people.[72] They can be used very well in combination with Usui Reiki. No wonder—both of these spiritual arts draw upon the same source for their power!

Beginning with the Second Degree, the symbols of the Reiki force can be used to achieve a specific effect. Whenever we draw the symbols, we do this with the *Abhaya Mudrâ* (Mudrâ of Giving Reiki), which means with the open, flat hand. This is as if a writing brush was coming out of the Palm Chakra, with which the symbols are written or drawn. This is also the first example of the importance reflected in the relationship between mudrâ, symbol, and mantra. After the initiation, the mudrâ is the hand gesture with which Reiki is given, the symbol determines the direction of the effect, and the mantra activates everything. The direction of the effect means the result attained by the individual symbol.

The following brief list summarizes the basic functions of the four Reiki symbols. The individual chapters of this book explain the large variety of additional functions that the symbols have:

ॐ CR for power-intensification and spatial orientation of the Reiki energy, as well as integrating spiritual powers into the material world and activating the other Reiki symbols.

ॐ SHK for mental healing and realization of the individual spiritual paths, as well as impregnating material objects and substances with spiritual power.

ॐ HS for distant healing, making medial contact, connecting with light beings, and awakening the Buddha consciousness that transcends time and space.

ॐ DKM for initiations and awakening the spirit of enlightenment and an individual's Buddha nature or the spiritual beingness.

[72] See pg. 391 in the chapter on the DKM Symbol for more information.

The Mudrâ of Giving and Taking

Yogan in, Segan in, Seyo in
(Skr.: *Varada mudrâ*; Chin.: *Shinyan Yin*)

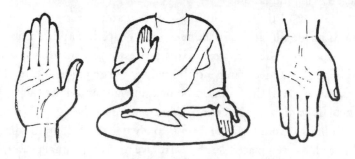

ILL. 51 – THE MUDRÂ OF GIVING AND TAKING

One or both hands are turned with the palms outward and the finger-tips pointing downward, sometimes held slightly forward. This mudrâ symbolizes sacrifice, giving, receiving, compassion, brotherly love, and sincerity. In addition, it stands for the fulfillment of the wish to achieve enlightenment in this lifetime. In Buddhism, this mudrâ usually appears in combination with the above-described mudrâ *Semui in* (the *Mudrâ of Giving Reiki*). When giving or receiving something within a spiritual context, the hands are always held in this mudrâ.

The combination of both mudrâs indicates giving and taking. As in all of nature, there is a fair exchange that takes place for everything. With the one hand we give and with the other we receive.[73] This obviously also tells us some things about the function of the Palm Chakra. Just as we can give and take with the hands, we can also give and receive energies with these chakras. Within this context, it is clearly also important to mention that traditional initiation methods in the Reiki system protect us from receiving disharmonious energies from the clients and also not

---

[73] In the old Nordic spiritual tradition, this principle is expressed by the rune *Gebo*. Just like everything that is divine in the narrower sense, there are various forms of manifestation throughout the world but the essence always remains unchanged. There is only one Creative Force and only one spiritual truth—and many paths lead to it.

195

transmitting any type of energies that would be harmful to them. This occurs through a type of energetic filter that is activated as soon as the client absorbs Reiki from our hands. This filter is permanently anchored in the Hand and Finger Chakras and securely protected against every type of negative manipulation.

The effect of these two mudrâs in numerous Reiki techniques and portions of the initiations is the reception of spiritual powers and their transmission to other people. In this process, as in Buddhism, the left hand is usually the receiving and the right is the giving hand. In terms of the receiving hand, this can also be held upward and downward. When it is held upward, in the direction of heaven, we receive currents of power from Father Heaven, *Dainichi Nyorai*. But when it is held in the direction of the earth or even placed on the earth, we receive spiritual powers from the goddess Mother Earth, which leads us directly to the next mudrâ.

The Mudrâ of Grounding

Goma in, Anzan in, Anchi in, Sokuchi in
(Skr.: *Bhûmisparsa mudrâ*; Chin.: *Chudi Yin*)

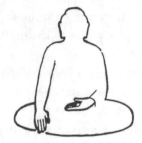

ILL. 52 – THE MUDRÂ OF GROUNDING

Here we touch the earth with one or both hands or fingertips. This mudrâ is literally translated as the "Gesture of Touching the Earth." It dates back to an episode in the life of the historical Buddha Shâkyamuni. When Buddha had achieved enlightenment under the Bodhi tree near Bodh-Gâya, he touched the earth with his right hand as evidence of his realization. Touching the earth is described as calling upon the Great Goddess Earth (Shakti) as a witness of enlightenment. However, it is also a symbol of unshakeable determination. There are some stories that also tell how the Earth Goddess sent an army of light beings to Buddha to protect him from the demons of *Mâra*, the King of Hell, who wanted to stop Buddha from achieving enlightenment. There is a great deal of wisdom in this story that has a very strong relationship to Reiki, which I would like to explain more extensively.

197

The term "grounding" or "to ground oneself" is now familiar to most people. Grounding is useful during an energy-work session when a person has been filled with strong yang forces and needs to be brought into balance through the appropriate yin influence. The demons of *Mâra* are an example or metaphor for this because enlightenment means a huge amount of energy. With the help of grounding, we also put ourselves under the protection of Mother Earth so that we can better process the experiences that we have had. This means that they are integrated into our daily lives and into the personality in a practical way. Otherwise, even though we may have experienced many things—nothing has changed and we therefore remain caught in the same lifestyle as before the healing.

When we give ourselves Reiki, this grounding is quite easy because we just need to place our hands on the soles of our feet. If the energy channels in the legs are blocked, then we also treat the knees and ankles.[74]

Here is another example: When a person has a headache, applying Reiki to the head and shoulders may make it even worse. The explanation for this is that blockages are dissolved by the spiritual life energy, but their contents cannot flow out of the body on their own because the appropriate energy channels do not function adequately. The result is that increasingly more released energies move in the area of the head and create headaches or feelings of unreality. If we support the body functions that are responsible for grounding by giving Reiki on the soles of the feet, especially from the toes to the middle of the foot (which is where the reflexology zones for the upper part of the body are located), the unusable energies will flow through the legs and feet to the earth within a short amount of time and the symptoms will disappear.

[74] See the chapter on the integration of spiritual experiences for more details.

The Mudrâ of Meditation

Jô in, Jôkai Jô in
(Skr.: *Dhyâna mudrâ*; Chin.: *Ding Yin*)

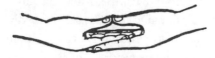

ILL. 53 – THE MUDRÂ OF MEDITATION

This mudrâ is used in wide areas of Asia for supporting meditation techniques. The hands are held in front of the lower belly, just below the navel, in this mudrâ. The fingers of one hand are placed on top of the fingers of the other hand so that the tips of the thumbs are touching lightly. The mystical triangle created between the fingers in this way is the symbol for the spiritual fire in Esoteric Buddhism. The same triangle can also be observed when someone sits in the lotus posture: We then see the head as the tip and the two knees as the base corners of the triangle. This *âsana* (spiritual body posture for focusing the life force) results in an increasing stability of body and mind. The high-frequency spiritual fire that develops through the lotus posture transforms blockages and low-frequency forces of all types within the body. In this manner, it opens human beings for the integration of the divine light. The shape of a flame, which also represents the light, usually has a triangular form when seen from the side in an undisturbed state. In addition, the triangle[75] is a symbol for the harmonious union between the mandalas of the two spiritual worlds, *Kongôkai* and *Taizôkai*, of *Dainichi Nyorai*. In the Womb World Mandala (*Taizôkai*), *Dainichi Nyorai* holds his hands in this mudrâ.

When the left hand is on top, this points to the enlightened state of the Buddha. When the right hand is on top, in the Buddhist schools this means that the meditating person is on the path to enlightenment or shows others the path to this divine state.

---

[75] see next page

There are many other variations in which we can recognize the individual Buddhas. However, we generally just see this hand position in the Great Buddhas who, as the central light beings, give spiritual orientation and divine healing to all the other beings. The historical Buddha Shâkyamuni also used this mudrâ while meditating shortly before his enlightenment. Even before that time, it had already been a widespread technique among the Brahmanic yogis for achieving divine consciousness. Shâkyamuni studied for many years with advanced Brahmanic masters and adepts before he created the new system of Buddhism from his insights and experiences.

[75] In the ancient Chinese oracle and wisdom book, the *I Ching—The Book of Changes* this symbol, the triangle, can also be found as the mountain in Chapter No. 52, *Gen*, the Mountain. The hexagram at the beginning of this chapter gives a detailed description of meditation, the required techniques, and their effects. Within this context, we can also compare the importance of mountains for the spiritual practice in Esoteric Buddhism, Shingon, and Japanese and Chinese shamanism. The sacred, divine fire is especially strong on a mountain. The shadow sign— all of the lines of the first hexagram turned into the exact opposite—for No. 52 is No. 51, the Shaking, the thunder. This tells how a direct encounter with the divine forces initially produces fear and then the motivation to advance on the path of one's own spiritual realization. Incidentally, these forces arise from within the earth: the Kundalinî experience: Shakti, the Great Goddess, rises through the energy channels of the spinal column to the sleeping Shiva, the Great God, in the Crown Chakra, to awaken him so that he releases his power for all beings. Those who practice meditation on a sacred mountain will undergo a shattering spiritual experience and cheerfully change their lives for the better after they have meaningfully integrated what they have experienced. It seems that there are astonishing parallels here! The Celts and Teutons in Europe frequently also liked to worship the gods on mountaintops.

The Mudrâ of the Paradise Buddha

Amida jô in

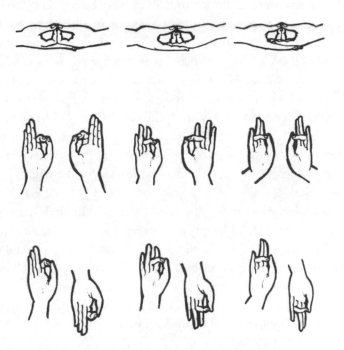

ILL. 54 – THE MUDRÂ OF THE PARADISE BUDDHA

The mudrâ of the Paradise Buddha *Amida Nyorai*, which is related to the SHK symbol, connects one or more fingers with the thumbs. Then it is called *Amida jô in*. This mudrâ is also an extension of the normal meditation mudrâ *Jô in*.

Altogether, there are nine combinations here that are related to the possibilities for gaining access to *Amida's* Paradise—the pure Land of the West—and the corresponding states of consciousness. The nine variations are the forms of *Amida* in Esoteric Buddhism. Connecting individual fingers with the thumbs always creates two circles, which symbolize the unity of the Womb World and the Diamond World. They are only separate from each other in the mudrâs because they are formed with different hands. At the same time, the right hand represents the world of the Buddhas and

201

the left symbolizes that of the sentient beings. The mudrâ—the bringing together of the hands—shows that the Buddhas and the sentient humans are in unity. We do not have to look far to find enlightenment since the Buddha consciousness is already present in every being. The nine mudrâ variations give us nine possibilities of accessing it. There is a connection here with *Dainichi Nyorai* since one of the virtues of *Amida Nyorai* is the Mirror-Like Wisdom that belongs to the five wisdoms of *Dainichi Nyorai*. The nine mudrâs also conceal a system of meditation. A round form is created when we connect individual finger with the thumb. The circle represents perfection in Zen Buddhism and the light-filled emanation of the Buddha in Esoteric Buddhism. In addition, each individual variation of this mudrâ with the two circles that it creates is a mandala clearly depicting the unity of the two worlds and/or the Great God and the Great Goddess.

Mandala is the Indian Sanskrit term for circle. The circle has neither a beginning nor an end. It is empty and yet enclosed. Its perfect form is the symbol for the Mirror-Like Wisdom of *Dainichi Nyorai*. The full moon also stands for the fusion of the Buddha consciousness and the individual self. In the many meditations of Esoteric Buddhism, the recognition of the Buddha consciousness inherent to an individual is often visualized as a *Siddham* symbol like the SHK on a moon disk.

The Mudrâ of the Connection between the Material and the Spiritual World

Hokkai jô in

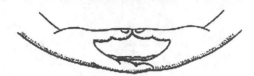

ILL. 55 – THE MUDRÂ OF THE CONNECTION
BETWEEN THE MATERIAL AND THE SPIRITUAL WORLD

With the term *Hokkai jô in* the mudrâ for the Meditation becomes the special illustration of the Great Sun Buddha *Dainichi Nyorai* in the Womb World, where he represents the Great Goddess (*Dai Marishi Ten*). It is the moon in the second character (*myô* 明) of the DKM symbol. Like the above described *Amida jô in* this mudrâ shows in form and symbolism the connection between the Paradise Buddha *Amida Nyorai* and the Great Sun Buddha *Dainichi Nyorai*. In addition, this mudrâ also stands for the connection between the material and the spiritual world and the exchange of energies in both realms. This is why the *Hokkai jô in* is also a mudrâ that represents the Reiki symbols CR and HS. One function of the CR symbol is the integration of spiritual energies into the material realm. One function of the HS symbols is to build a bridge between the material and the spiritual world that makes it possible for us to discover the Buddha nature within ourselves. The Medicine Buddha *Yakushi Nyorai* also holds his hands in this mudrâ. He holds a medicine bowl in them, which is equally nourished by the Great Goddess and the Great God.

The Mudrâ of the Pagoda

Dainichi Ken in, Musho fushi in, Rito in, Biroshana in, Sanmitsu in
(Chin.: *Wusobuzhi Yin*)

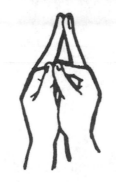

ILL. 56 – THE MUDRÂ OF THE PAGODA

The ring finger, little finger, and middle finger are pointing upward and the fingertips slightly touch each other. The index fingers are bent to form right angles and the fingertips also touch each other here. The thumbs are vertical, pointing upward, and touch each other, as well as the tips of the index fingers. As the name already implies, this is a mudrâ that solely represents *Dainichi Nyorai* of the Womb World (*Taizôkai*). Depending on the school of Esoteric Buddhism, there are various names for this mudrâ. The individual names reflect the various aspects and meanings.

The three upward stretched fingers symbolize the three mysteries (Jap.: *Sanmitsu*; Skr.: *triguhya*) of body, speech, and mind. The mudrâ relates to an practice where the practitioner determines that his own body, speech, and consciousness are identical with *Dainichi Nyorai* and that enlightenment is therefore inherent in him. This is why it is also associated with the mantra from the *Siddham* symbols *om a hûm* and the colors of white, red, and blue.

As a physical gesture that corresponds with a pagoda[76], this mudrâ also has a close relationship to the HS symbol, which also depicts a stylized pa-

---

[76] Architectonically symbolic portrayal of the spiritual structure of the universe in its five archetypal elements of earth, fire, water, wind, and ether (emptiness).

goda, as described in the appropriate chapter. On the one hand, *Dainichi Nyorai* is enlightenment in person. On the other hand, the HS and the pagoda are also a bridge to enlightenment. The monk Kûkai frequently emphasized that enlightenment can be found in this lifetime. The reason for this is mentioned in various places in the sutras of Esoteric Buddhism. *Dainichi Nyorai*, or the pagoda symbolizing him, dwells at the center of the universe, which is also a mandala. A mandala of Esoteric Buddhism is nothing other than the depiction of the universe, the Creation in its entirety. *Dainichi Nyorai's* pores radiate the light that enlightens the entire cosmos. If these light rays are enlarged, it becomes obvious that they are the infinite numbers of *Dainichi Nyorais*. The translation of the mudrâ *Musho fushi in* means: "There is no place that is not reached (by him)." If *Dainichi Nyorai* reaches and illuminates every place, and his emanations are he, then every place and every being is a part of *Dainichi Nyorai*. When we recognize this, there is great joy and the spiritual awakening to beingness occurs as a natural consequence.

There is an entire series of additional names for the mudrâ *Musho fushi in*. One attribute of *Dainichi Nyorai* is the Sword of Wisdom. When he manifests himself as the Imperturbable Wisdom King *Fudô Myôô*, he carries this sword in order to cut away the obstacles such as anger and envy. If the situation involves practices in *Dainichi Nyorai Kidô*, where such obstacles are dissolved, the same mudrâ is called *Dainichi ken in* (Sword Mudrâ of the Great Sun Buddha).

It becomes clear here that several applications are possible with one mudrâ and that not only the mudrâ but also the initiation, the mantra, the symbol, and the visualization in combination have important functions to achieve a specific effect.

The Mudrâ of Spiritual Wisdom

Chiken in, Kakusho in, Daichi in
(Chin.: *Zhiquan Yin*)

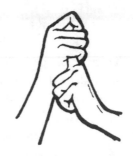

ILL. 57 – THE MUDRÂ OF SPIRITUAL WISDOM

The upward-pointing index finger of the right hand is enclosed by the fingers of the left hand. The tip of the thumb of the left hand touches the end of the right index finger. Depending on the intention, it is also possible to hold the hands the other way around or letting other fingers touch the thumb.

This mudrâ is also a mudrâ for *Dainichi Nyorai*, but in this case it refers to the Diamond World (*Kongôkai*), the guiding and channeling active power of wisdom. This mudrâ contains the wisdom of using power in such a way that it serves the highest good for the whole and that the suffering in this world is dissolved. It is also called the Mudrâ of the Six Elements or the Mudrâ of the Fist of Wisdom. It relates to the importance of insight in the spiritual world. The five fingers of the right hand represent the five elements of earth, water, air, fire, and emptiness that protect the sixth element, human beings. In addition, the upright index finger represents the knowledge that is concealed by the world of illusions.

Why are human beings the sixth element? Although we are influenced by the other elements, our own karma, and our individual constitution, as well as the actions of others, we have the greatest amount of free will in relation to all of the beings that live on the earth. This free will and our ability to translate it into action with the help of other resources of all types make us an essential factor of influence that constantly effects the world. Instead of "human beings," this element could also be called "conscious mind" or "consciousness." So this means the individual, conscious form of existence that can play a creative part in the world by virtue of its own power of decision and can develop from within itself the complete divine qualities: to be able to permeate everything and merge into oneness. Dainichi Nyorai symbolically personifies this enlightened, divine consciousness. *Kûkai* wrote the following about the nature of the elements: "In the various worldly teachings, the elements are as seen as inanimate, as not endowed with perception. The esoteric teachings (of Shingon) explain them as the secret, all-permeating body of the Buddha. These… elements are not separate from (divine) consciousness; even when the mind and form are different, they are still one in their nature because form is mind and mind is form, without any obstacles and without boundaries."

Another important meaning is the union between the Goddess and the God, *Shakti* and *Shiva,* in the Sacred Marriage that constantly creates life anew and imbues it with spiritual power. The chapter on Spiritual Cosmology provides a precise explanation of this.

The meanings of the Sacred Marriage are especially related to the last character of the DKM symbols (sun/moon) and the HS symbol as the connection between heaven and earth. As mentioned above, the moon and the sun express the union of the masculine and the feminine. One example of this is *Wu* shamanism and its central spiritual source of power, the union between the divine powers of the earth and the divine powers of heaven in the heart. The newly constellated power that has been acquired in this manner is then translated into practice through the Fifth Chakra. The mantra that represents this act and whose practice enables this ability is the personal mantra of Dainichi Nyorai and all of Esoteric Buddhism. It is the a, the primal sound that is the first and most important letter of the *Siddham* alphabet.

The sûtra of *Shobutsu kyô gaishô shinjitsu kyô* states: "The thumb of the right hand touches the index finger of the left hand. This is held in front of the chest. It is the *Mudrâ of the Wisdom Fist* that leads to enlightenment. Through the spiritual empowerment (*kaji*), the various Buddhas bring the adepts to perfect enlightenment—the wisdom of *Dainichi Nyorai's* mudrâ. "With this mudrâ, we can enter into the world of the wisdom of all Buddhas and learn from them by merging with them."

207

The Mudrâ of Heart Work

Gasshô in, Renge Gasshô in, Sashu Gasshô in, Kimyô Gasshô in
(Skr.: *Anjali mudrâ*; Chin.: *Hezhang Yin*)

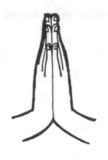

ILL. 58 – THE MUDRÂ OF HEART WORK

The hands are held on top of each other directly in front of the heart or at a small distance from it. Depending on the school, there are a number of variations. *Gasshô* is one of the mudrâs that is used by a Buddha who manifests as a Bodhisattva in order to help the beings. It is usually used as a greeting, during prayer, and when making offerings.

The union of both hands also represents the union of the God and the Goddess here, which is depicted in Esoteric Buddhism as the Mandalas of the Diamond World and the Womb World. The Goddess is the Womb World Mandala (*Taizôkai*) and the God is the Diamond World Mandala (*Kongôkai*). Moreover, the left hand represents the world of the beings and the right hand stands for the Buddha. This means that enlightenment is not far away from the beings.

In Reiki, this mudrâ is assumed during the initiations, during the *Gasshô* meditation, and at the beginning and the end of a treatment when we request and give thanks for being allowed to be a Reiki channel. It helps in strengthening the connection to *Dainichi Nyorai*, which is why the *Gasshô* meditation already presents an effective means of power-intensification in the First Degree. If this mudrâ is understood and performed as a process, it has a much stronger and more profound effect. When we do it, we should very slowly and consciously bring the palms of our hands together in front of our heart and feel the increasing power of the energy flow between them. This is the attraction between the two poles of the divine Oneness that longs for union. Then we can enjoy the rising of the opposites in the contact between the two polarities that is made possible through the loving power of the heart.

Fukû Kensaku Kannon, a special manifestation of the Bodhisattva *Kannon* (Skr.: *Avalokitesvara*; Chin.: *Kuan Yin*) holds the hands at a distance of about one to two centimeters (about 5 to 1 inch). Between them she holds a little crystal quartz ball. Through the strong flow of energy between the oppositely poled palms, the crystal quartz ball becomes energetically activated and receives a greater healing power. This hand position is also suitable as a meditation if it is held for a longer amount of time such as 15-20 minutes. With this technique, the power of the crystal quartz is directed through the hand reflex zones into the body and the energy flow between the hands is increased at the same time as the power of the stone. This meditation technique was described for the first time in the West in *The Complete Reiki Handbook* (Lotus Press).

We now know that Dr. Usui used crystal balls that he had charged with Reiki as support for Reiki treatments and also sent them home with his clients. It is quite likely that incorporated this method into the Reiki System from the cult of the *Fukû Kensaku Kannon*. This effective technique can also be done with other crystals such as rose quartz (strengthens the power of the heart), amethyst (helps achieve resonance with our spiritual path), fluorite (supports a new beginning and an active life in the sense of the divine order), smoky quartz (relieves stress and supports overcoming blockages inside and outside) or moonstone (strengthens the development of medial abilities, increases our own vibration, and stabilizes the feminine side of a human being).

If the hands are held without a crystal between them so that the fingers touch each other but there is an empty space between them, this area is called the "empty heart." This is the bridge between the material world and spiritual world, which means that it is closely connected with the HS and CR symbol. Another variation of this mudrâ consists of holding the hands even further apart. In this case, the mudrâ then facilitates energy transmission during the distant treatment.

The Mudrâ of the Great Goddess Dai Marishi Ten

Ongyô in, Hôbyô in
(Chin.: *Yinxing Yin*)

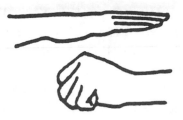

ILL. 59 – THE MUDRÂ OF THE GREAT GODDESS DAI MARISHI TEN

The left hand, shaped into a fist, is held slightly open so that a hollow is created. The right hand is held somewhat above it. This is the mudrâ of the Goddess of Light and the Gloria *Dai Marishi Ten*. It is one of the active energy-work mudrâs of Esoteric Buddhism. Depending upon the application, it can be used to protect someone, to heal, to transform encapsulated neurotic structures or to become invisible (difficult to perceive). This last point has led to *Dai Marishi Ten* and this mudrâ becoming especially popular with the *Ninja*, the Japanese shadow warriors who practice the martial art of *Ninjutsu*.[77]

The purpose of holding the right hand above the left fist is to conceal the body. *Dai Marishi Ten*—the spiritual mother of *Dainichi Nyorai*—is both his beloved and his protectress. This idea comes from the Indian Sun God Sûrya, who she also accompanies as a protectress. As such, she circles so quickly around *Dainichi Nyorai* that she can no longer be perceived. She protects the sun and the moon to the same degree, which means both the feminine and the masculine aspect of *Dainichi Nyorai*, which is concealed within the DKM. As a result, she is also known in Tibet as the

---

[77] Anyone interested in *Ninjutsu*, a spiritual inner martial art with a high emphasis on healing for the body, mind, and soul, can contact me (Mark). In addition to Reiki, *Ninjutsu* is one of the focal points of my work. Since 1987, I have studied inner martial arts with various Japanese masters up to the Master Degree and have developed my own spiritually-oriented style on this basis.

Goddess of the Sunrise. In a sense, she decides whether the (real, divine) world will become bright and visible. In Japan, people also assume that she resides in one of the seven stars of the Great Bear. It is possible to become invisible in a certain sense with the help of the *Dainichi Nyorai Kidô* practices through initiation, mudrâ, and mantra. This means that we are no longer seen by those who could make life unpleasant for us.

With the *Ongyô hô* ritual of Esoteric Buddhism, states of possession (foreign energies, ways of thinking, trauma, emotional states) can be removed by means of a spiritual power current from the goddess *Dai Marishi Ten* and her mudrâ.

The *Sûtra of the Goddess Dai Marishi Ten* (Jap.: *Marishiten kyô*) describes how the Buddha once spoke to his students: "There is a goddess called *Dai Marishi Ten*. She has supernatural powers. She rushes ahead of the Gods of the Sun and the Moon, but they cannot she her. Yet, *Dai Marishi Ten* can see the gods. We cannot see her with our eyes, catch her, or bind her. She cannot be hurt or harmed in any way. And those who attempt to do this cannot expect to receive her help."

"If you keep the name of *Dai Marishi Ten* in your mind, no one can perceive, capture, or injure you. The beings who do not act for the greatest good of all participants do not receive help from her."

The mudrâ *Ongyô in* is also described in this sûtra: "The *Ongyô in* is the mudrâ for concealing the form. The left hand forms an empty fist (it is hollow). The thumb lightly touches the tip of the index finger. The other three fingers are closed like a fist. Hold the hand in front of you heart. Then meditate on someone climbing into the hollow of the hand and staying there. Hold the right hand above it as protection. The *Mudrâ of the Goddess Dai Marishi Ten* herself is what protects you in her heart. You achieve this protection under the precondition that we act for the greatest good of the whole. Then you will be protected on the divine level, then you will become invisible and can avoid all misfortune."

The Mudrâ of Initiation

Kanjô in
(Skr.: *Abhiseka mudrâ;* Chin.: *Guanding Yin*)

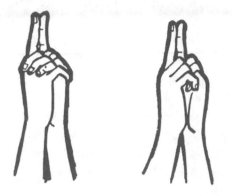

ILL. 60 – THE MUDRÂ OF INITIATION

Kanjô in is the mudrâ of initiation for magical rituals in Esoteric Buddhism that involve the transmission of very specific abilities. In contrast to most mudrâs, it is never used by Buddhas or Bodhisattvas. It is solely intended for the recipient of a spiritual empowerment (*kanjô*). In addition to magical initiations, it is beneficial to use this mudrâ in *Dainichi Nyorai Kidô* when we are receiving something from a light being after an offering, such as Reiki, has been made.

The fingers are interlaced for the Mudra of Initiation, except for the index fingers. The latter are raised and resting against each other as they point upward.

CHAPTER 11

Kuji Kiri
九字切

Introduction to the Kuji Kiri

In the secret teachings (Jap.: *mikkyô*) of Japan's Esoteric Buddhism and in Shugendô—Japanese magic—there are quite a few methods of spiritual healing and personality development that are centered around the great Sun Buddha *Dainichi Nyorai* and the Goddess of Light *Dai Marishi Ten*. *Dainichi Nyorai* is the essence of all light beings and can appear in many forms. In addition to the friendly-looking manifestations of the Sun Buddha, there are also some that have a more fierce or even angry facial expression. However they may look, they always use their power for the highest good of all. The facial expression is just the outer appearance in order to lead the beings who need it to the good or to protect the weak.

There are no evil light beings, even if they are often referred to. This is simply because people ascribed certain diseases or phenomena to supposedly existing evil spirits when they did not know what to call them. In addition, individuals who have not achieved spiritual realization more or less have the tendency to consider the problems in their lives as being caused by something outside of themselves so that they are not responsible for them. This tendency appears to exist in all cultures. However, when we turn to those who are knowledgeable about spirituality, they can confirm that there are only light beings who support life. All of the great spiritual teachings emphasize that it is important to also cultivate the divine qualities within ourselves in order to develop our divinity. This absolutely also includes taking responsibility for our own destiny. Imagine God saying that he is not to blame, that he is not doing well because this is someone else's fault. How would we respond to this in terms of omnipotence and wisdom?

213

The Role of the Imperturbable
Wisdom King Fudô Myôô

The wrathful manifestation of *Dainichi Nyorai* that is probably most familiar in Japan is the Imperturbable Wisdom King *Fudô Myôô*. I (Mark) first became acquainted with this light being in Japan and was able to have many good experiences as a result. Within the scope of my research on esoteric rituals and Reiki symbols, I had the opportunity to practice ascetic exercises with some mountain ascetics, as well as high-ranking monks in the Japanese forests, and participate in their rituals.

In order to become a monk in the Tendai School of Esoteric Buddhism, a person must first spend a period of 1000 days and nights without interruption on a pilgrimage on Mount Hiei, independent of the season. This includes meditating under waterfalls, walking 30-64 kilometers every day, and performing numerous rituals with light beings, mantras, mudrâs, sutras, and symbols. This ultimately has the effect of allowing the person to merge with the Imperturbable Wisdom King *Fudô Myôô*. One of my teachers even carried out this ritual for 4000 days (12 years) without interruption. He initiated me into the power of *Fudô Myôô* and then I was allowed to go on a pilgrimage for some days and nights through the mountains. This experience, together with some fire rituals with *Fudô Myôô*, solved my greatest problems at that time—a number of traffic accidents in a row.

Up to that time, I had always put the SHK symbol over me like a bell to protect me from accidents and the like. At the time that I learned this method, which is unfortunately not very effective, from a Reiki Master in the Northern part of Germany, I believed that it would work. But the experience with it has abundantly shown that neither the belief nor the possible placebo effect have any type of result. The SHK symbol simply does not have the function of a protective bell. Like the other symbols, it must be used within the scope of a technique for personality development or healing in order to have the appropriate effects. Just slipping on a symbol is not a technique and is comparable to a prejudice that was widespread in the past in developing countries: The contraceptive pills just had to be placed on the house altar to prevent the calamity of unwanted conception. In order to discover this principle, I had to take a very close look at the inside of an ambulance, as well as asphalt, concrete ditches, and the hoods of cars.

This taught me that experience is better than just believing. The more intensively we examine a method, the more we should realize (have the experience) that it functions properly. If it does not function or does not function well or only works sometimes, then we should think about the reason for this in order to find out how we can do better. This is why I am endeavoring in this book to describe everything in detail and to explain how truly practical effects with a high degree of effectiveness can be achieved with the traditional Reiki symbols of Dr. Usui. Since the fire ritual with *Fudô Myôô*, with which the karmic connections and causes for the traffic accidents were severed, I have had no more problems in this regard. The effect took hold immediately because the right technique was combined with the proper consciousness in an appropriate way by a person (my teacher) who was empowered to do this.

When I did the pilgrimage of the 88 temples of Shikoku in the Japanese primeval forest, the ice-cold mountain streams sometimes called to me as I dripped in sweat. These are so cold that people can usually just stay in for a few seconds. But with the help of the Mantra of *Fudô Myôô*, that extensively activated the spiritual fire force of my energy system, as my master had transmitted it to me, I could stay there for a long time without any effort. This is a fantastic method.

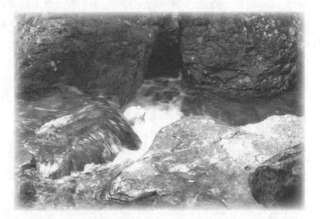

ILL. 61 – MARK HOSAK MEDITATING IN THE WATERFALL

However, completely different things are possible with the power of *Fudô Myôô*. With his sword, he symbolically cuts off the attachments to what is useless and he rescues the good with his lasso. The deep wrinkles on his forehead wash away evil and his fierce facial expression is so terrifying that anyone would turn away from bad intentions.

A friend of mine whom I met in a temple of the Paradise Buddha *Amida* had been the leader of a somewhat unpleasant motorcycle gang in his youth. One day, he discovered that his path at that time with power struggles and baseball bats hardly got him any further in life. In addition, he had to think about how he could develop his personality and use his potential in a meaningful way. He actually had very few possibilities to choose from since the police were after him and wanted to make sure that he could advance his development in prison. So he fled to the mountains to see the highest monk of the Tendai School and asked him for advice as to what he could do with his ruined life and if there was any chance at all for him. The monk explained to him that the historical Buddha *Shâkyamuni* had taught that even the most evil and cruel human being can achieve enlightenment if he sincerely performs the special practices of Esoteric Buddhism with which he can dissolve the bad karma of the past in just one lifetime and sow good seeds for the future. So he began the 1000-day meditation in the Japanese primeval forest, dissolved the karma of his past, and became a monk. This was also very good for his figure. He weighed 480 pounds before, but just 160 pounds at the end of the 1000 days. Today he weighs about 290 pounds. With this ideal weight and his life as a monk living in the temple, the police absolutely could not find him. In addition to the everyday rituals in the temple for the light beings and the daily visitors, he once saved the life of the Japanese Tennô. A time bomb had been hidden beneath the Paradise Buddha *Amida* with the intention of sending the ruler to the next world. However, the monk discovered the bomb during a preparatory ritual and took it into the forest. His temple and the Paradise Buddha *Amida* were not destroyed thanks to the imperturbable power of the *Fudô Myôô* who works through him. And the Japanese Tennô escaped the attempt on his life.

In the inner martial art of *Ninjutsu*, *Fudô Myôô* also plays an important role. Among other things, this is because the *Ninja* (practitioners of *Ninjutsu*) protected the temples of Esoteric Buddhism and taught the monks the fighting techniques. Many *Ninja* became monks themselves and integrated the secret teachings of Esoteric Buddhism into *Ninjutsu*. In this way, the so-called warrior monks in Buddhism and the *Ninja* magic in *Ninjutsu* came into being on Mount Hiei (across from Mount Kurama close to the wonderful garden city of Kyoto). However, because this phenomenon has been a thorn in the eye of the Japanese historiography and a bogey-man always has to be found, the noble *Ninja* are now frequently called forest spirits with long noses (Jap.: *tengu*) and both spies and perpetrators are classified as *Ninja*. *Yoshitsune*, the most famous samurai in Japan, grew up in the Kurama temple and secretly learned the Japanese art of sword fighting—*Kenjutsu*—from a *Tengu*. There was another mutual influence between the mountain ascetics (*Yamabushi*) of *Shugendô* and the *Ninja* since both lived in the mountains, learned from each other, and reciprocally protected each other.

The Nine Characters of the Kuji Kiri

The best-known practice in *Ninjutsu* from the secret teachings (*mikkyô*, Esoteric Buddhism and Taoism in Japan; in China, this was originally a ritual of Taoism from the 3rd-4th Century B.C.) is the "Protection Meditation of the Nine Signs" (Jap.: *Kuji goshin hô*. or also commonly called "The Cutting of the Nine Signs" (Jap.: *Kuji kiri*). The nine signs are the nine Chinese characters (臨兵鬪者皆陣列在前), with which nine mudrâs and mantras are associated. Integrated into a meditation and ritual cycle, they improve the personality on many levels. In addition, through the power of several light beings related to *Dainichi Nyorai* such as *Fudô Myôô, Dai Marishi Ten, Nitten,* and *Bishamonten,* they ensure protection against dangers and guidance on the path.

Additional possibilities for applications include removing states of possession, protecting places and people, the art of walking on fire without getting burned, meditating under half-frozen waterfalls without suffering from hypothermia, becoming invisible to those by whom we do not want to be seen, seeing things that cannot be perceived with the five senses, traveling in astral worlds to learn from them, or accepting light beings into ourselves in order to prepare for interstellar communication. In addition, this dissolves our own fears, which is a good precondition for protecting and healing other people, as well as helping them in finding their individual path. Once we are freed from our fears, we can expand our own heart power (love) that connects the spiritual and the material into a meaningful whole and makes developing our divinity in this world possible in the first place. In my opinion, this last effect of the *Kuji kiri* is the most important since it helps us to realize the divine within ourselves.

In order to achieve these abilities, the three areas of being—body, speech, and mind—with which the seeds can be sown for the future are purified, developed, and strengthened on three levels. The number nine represents the wholeness and perfection of the cosmos. It is the number of fields in the Diamond World Mandala (Jap.: *kongôkai*) of Esoteric Buddhism, a graphic depiction of the entire cosmos. It consists of the eight directions and the center. This pattern is reflected in the Chinese Feng Shui, in the ritual worship of the nine heavens (spiritual sources of power) of the *Wu* shamans, and many other esoteric techniques throughout the world. The number nine consists of three times three. Three is the necessary number of archetypal spiritual powers for an act of creation in the material world. By means of the three times three, this creation expresses in a perfect way the divine order in the material world. Even today, witches in the Western world swear by the power of the three times three. Within the scope of a spiritual path, this can be understood to mean that human beings, who were conceived on the basis of the three powers, first turn to the material world through the means of our own creativity. Then, when we have had enough of it, we turn to the spiritual other world. In conclusion, when we have understood that this is also not the right way, we discover the divine state of being that has always been within us. And this means that we have finally "arrived."

The nine signs come from Taoism. In Japan, they are combined with Esoteric Buddhism and Shintô into the methods introduced here. The pronunciation of each of the characters is the mantra itself, and all nine together also result in a mantra. Although this sounds complicated, it is very similar to the structure of the HS symbol in its essence. The only difference is in the type of the application and the great variety of effects. If the HS symbol is just reduced to the function of distant healing, the parallels can hardly be recognized. However, if we consider the teaching of the five elements and other concealed functions within the HS symbol, we discover a method that is similar in its complexity to the protection meditation of the Nine Signs. In my opinion, there is a deep connection between the Nine Signs and the HS symbol in terms of ritual applications.

In the customary order of the Nine Signs, they result in the Chinese sentence "臨兵鬭者皆陣列在前", which has the following meaning: "Advance toward the army. The warriors fight. They are all in front and destroy the ranks of the army." This sentence is, as also applies to the HS symbol, an encoding of the method itself. Non-initiates see the meaning of the sentence in it, but not the method that it conceals. The individual characters actually correspond more with the pronunciation of the mantras and are placed together in this sentence to confuse the uninitiated. But the content is still somewhat related to the ritual itself.

For the initiated, the Nine Signs are an aid in remembering how to perform the ritual. While the individual mantras in the sequence of the sentence are pronounced, the mudrâ for each mantra is assumed according to the appropriate light being that is concealed behind it. In addition, the associated symbol is visualized. The three actions of mantra, mudrâ, and symbol speak directly to the three areas of being—body, speech, and mind—in order to be effective there. Each individual symbol, as well as all of the symbols together, has effects both on the outside (surroundings) and inside (development of the inner powers). This is repeated nine times (nine mantras, nine mudrâs, and nine symbols). Afterward, all nine signs are summarized into one symbol, the so-called "Nine-Sign Protective Grid" or the "Nine-Sign Protective Star," which is drawn in the air like the Reiki symbols and activated with the mantra. Then an additional symbol can be drawn and activated. The symbol selected at the very end varies depending upon the intention, from which many types of application possibilities can result.

It is useful to prepare for the *Kuji kiri* beforehand. The five brief meditations (*Goshinbô*) and some additional preparation practices are helpful in doing this. They help us purify ourselves of karmic influences and strengthen ourselves for the actual practice so that we can deal with the energies in a good way.

The Five-Fold Protective Method
(Goshinbô)

In this practice series, there is an entire sequence of mantras, as they are found in the sutras of Esoteric Buddhism. There are also no translations of the meanings. When the sutras were translated into Chinese from Sanskrit, all of the texts were translated but the mantras were left in the Siddham script. Chinese characters that had a similar sound were written next to them as an aid in pronunciation. Even today, the mantras in *Siddham* can still be found between the Chinese texts. As Buddhism came to Japan in a number of waves during the course of the centuries, the sutras from China were transmitted to Japan unchanged. So the pronunciation of the following mantras is the traditional Sino-Japanese reading of Chinese characters. Although words appear next to the *Siddham* symbols in the mantras that have an inner meaning, the significance of the mantras for the practice is less important or may not even be useful. Furthermore, most of the Japanese monks who I got to know in Japan do not know the meaning of the mantra. The effect occurs through the audible intoning, which means through the sound and the vibration of the individual syllables that are created in this way.

Purifying Karma

Jôsangô 浄三業

This practice helps purify karmic actions on the levels of body, speech, and mind in order to attain an inner level of consciousness.

ILL. 62 – LOTUS BLOSSOM MUDRÂ RENGE GASSHÔ

Fold the hands into the *Renge Gasshô* (Lotus Blossom Mudrâ of the Heart Work) and bless the forehead, right shoulder, left shoulder, chest, and throat by touching them. While you do this, recite the following mantra five times:

Om sohahanba, shuda, saraba, tarama, sohahanba shudo kan

Purifying the Body with the Power
of the Buddha of the Ten Directions and Three Times

Butsubu sanmaya 佛部三昧耶

Assume the *Bucchô no in* mudrâ. Keep the little finger, ring finger, and middle finger next to each other. Cross the index fingers over the middle fingers. Place the thumbs next to the index fingers. Hold your holds like a bowl.

ILL. 63 – BUDDHA'S CROWN BUCCHÔ NO IN

Visualize how *Dainichi Nyorai* comes to bless you. From his Third Eye (6th Chakra), clear white-golden light flows into your Third Eye and fills you up completely. As a result, the karma of your actions is purified, your offences and obstacles are eliminated, and the seeds for service and wisdom are sowed.

During the visualization, recite the following mantra 108 times or a multiple thereof:

Om tatagyato, dohanbaya sowaka

The Purification of Speech
with the Power of the Eight-Petaled Lotus

Rengebu sanmaya 蓮華部三昧耶

Assume the *hachiyô no in* mudrâ.

ILL. 64 – EIGHT-PETALED LOTUS HACHIYÔ NO IN

Visualize the Goddess of Great Compassion *Kannon* and the many companions coming to you. From her Fifth Chakra, a brilliant red light radiates into your Fifth Chakra and fills you up completely. As a result, the karma that has been created as a result of words is purified. Your words will be distinguished by eloquence so that they make others happy. You will become a master in the teachings for the highest good of all participants. Recite the following mantra 108 times or a multiple thereof:

Om handobo, dohanbaya sowaka

The Purification of the Mind with the Power of the Triple Vajra
(Thunderbolt)

Kongôbu samaya 金剛部三昧耶

Assume the *Sanko no in* mudrâ.

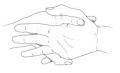

ILL. 65 – THUNDERBOLT WITH THREE PRONGS SANKO NO IN

The back sides of the hands lie on each other. The little finger of the right hand touches the left thumb, while the little left finger touches the right thumb. The other fingers form the triple *Vajra*. Visualize *Kongôsatta* and all of *Vajra* holders. From his heart, a powerful luminous blue light radiates into your chest and fills up your entire body. This will give you the power to quickly purify the karma of the mind. It helps in awakening the spirit of enlightenment, imparts abilities and freedoms, liberates from disease, and strengthens the body through the mind. Recite the mantra 108 times or a multiple thereof:

Om bazoro dohanbaya sowaka

Putting On the Armor

Hikô 被甲

Assume the *hikô goshin* mudrâ.

ILL. 66 – PUTTING ON THE ARMOR HIKÔ GOSHIN

Cross your index fingers over the middle fingers. Place your thumbs behind your middle fingers and fold the remaining fingers inward. The balls of the thumbs touch each other. Bless the five areas of the body with this mudrâ. Visualize yourself wearing the armor of great compassion and love. Golden light radiates from your pores and you are in a golden halo so that your karma will no longer be tarnished. This is how you can free yourself from suffering and the eternal cycle of rebirth, quickly attaining the state of great enlightenment. Recite the following mantra 108 times or a multiple thereof:

Om bazara, gini, harachi, hataya sowaka

Preparation Practices for the Kuji Kiri

You can have many wonderful experiences with the following practices, but I recommend that you follow the sequence recommended here. This is necessary so that you can develop the effect of these practices in their full power. Remain with an practice until you can do it in a confident and successful way before you attempt the next.

The monk *Kûkai* said about these practices: "If you do this meditation with a pure heart and complete trust, the highest teaching will be revealed to you."

In addition to your ability to visualize, the following four preparation practices also promote your powers of perception. They are an aid with which you can learn to orient yourself in many levels of existence. With the meditation on the *Siddham* symbol of "a" at the conclusion of the preparation, it will be easier for you to awaken the concealed powers and recognize your own mind. Through the direct contact with *Dainichi Nyorai*, your mind will be purified and stabilized on a first level. The more often you do this practice, the more the purifying process will penetrate into the deeper layers.

Meditation of Gazing at the Moon Disk

Go to a calm place that is neither too light nor too dark. Sit in a full or half-lotus posture or in Japanese Seiza position on your knees. Your eyes should be half-open.

Place your hands together in front of your heart in the way that you know from the initiations or the Gasshô meditation. Calm your mind by concentrating for a while on breathing into the Hara and the Reiki power in your hands.

*Now use the distant contact to connect with **Dainichi Nyorai**. Greet him with the words: "Dear **Dainichi Nyorai**, I come to you as a sick person and request healing. I come to you as an ignorant person and request teaching. I come to you as someone who does not know the way and ask for protection and guidance. I come to you as someone who is helpless and ask you for power in order to better serve. As compensation, I send you Reiki. Please use it as you wish for the benefit of all." Then draw several CR symbols and activate each of them with the mantra for intensifying the Reiki flow of power.*

Use your inner eye to draw a moon disk in front of you. The outline is black and the surface is white. Look at the disk as long as you need to see it clearly. Now imagine that the power of *Dainichi Nyorai* flows into you from the moon disk as you inhale. When you exhale, everything that is impure leaves your body and is purified by the moon disk. Continue to look at the white moon disk in front of your inner eye as you do this.

*

Now take leave of **Dainichi Nyorai** *by quietly saying or thinking: "Dear* **Dainichi Nyorai,** *I thank you for the beautiful meditation and ask permission to call on you again soon. I wish you the blessing and protection of the Creative Force on your path."*

Blow strongly between your hands and then rub them together in order to detach yourself from the contact.

Meditation of Gazing at the Moon Disk in the Heart

Go to a calm place that is neither too light nor too dark. Sit in a full or half-lotus posture or in Japanese **Seiza** *position on your knees. Your eyes should be neither opened nor closed.*

Place your hands together in front of your heart in the way that you know from the initiations or the Gasshô meditation. Calm your mind by concentrating for a while on breathing into the Hara and the Reiki power in your hands.

Now use the distant contact to connect with **Dainichi Nyorai.** *Greet him with the words: "Dear* **Dainichi Nyorai,** *I come to you as a sick person and request healing. I come to you as an ignorant person and request teaching. I come to you as someone who does not know the way and ask for protection and guidance. I come to you as someone who is helpless and ask you for power in order to better serve. As compensation, I send you Reiki. Please use it as you wish for the benefit of all." Then draw several CR symbols and activate each of them with the mantra for intensifying the Reiki flow of power.*

*

Use your inner eye to draw a moon disk in front of you. The outline is black and the surface is white. Then draw the moon disk into you. It is now in your chest. Look at the moon in your chest as long as you need to

225

see it clearly. Now imagine that golden light is radiating from the moon disk and filling your entire body. Continue to look at the white moon disk in your chest.

*

Now take leave of **Dainichi Nyorai** *by quietly saying or thinking: "Dear* **Dainichi Nyorai,** *I thank you for the beautiful meditation and ask permission to call on you again soon. I wish you the blessing and protection of the Creative Force on your path."*

Blow strongly between your hands and then rub them together in order to detach yourself from the contact.

Meditation of Enlarging the Moon Disk in the Heart

Go to a calm place that is neither too light nor too dark. Sit in a full or half-lotus posture or in Japanese **Seiza** *position on your knees. Your eyes should be neither opened nor closed.*

Place your hands together in front of your heart in the way that you know from the initiations or the Gasshô meditation. Calm your mind by concentrating for a while on breathing into the Hara and the Reiki power in your hands.

Now use the distant contact to connect with **Dainichi Nyorai.** *Greet him with the words: "Dear* **Dainichi Nyorai,** *I come to you as a sick person and request healing. I come to you as an ignorant person and request teaching. I come to you as someone who does not know the way and ask for protection and guidance. I come to you as someone who is helpless and ask you for power in order to better serve. As compensation, I send you Reiki. Please use it as you wish for the benefit of all." Then draw several CR symbols and activate each of them with the mantra for intensifying the Reiki flow of power.*

*

Use your inner eye to draw a moon disk in front of you. The outline is black and the surface is white. Then draw the moon disk into you. It is now in your chest. Look at the moon in your chest as long as you need to see it clearly. Now imagine that the moon disk is expanding. At first, it is the size of your own body. Then it becomes the size of a house, of the city in which you live, of your country, of your continent, of the earth, and finally, the size of the universe. Focus your attention on each size until you can fully perceive it.

*

*Now take leave of **Dainichi Nyorai** by quietly saying or thinking: "Dear **Dainichi Nyorai**, I thank you for the beautiful meditation and ask permission to call on you again soon. I wish you the blessing and protection of the Creative Force on your path."*

Blow strongly between your hands and then rub them together in order to detach yourself from the contact.

Meditation of Enlarging and Decreasing the Size of the Moon Disk

*Go to a calm place that is neither too light nor too dark. Sit in a full or half-lotus posture or in Japanese **Seiza** position on your knees. Your eyes should be neither opened nor closed.*

Place your hands together in front of your heart in the way that you know from the initiations or the Gasshô meditation. Calm your mind by concentrating for a while on breathing into the Hara and the Reiki power in your hands.

*Now use the distant contact to connect with **Dainichi Nyorai**. Greet him with the words: "Dear **Dainichi Nyorai**, I come to you as a sick person and request healing. I come to you as an ignorant person and request teaching. I come to you as someone who does not know the way and ask for protection and guidance. I come to you as someone who is helpless and ask you for power in order to better serve. As compensation, I send you Reiki. Please use it as you wish for the benefit of all." Then draw several CR symbols and activate each of them with the mantra for intensifying the Reiki flow of power.*

*

Use your inner eye to draw a moon disk in front of you. The outline is black and the surface is white. Then draw the moon disk into you. It is now in your chest. Look at the moon in your chest as long as you need to see it clearly. Now imagine that the moon disk is expanding gradually into the universe. Slowly reduce the size of the moon disk again. The more slowly it becomes smaller, the more effective this practice will be. It

227

should once again be as large as the original moon disk in the heart. Now allow it to become even smaller until just a tiny point is visible. Imagine that you go into this point and both of you become even smaller together with it. Intensify this state every time you practice.

*

*Now take leave of **Dainichi Nyorai** by quietly saying or thinking: "Dear **Dainichi Nyorai**, I thank you for the beautiful meditation and ask permission to call on you again soon. I wish you the blessing and protection of the Creative Force on your path."*

Blow strongly between your hands and then rub them together in order to detach yourself from the contact.

Dainichi Nyorai Meditation of the Siddham Symbol A

Wash your hands and rinse out your mouth. Draw the *Siddham* syllable *a* in a circle that symbolizes the moon disk.

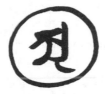

ILL. 67 – SIDDHAM A ON A MOON DISK

Go to a calm place that is neither too light nor too dark. Sit in a full or half-lotus posture or in Japanese Seiza position on your knees. Your eyes should be neither opened nor closed.

Place your hands together in front of your heart in the way that you know from the initiations or the Gasshô meditation. Calm your mind by concentrating for a while on breathing into the Hara and the Reiki power in your hands.

*Now use the distant contact to connect with **Dainichi Nyorai**. Greet him with the words: "Dear **Dainichi Nyorai**, I come to you as a sick person and request healing. I come to you as an ignorant person and request teaching.*

I come to you as someone who does not know the way and ask for protection and guidance. I come to you as someone who is helpless and ask you for power in order to better serve. As compensation, I send you Reiki. Please use it as you wish for the benefit of all." Then draw several CR symbols and activate each of them with the mantra for intensifying the Reiki flow of power.

*

Place your hands in *Gasshô* and bow three times so that your hands and elbows touch the ground. Calm your mind by concentrating for a while on breathing into the Hara and the Reiki power in your hands.

Continue to hold the hands in *Gasshô* and use your middle fingers to touch the forehead, the right and left shoulder, chest, and throat for the purification of body, speech, and mind. As you do this, recite the following mantra three times: *Om sohahanba, shuda, saraba, tarama, sohahanba shudo kan*

To development the potential for enlightenment (*bodhicitta*), keep your hands in *Kongô Gasshô* (similar to *Gasshô* but the fingertips are crossed).

ILL. 68 – KONGÔ GASSHÔ

Recite the following mantra seven times: *Om bodhicittam utpâdayâmi.*

Then recite the following mantra seven times: *Om sanmayas tvam.*

Recite the five great rules of the Bodhisattvas or Dr. Usui's life principles: "Living beings are infinite in their number. I promise to lead all of them to happiness. Merits and knowledge are infinite in their number. I promise to gather all of them. The teachings of the Dharma are countless. I promise to master all of them. The light beings are countless. I promise to serve all of them. Enlightenment is unique. I promise to attain it."

Recite the following mantra seven times: *Om a bi ra un ken.*

Now assume the *Hokkai jô-in* Mudrâ of the Meditation of the Great Sun Buddha *Dainichi Nyorai.*

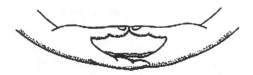

ILL. 69 – HOKKAI JÔ IN

Concentrate on your breathing. Exhale powerfully twice through your mouth and then continue to breathe calmly through your nose.

Slightly open your eyes and look at the *Siddham* symbol *a*. As you do this, imagine that you are looking into a mirror. Visually that you are drawing the *a* with the moon disk into your chest. Keep your attention there for a while. Now imagine that the moon disk has turned into a crystal ball. The *a* is floating in it. Also remain in this state as long as you can. A white-golden light is now radiating from the *a* in the crystal ball and fills your whole body.

Now push the syllable *a* with the moon disk back out of your chest into the image in front of you. Then ask *Dainichi Nyorai* that the powers of the *Kuji kiri* may be actualized to a degree that is appropriate for you and for the highest good of all beings. Recite the following mantra five times: *Om vajrâgni pradiptâya svâhâ.*

Imagine that you are protected by the armor of great compassion and all spiritual merits for the benefit of all beings by *Dainichi Nyorai*. Your body radiates flames that catch everything that disrupts and transforms it into love, wisdom, and peace.

*

*Now take leave of **Dainichi Nyorai** by quietly saying or thinking: "Dear **Dainichi Nyorai**, I thank you for the beautiful meditation and ask permission to call on you again soon. I wish you the blessing and protection of the Creative Force on your path."*

Blow strongly between your hands and then rub them together in order to detach yourself from the contact.

Performing the Kuji Kiri

In addition to the realized personality development, the success of the *Kuji kiri* also depends upon how intensively the preparatory practices have been performed. The basic preconditions are good visualization abilities and a fluid approach to the fundamental practices. Upon this basis, the actual *Kuji kiri* follows in a number of levels, which will now be presented in order here.

Practice 1: The Nine-Sign Sword

Purpose of the practice: On the one hand, this practice will lead you closer to the essence of the effective power of the *Kuji kiri*; and on the other hand, you can employ the Cutting of the Nine Sign very well later in rituals. By performing the Cutting of the Nine Signs, you can purify the place where a ritual is to take place with the power of the Imperturbable Wisdom King *Fudô Myôô* and/or build up a certain protection from disruptive influences. As a result, rituals will become stronger and healing is intensified. If the *Kuji kiri* is used directly for people, it is an effective means of removing any type of state of possession. The latter is generally one of the main functions of the *Fudô Myôô*.

Applications:

*Use the distant contact to connect the Imperturbable Wisdom King **Fudô Myôô** (a wrathful emanation of **Dainichi Nyorai**). Greet him with the words: "Dear **Fudô Myôô**, I come to you as a sick person and request healing. I come to you as an ignorant person and request teaching. I come to you as someone who does not know the way and ask for protection and guidance. I come to you as someone who is helpless and ask you for power in order to better serve. As compensation, I send you Reiki. Please use it as you wish for the benefit of all." Then draw several CR symbols and activate each of them with the mantra for intensifying the Reiki flow of power.*

*

Assume the Mudrâ of the Sword Hand (*Shutô in*). This means that the right hand forms the sword and the left hand is the chain of the Imperturbable Wisdom King *Fudô Myôô*. Here are the instructions: Extend the index and middle finger of the right hand (sword) upward. Bend the little finger and ring finger. Touch the fingernails both of these fingers with the tip of the thumb. Do the same with the left hand (chain). Now stick the fingertips of the extended index and middle finger of the right hand from below into the hole created by the thumb, ring finger, and little finger of the left hand.

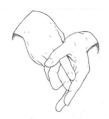

ILL. 70 – MUDRÂ OF THE SWORD HAND

Visualize a lotus blossom in front of you, upon which a standing moon disk rests. Use your inner eye to draw the symbol *kanman* of *Fudô Myôô* on it.

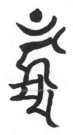

ILL. 71 – SIDDHAM KANMAN

To activate the symbol, recite three times the medium-long mantra of *Fudô Myôô*: *Namaku samanda basara nan senda makaroshana sowataya untarata kanman.*

Now draw the lotus blossom, moon disk, and symbol into your chest and visualize them there. Red-golden light radiates from the symbol until your entire body is filled with it.

Now draw the right hand (the sword) out of the left and move the left hand, without releasing the mudrâ, to the hip. As shown in the illustration, cut five horizontal and four vertical lines in the air.

232

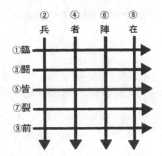

ILL. 72 – CUTTING DIRECTION OF THE 9 SIGNS

With each cut, intone the nine symbols *Rin – byô – tô – sha – kai – jin – retsu – zai – zen* (臨兵闘者皆陣列在前) like a *Kiai*[78] and visualize your sword hand as if it had a genuine blade emitting light and cutting through any type of disruptive influences.

Move your right sword hand back into the left chain hand as it was before so that the opening mudrâ is created. Now the forms in your chest dissolve.

*

*Feel what is happening within you for another moment and then take leave of the distant contact with **Fudô Myôô** by quietly saying or thinking: "Dear **Fudô Myôô**, I thank you for the beautiful meditation and ask permission to call on you again soon. I wish you the blessing and protection of the Creative Force on your path."*

Blow strongly between your hands and then rub them together in order to detach yourself from the contact.

If necessary, ground yourself for a while by giving yourself Reiki on the soles of your feet and then doing some physical exercises.

---

[78] *Kiai* (気合) is the term used in martial arts for the battle cry with which the energies of the body, speech, and mind are attuned to each other. As a result, the energy is so directed at one point that a maximal focusing of the force becomes possible.

Practice 2: The Nine Mudrâs and the Kuji Kiri

Each mantra of the Nine Symbols also has a mudrâ. When these are applied correctly, you can use them to invite the light beings to come into you and attain their individual powers and abilities by merging with them. Then the healing powers of the light beings can have an internal and external effect. "Internal" represents your own development and "external" means the possibility of making these powers available to other beings and places.

All nine mantras, mudrâs, and symbols have unique effects that as a whole lead to getting to know yourself in the deepest part of your being. This is also one of the reasons why the *Kuji kiri* was so popular with the *Ninja* and some of the Samurai; it was said that only those who know themselves can also know the enemy and become one-hundred times more dangerous than the enemy himself as a result. Through self-perception, it is possible to know the enemy and recognize in advance what he is planning to do and when he will do it. This means that you can avoid the dangers in advance. Through the protection of the Great Goddess of Light *Dai Marishi Ten*, this protection can also take place unconsciously in that things happen to make sure that you are increasingly in the right place at the right time.

Applications

Connect through the distant contact with the Imperturbable Wisdom King **Fudô Myôô***. Welcome him with the words: "Dear* **Fudô Myôô***, I come to you as a sick person and request healing. I come to you as an ignorant person and request teaching. I come to you as someone who does not know the way and ask for protection and guidance. I come to you as someone who is helpless and ask you for power in order to better serve. As compensation, I send you Reiki. Please use it as you wish for the benefit of all." Then draw several CR symbols and activate each of them with the mantra for intensifying the Reiki flow of power.*

Connect through the distant contact with the Great Goddess of Light **Dai Marishi Ten***. Greet her with the words: "Dear* **Dai Marishi Ten***, I come to you as a sick person and request healing. I come to you as an ignorant person and request teaching. I come to you as someone who does not know the way* *and ask for protection and guidance. I come to you as someone who is help-less and ask you for power in order to better serve. As compensation, I send you Reiki. Please use it as you wish for the benefit of all."* Then draw several CR *symbols and activate each of them with the mantra for intensifying the Reiki flow of power.*

*

Visualize a lotus blossom in front of you, upon which a standing moon disk rests. With your inner eye, draw the symbol *ma* of *Dai Marishi Ten* on it.

To activate the symbol, recite the mantra of *Dai Marishi Ten: Namaku samanda bodanan om Sutras ei sowaka* three times.

Now pull the lotus blossom, moon disk, and symbol into your chest and visualize them there. Red-gold radiant light now emanates from the symbol until it completely fills your body.

Now draw the first symbol in the air with the palm of your hand. Assume the appropriate mudrâ and recite the appropriate mantra with it once by saying it with *ki*. Go through all nine symbols, mantras, and mudrâs in this way. (The stroke sequences of the symbols can be found with the individual mudrâs.)

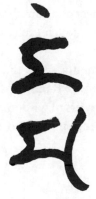

ILL. 73 – STROKE SEQUENCE FOR THE SIDDHAM MA

臨 *Rin* – The Mudrâ of the Old Loneliness
(Jap.: *Toko in* 獨古印)

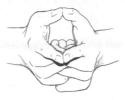

ILL. 74 – MUDRÂ OF THE OLD LONELINESS

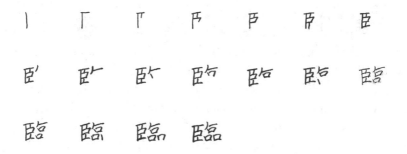

ILL. 75 – STROKE SEQUENCE FOR RIN

Hand Position: The index finger and thumb of the right and left hand are extended so that the fingertips touch each other. The other fingers form rings that fit into each other.

Esoteric Meaning: The mudrâ *rin* is the physical expression for the thunderbolt *Vajra* (Jap.: *kongô*; a Buddhist scepter that is used for rituals). The *Vajra* depicts the powers of wisdom that destroy ignorance. The mudrâ is used to build up the strength to overcome both mental and physical obstacles.

兵 *Byô* – **The Mudrâ of the Great Vajra Wheel**
(Jap.: *Daikongôrin in* 大金剛輪印)

ILL. 76 – MUDRÂ OF THE GREAT VAJRA WHEEL

ILL. 77 – STROKE SEQUENCE FOR BYÔ

Hand Position: The little fingers and the ring fingers are wrapped around into each other. The index fingers and thumbs are positioned so that the fingertips of both hands touch. The middle fingers are placed across the back of the index fingers and touch each other at the fingertips.

Esoteric Meaning: *Byô* is the mudrâ for the great Vajra Wheel. It is the symbol of the knowledge that transcends all worldly limitations. It can be used to bring channeled energies into various levels of consciousness.

鬪 *Tô* – **The Mudrâ of the Outer Lion**
(Jap.: *Gejiji in* 外獅子印)

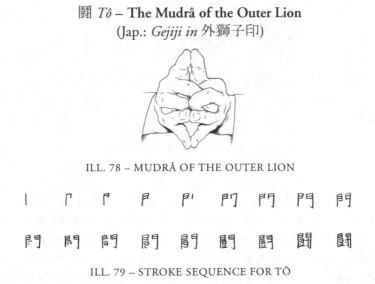

ILL. 78 – MUDRÂ OF THE OUTER LION

ILL. 79 – STROKE SEQUENCE FOR TÔ

Hand Position: The right index finger is extended between the middle and ring finger of the left hand. The left index finger is extended in the same way between the middle and ring finger of the right hand. The middle fingers are placed in the opening between the ring and index finger so that they wrap around the index finger. The fingertips point downward and touch each other at the fingernails. The ring fingers and the little fingers are extended and placed together. The distance between the little fingers and the ring fingers should remain open a little. This is the mouth. The thumbs are the ears and the tips of the index fingers are the eyes of the lion.

Esoteric Meaning: *Tô* is the Mudrâ of the Outer Lion. This refers to the roaring of this mighty animal. Concentrating the power to one point by roaring (*kiai*) can considerably intimidate the opponent and lead to victory. It can also be helpful in waking up in order to let go of certain structures in the personality. The intuition, mind, and charisma are strengthened.

者 *Sha* – The Mudrâ of the Inner Lion
(Jap.: *Naijiji in* 內獅子印)

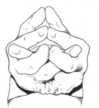

ILL. 80 – MUDRÂ OF THE INNER LION

一　十　土　耂　耂　者　者　者

ILL. 81 – STROKE SEQUENCE FOR SHA

Hand Position: The tip of the right ring finger is extended between the left middle and index finger. The tip of the left ring finger is extended in the same way between the right middle and index finger. The middle fingers of the right and left hand wrap around the ring fingers so that the fingertips point downward. The thumbs, little fingers, and index fingers are extended and placed together. The little fingers form the ears. The

238

distance between the thumbs and index fingers are the mouth. The tips of the ring fingers are the eyes of the lion.

Esoteric Meaning: *Sha* as the symbol of the inner lion awakens the inner powers and the perception directed inwards. Negative thoughts dissolve and the will is strengthened. This promotes the ability to heal others and the powers of self-healing.

皆 *Kai* – **The Mudrâ Wrung to the Outside**
(Jap.: *Gebaku in* 外縛印)

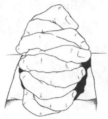

ILL. 82 – MUDRÂ WRUNG TO THE OUTSIDE

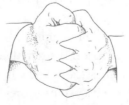

ILL. 83 – STROKE SEQUENCE FOR KAI

Hand Position: The fingers of both hands are folded.

Esoteric Meaning: With *kai,* the connections and illusions that disturb our recognition of our own divinity are stripped away. The more we recognize and integrate our own divinity, the most easily we can develop our subtle abilities.

陳 *Jin* – **The Mudrâ Wrung to the Inside**
(Jap.: *Naibaku in* 内縛印)

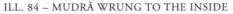

ILL. 84 – MUDRÂ WRUNG TO THE INSIDE

239

マ　了　ド　ド　ド　阡　阡　阽　阽　陣

ILL. 85 – STROKE SEQUENCE FOR JIN

Hand Position: The ten fingers of the right and left hand are interlaced with each other toward the inside.

Esoteric Meaning: With *jin,* we can strengthen our self-confidence in our own intuitive abilities and the effect of our charisma on others.

列 *Retsu* – **The Mudrâ of the Wisdom Fist**
(Jap.: *Chiken in* 智拳印)

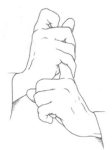

ILL. 86 – MUDRÂ OF THE WISDOM FIST

一　丁　歹　歹　列　列

ILL. 87 – STROKE SEQUENCE FOR RETSU

Hand Position: The four fingers of the left hand wrap around the extended index finger of the right hand. The four remaining fingers of the right hand form a fist. The tip of the left thumb touches the tip of the right index finger.

Esoteric Meaning: The unity of the two hands in *retsu* symbolizes perfection through the union of the God and the Goddess of the Diamond World and Womb World of Dainichi Nyorai. The mudrâ helps in the liberation from time and space. It strengthens the abilities of distant healing and orientation in the astral worlds. It is an outstanding means for the transmission of consciousness into other worlds, just like the light of *Dainichi Nyorai* shines everywhere.

在 *Zai* – The Sun-Wheel Mudrâ
(Jap.: *Nichi rin in* 日輪印)

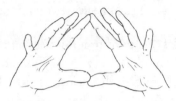

ILL. 88 – SUN-WHEEL MUDRÂ

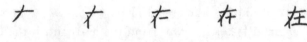

ILL. 89 – STROKE SEQUENCE FOR ZAI

Hand Position: The tips of the right and left index fingers, as well as those of the thumbs, are touching each other so that a circle is created that looks like the sun (Sun Wheel). The other fingers are extended to the side. They form the halo of the sun.

Esoteric Meaning: A triangle is created between the fingers when the hands form the mudrâ *zai*. The triangle, as it also appears in the Mandala of the Womb World, symbolizes the fire that destroys all impurities. At the same time, it is like a type of gateway and especially helpful in becoming one with other beings and things.

前 *Zen* – The Mudrâ of the Concealed Form
(Jap.: *Ongyô in* 隱形印)

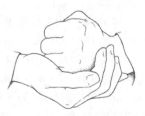

ILL. 90 – MUDRÂ OF THE CONCEALED FORM

241

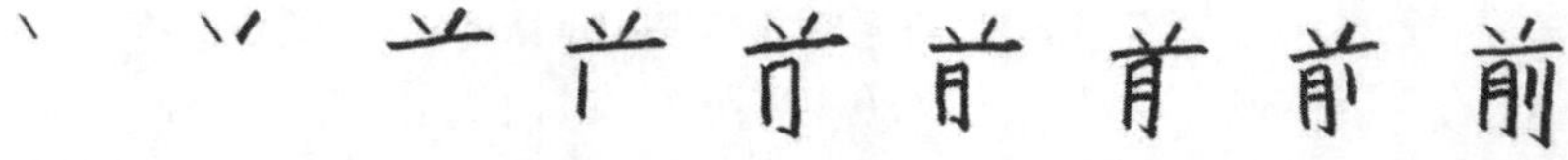

丶　丷　亠　广　䒑　䒑　𦣻　前　前

ILL. 91 – STROKE SEQUENCE FOR ZEN

Hand Position: The left hand forms a fist, leaving a hollow space inside. In this variation of the mudrâ *Ongyo,* the right hand is not held above the fist (cf. page 241) but protectively encloses it from below.

Esoteric Meaning: Zen offers the necessary protection in every accustomed or even a foreign environment by making us invisible and inviolable to the disturbing influences.

Assume the Mudrâ of the Sword Hand (*Shutô in*). When we do this, the right hand forms the sword and the left hand is the chain of the Imperturbable Wisdom King *Fudô Myôô*. Here is how to do it: Extend the index and middle fingers of the right hand (sword) upward. Bend the little finger and ring finger. Touch the fingernails of the two fingers with the tip of the thumb. Do the same with the left hand (chain). Stick the fingertips of the extended index and middle fingers of the right hand from below into the hole between the thumb, ring finger, and little finger of the left hand.

Visualize a lotus blossom in front of you, upon which a standing moon disk rests. With your inner eye, draw the symbol *kanman* of *Fudô Myôô* on it.

To activate the symbols, recite three times the medium-long mantra of *Fudô Myôô*: *Namaku samanda basara nan senda makaroshana sowataya untarata kanman.*

Now pull the lotus blossom, moon disk, and symbol into your chest and visualize them there. A red-golden light emanates from the symbol until it completely fills your body.

Now pull the right hand (the sword) out of the left hand and move the left hand, without undoing the mudrâ, to your hip. As shown in the graphic, use the right hand to cut five horizontal and four vertical lines in the air. With each cut, sound the Nine Symbols *Rin – byô – tô – sha – kai – jin – retsu – zai – zen* (臨兵闘者皆陣列在前) like a *Kiai* and visualize your sword hand as if it was a real blade that has light radiating from it and cuts through every disturbing influence.

Move your right sword hand back into the left chain hand like it was before so that the initial mudrâ is created. Now the forms within you dissolve. Stay with this feeling for another moment and then take leave from the distant contact to **Fudô Myôô** *and* **Dai Marishi Ten** *by quietly saying or thinking: Dear* **Fudô Myôô** *and dear* **Dai Marishi Ten**, *I thank you for the beautiful meditation and ask permission to call on you again soon. I wish you the blessing and protection of the Creative Force on your path."*

Blow strongly between your hands and then rub them together in order to detach yourself from the contact.

If necessary, ground yourself for a while by giving yourself Reiki on the soles of your feet and then doing some physical exercises.

Practice 3: Worshipping the Sun God Nitten 日天

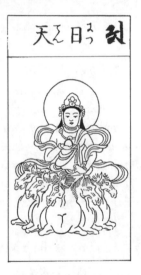

ILL. 92 – THE SUN GOD NITTEN

The Sun God *Nitten* was originally the Indian Sun God *Sûrya* and also has a close connection with *Dainichi Nyorai* and *Dai Marishi Ten* because of the similar *Siddham* symbol. With the exception of Japan, the Sun God *Nitten* very rarely appears in Buddhism. *Nitten* sits on a lotus disk on top of five or eight horses. In the Diamond World Mandala (*kongôkai*), *Nitten* sometimes rides a horse and holds a ball of the sun in front of his heart.

Assume the *Gasshô* mudrâ, breathe into your hara and bow three times in the direction of the East, where the sun rises. (An especially good time for this practice is at sunrise.)

*Connect with the Sun God Nitten through the distant contract. Greet him with the words: "Dear Sun God **Nitten**, I come to you as a sick person and request healing. I come to you as an ignorant person and request teaching. I come to you as someone who does not know the way and ask for protection and guidance. I come to you as someone who is helpless and ask you for power in order to better serve. As compensation, I send you Reiki. Please use it as you wish for the benefit of all." Then draw several CR symbols and activate each of them with the mantra for intensifying the Reiki flow of power.*

*

Reassume the *Gasshô* mudrâ and recite the mantra of the Sun God *Nitten* three times:

Om ajichi ya sowaka.

*

*Connect with **Dai Marishi Ten** through the distant contact. Greet her with the words: "Dear **Dai Marishi Ten**, I come to you as a sick person and request healing. I come to you as an ignorant person and request teaching. I come to you as someone who does not know the way and ask for protection and guidance. I come to you as someone who is helpless and ask you for power in order to better serve. As compensation, I send you Reiki. Please use it as you wish for the benefit of all." Then draw several CR symbols and activate each of them with the mantra for intensifying the Reiki flow of power.*

*

Return your hands to *Gasshô* and recite the mantra three times:

Om Sûtrasei sowaka.

Also recite the following mantra three times:

Namu kimyô chôrai, dainittenshi, amaterashi mashimasuhi no ongami, ido shujôko, fushô shitenge.

*

*Connect with **Dainichi Nyorai** through the distant contact. Greet him with the words: "Dear **Dainichi Nyorai**, I come to you as a sick person and request healing. I come to you as an ignorant person and request teaching. I come to you as someone who does not know the way and ask for protection and guidance. I come to you as someone who is helpless and ask you for power in order to better serve. As compensation, I send you Reiki. Please use it as you wish for the benefit of all." Then draw several CR symbols and activate each of them with the mantra for intensifying the Reiki flow of power.*

*

Now assume the Mudrâ of the Hands Folded to the Outside (*Gebaku in*) and recite the first short mantra of Dainichi Nyorai for the "Destruction of the Seven Difficulties" three times:

Om abira unken

Now assume the Mudrâ of the Hands Folded to the Inside (*Naibaku in*) and intone the first short mantra of *Dainichi Nyorai* for "Reviving the Seven States of Happiness" three times:

Om bazara dadoban

Now assume the mudrâ *Kongô Gasshô* by placing the palms of the hands together and slightly crossing the fingertips.

Visualize the Great Sun Buddha *Dainichi Nyorai* in front of you, as well as the Sun God *Nittenshi* and the Goddess of Light *Dai Marishi Ten* to the right and left of him or their *Siddham* symbols at the same time on lotus blossoms and moon disks.

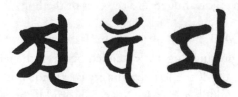

ILL. 93 – SIDDHAM A FOR NITTENSHI – SIDDHAM VAM FOR DAINICHI
NYORAI – SIDDHAM MA FOR DAI MARISHI TEN

Recite the following mantra three times:

Om ajichi ya marishiei sowaka

Now draw the first of the Nine Symbols with the palm of your hand in the air. Assume the appropriate mudrâ and recite the appropriate mantra with it one time by saying it with *ki*. Go through all of the Nine Symbols, mantras, and mudrâs in this way.

臨 *Rin* – The Mudrâ of the Old Loneliness (Jap.: *Toko in* 獨古印)

The index fingers and thumbs of the right and left hand are extended so that the fingertips touch each other. The other fingers form rings that fit into each other.

兵 *Byô* – The Mudrâ of the Great Vajra Wheel
(Jap.: *Daikongôrin in* 大金剛輪印)

The little fingers and the ring fingers are wrapped around each other. The index fingers and thumbs are positioned so that the fingertips of both hands touch. The middle fingers are placed across the back of the index fingers and touch each other at the fingertips.

闘 *Tô* – The Mudrâ of the Outer Lion (Jap.: *Gejiji in* 外獅子印)

The right index finger is extended between the middle and ring finger of the left hand. The left index finger is extended in the same way between the middle and ring finger of the right hand. The middle fingers are placed in the opening between the ring and index finger so that they wrap around the index finger. The fingertips point downward and touch each other at the fingernails. The ring fingers and the little fingers are extended and placed together. The distance between the little fingers and the ring fingers should remain open a little. This is the mouth. The thumbs are the ears and the tips of the index fingers are the eyes of the lion.

者 *Sha* – The Mudrâ of the Inner Lion (Jap.: *Naijiji in* 内獅子印)

The tip of the right ring finger is extended between the left middle and index finger. The tip of the left ring finger is extended in the same way between the right middle and index finger. The middle fingers of the right and left hand wrap around the ring fingers so that the fingertips point downward. The thumbs, little fingers, and index fingers are extended and placed together. The little fingers form the ears. The distance between the thumbs and index fingers are the mouth. The tips of the ring fingers are the eyes of the lion.

246

皆 *Kai* – **The Mudrâ Wrung to the Outside**
(Jap.: *Gebaku in* 外縛印)

The fingers of both hands are folded.

陳 *Jin* – **The Mudrâ Wrung to the Inside** (Jap.: *Naibaku in* 内縛印)

The ten fingers of the right and left hand are interlaced with each other toward the inside.

列 *Retsu* – **The Mudrâ of the Wisdom Fist** (Jap.: *Chiken in* 智拳印)

The four fingers of the left hand wrapped around the extended index finger of the right hand. The four remaining fingers of the right hand form a fist. The tip of the left thumb touches the tip of the right index finger.

在 *Zai* – **The Sun-Wheel Mudrâ** (Jap.: *Nichi rin in* 日輪印)

The tips of the right and left index fingers, as well as those of the thumbs, are touching each other so that a circle is created that looks like the sun (sun-wheel). The other fingers are extended to the side. They form the halo of the sun.

前 *Zen* – **The Mudrâ of the Concealed Form**
(Jap.: *Ongyô in* 隱形印)

The left hand forms a fist, leaving a hollow space inside. The right hand protectively covers the left fist.

Assume the Mudrâ of the Sword Hand (*Shutô in*). When we do this, the right hand forms the sword and the left hand is the chain of the Imperturbable Wisdom King *Fudô Myôô*. Here is how this is done: Extend the index and middle fingers of the right hand (sword) upward. Bend the little finger and ring finger. Touch the fingernails of the two fingers with the tip of the thumb. Do the same with the left hand (chain). Stick the fingertips of the extended index and middle fingers of the right hand from below into the hole between the thumb, ring finger, and little finger of the left hand.

Visualize a lotus blossom in front of you, upon which a standing moon disk rests. With your inner eye, draw the symbol *kanman* of *Fudô Myôô* on it.

To activate the symbols, recite three times the medium-long mantra of *Fudô Myôô*: *Namaku samanda basara nan senda makaroshana sowataya untarata kanman*.

Now pull the lotus blossom, moon disk, and symbol into your chest and visualize them there. A red-golden light emanates from the symbol until it completely fills your body. Then pull the right hand (the sword) out of the left and move the left hand, without undoing the mudrâ, to your hip. As shown in the graphic, use the right hand to cut five horizontal and four vertical lines in the air. With each cut, sound the Nine Symbols *Rin – byô – tô – sha – kai – jin – retsu – zai – zen* (臨兵鬪者皆陣列在前) like a *Kiai* and visualize your sword hand as if it was a real blade that has light radiating from it and cuts through every disturbing influence.

Move your right sword hand back into the left chain hand like it was before so that the initial mudrâ is created. Now place both hands into *Gasshô* and recite the following mantra one time:

Goji mukô, aimin nauju

*

Take leave from the distant contact to all the light beings individually by quietly saying or thinking: "I thank you for the beautiful meditation and ask permission to call on you again soon. I wish you the blessing and protection of the Creative Force on your path." Blow strongly between your hands and then rub them together to detach yourself from the contact.

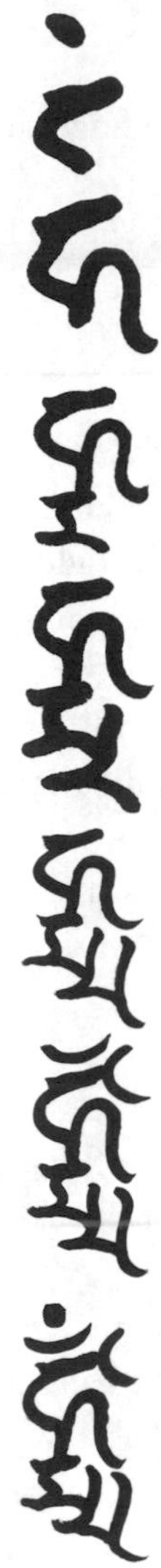

ILL. 94 –
STROKE
SEQUENCE FOR
THE SIDDHAM
KANMAN

CHAPTER 12

Dainichi Nyorai Kidô

In the second half of the 1990s, my research led me (Walter) through the origins of Reiki to the transcendental Buddha *Dainichi Nyorai*. The more I learned about him, the more impressed I was. The desire grew within me to learn directly from him. Since there are a variety of possibilities in Rainbow Reiki for establishing a connection with a light being, this was actually not difficult. The first contacts with *Dainichi Nyorai* already changed my entire view of Reiki—I began to have a premonition of the immense dimensions of this spiritual art of healing that extended far beyond everything I knew about Reiki at this time. *Dainichi Nyorai* was very friendly. He generously taught me how his powers can be used for healing and personality development. I also began to remember many things because I had already frequently worked with him, as I soon recognized.

As soon as I became confident enough through my personal experience, I began to pass on simple blessings and practices that he had taught me to my students. Knowledge must flow in order to be useful. At the beginning of the new millennium, I started to also transmit the more profound teachings to my students under the title of *Dainichi Nyorai Kidô* in the form of special seminars. The deep spiritual experiences that people had with the practices encouraged me to expand this area of Rainbow Reiki.

As a result of my cooperation with Mark, many more exciting details of *Dainichi Nyorai*'s teaching came to light. *Dainichi Nyorai Kidô* is now an integral component of Rainbow Reiki, which is taught up to the Teacher Degree and is quickly finding increasingly more friends throughout the world.

The central practices and teachings of *Dainichi Nyorai Kidô* are being imparted for the first time in this book. Anyone trained in Reiki can perform them without the additional initiations that are required for many other methods.

I would first like to introduce the *Mahâ Mudrâ* practice that is one of the foundations of *Dainichi Nyorai Kidô*.

Dainichi Nyorai and Mahâ Mudrâ, the Great Light

Dainichi Nyorai, the Transcendental Buddha, is also known in India as *Buddha Vairocana.* (Be careful when looking for sources! There are two different deities who have this name.)

He is the spiritual sun, the Great Light. The Great Light symbolizes the state of non-duality (*Sat-Chit-Ânanda*). In Japan, he has been equated for many centuries with the Sun Goddess (Shintô) *Amaterasu O Kami.*

Dainichi Nyorai unites all the elements of the universe within himself.

He resonates profoundly with the Reiki Master Symbol.

He is the source of all types of power flowing from Reiki.

If you have the proper inner attitude (this is imparted by *Sei Heki* in the Reiki System), which is attained through the technique explained below and an understanding of the spiritual philosophy, as well as the appropriate action, the result will be *Kaji.* This is a spiritual flow of power (this is imparted by *Choku Rei* in the Reiki System) from *Dainichi Nyorai* and the rest of the world to you. This awakens the Buddha within you (this is imparted through the Master Symbol in the Reiki System).

The Mahâ Mudrâ Practice

This practice supports the experience of the unity of individual consciousness with the cosmic consciousness of the One.

1. Sit with extended legs on the floor. Place the right foot with its sole on the left lower leg.

2. Inhale deeply. When exhaling, move the forehead as far as possible in the direction of the knees.

3. Move the hands forward next to the feet.

4. Relax, contract the anal sphincter, inhale deeply and lower the chin to the chest.

5. Remain in this position until it becomes unpleasant, continuing to hold the breath.

6. Repeat the practice on the other side.

7. The practice cycle should include nine times on each side.

Additional Practices from Dainichi Nyorai Kidô

It is useful to perform the following practices in the order listed here since they are technically based upon each other on the one hand and develop mental and spiritual abilities on the other hand that are preconditions for the subsequent practices. Do each of the practices until you feel confident about them.

Practice 1: Meditation on the Goddess Dai Marishi Ten

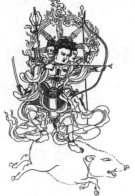

ILL. 95 – DAI MARISHI TEN

*Establish a connection with the Goddess **Dai Marishi Ten** through the distant contact. Greet her with the words: "Dear Goddess **Dai Marishi Ten**, I come to you as a sick person and request healing. I come to you as an ignorant person and request teaching. I come to you as someone who does not know the way and ask for protection and guidance. I come to you as someone who is help-less and ask you for power in order to better serve. As compensation, I send you Reiki. Please use it as you wish for the benefit of all." Then draw several CR symbols and activate each of them with the mantra for intensifying the Reiki flow of power.*

*

Assume the mudrâ *Ongyô in* (Mudrâ of the Great Goddess Dai Marishi Ten).

251

Visualize yourself as *Dai Marishi Ten* in a red color and as brilliant as a ruby with three faces, three eyes, and six arms. In your hands you hold a *Vajra* and an *Ashoka* branch, bow and arrow, as well as a needle and a noose. Imagine that your red body is empty on the inside. You are gradually becoming larger and larger. From your normal size, you expand to that of a house, a mountain, the earth, and finally, the universe. Keep your attention there. Then reduce yourself to the size of a sesame seed. However, the figure of *Dai Marishi Ten* should still be fully visible. Keep your attention on it.

While you alternate between large and small, recite the mantra: *Om ajiteiya Dai Marishi Ten* 108 times or a multiple thereof.

*

Take leave from the distant contact in your usual way.

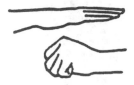

ILL. 96 – ONGYÔ IN

Practice 2: Meditation on the Energy Column of the Great Goddess Dai Marishi Ten

Establish a connection with the Great Goddess **Dai Marishi Ten** *through the distant contact. Greet her with the words: "Dear Great Goddess* **Dai Marishi Ten,** *I come to you as a sick person and request healing. I come to you as an ignorant person and request teaching. I come to you as someone who does not know the way and ask for protection and guidance. I come to you as someone who is helpless and ask you for power in order to better serve. As compensation, I send you Reiki. Please use it as you wish for the benefit of all." Then draw several CR symbols and activate each of them with the mantra for intensifying the Reiki flow of power.*

*

Assume the mudrâ *Ongyô in.*

Visualize your body as *Dai Marishi Ten* in the size of your own body and look at yourself from the outside by leaving yourself through the Crown Chakra. At the center of your hollow body you now see a red luminous energy column[79] that is also hollow.

Enlarge this energy column from the height of a high-rise to that of a mountain and then into expand it into the universe. In addition, extend it into the tips of fingers and feet. Let it reduce in size again until it looks as thin as a hair. At the end, visualize everything as empty.

Take leave from the distant contact in your usual way.

Practice 3:
Protective Meditation with Dainichi Nyorai and Fudô Myôô

*Establish a connection with the Great Sun Buddha **Dainichi Nyorai** through the distant contact. Greet him with the words: "Dear **Dainichi Nyorai**, I come to you as a sick person and request healing. I come to you as an ignorant person and request teaching. I come to you as someone who does not know the way and ask for protection and guidance. I come to you as someone who is help-less and ask you for power in order to better serve. As compensation, I send you Reiki. Please use it as you wish for the benefit of all." Then draw several CR symbols and activate each of them with the mantra for intensifying the Reiki flow of power.*

*Also connect with the Wisdom King **Fudô Myôô** through the distant contact. Greet him with the words: "Dear Wisdom King **Fudô Myôô**, I come to you as a sick person and request healing. I come to you as an ignorant person and request teaching. I come to you as someone who does not know the way and ask for protection and guidance. I come to you as someone who is helpless and ask you for power in order to better serve. As compensation, I send you Reiki. Please use it as you wish for the benefit of all." Then draw several CR symbols and activate each of them with the mantra for intensifying the Reiki flow of power.*

*

[79] Skr.: *Sushumnâ nâdi* = Rising energy channel through the center of the spinal column.

Assume the mudrâ *Dainichi Nyorai Ken in* (Mudrâ of the Pagoda).

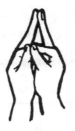

ILL. 97 – DAINICHI NYORAI KEN IN

Fill your lungs completely with air by first inhaling deep into your Hara. Contract the diaphragm and hold this state as long as possible. Then exhale completely (at least three times).

While exhaling, visualize that light is emanating from all of your pores. During the first seven breaths, the light is black (wind). During the next seven breaths, it is blue-green (emptiness), followed by red (fire), white (water), and yellow (earth). These lights radiate out into the whole world and illuminate every place. When you inhale, the rays come back again through the pores and fill up the body (7 times).

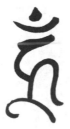

ILL. 98 – SIDDHAM HÛM

Visualize that the rays are now coming out of the pores in the five colors as the *Siddham hûm*. They also fill up the entire world and every place. When you inhale, they return to you again and fill up the entire body (7 times).

Now the *hûm* syllables are transformed into the fierce-looking light being *Fudô Myôô*.

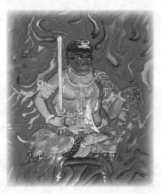

ILL. 99 – FUDÔ MYÔÔ

They have one face and two arms. In the right hand, they hold a *Vajra* sword and a lasso in the left hand. All of them have a fierce expression and are in the five colors, yet they are not larger than a sesame seed. When you exhale, they fill the world. When you inhale, they fill your body (7 times).

Now visualize a wrathful light being in each pore. All of them are looking out from the pores and form a type of protective cloak.

*

Take leave from both distant contacts in your usual way.

Practice 4: Opening the Energy Channels for Letting the Ki Flow in a Controlled Way

*Establish the connection with the Goddess **Dai Marishi Ten** through the distant contact. Greet her with the words: "Dear Goddess **Dai Marishi Ten**, I come to you as a sick person and request healing. I come to you as an ignorant person and request teaching. I come to you as someone who does not know the way and ask for protection and guidance. I come to you as someone who is helpless and ask you for power in order to better serve. As compensation, I send you Reiki. Please use it as you wish for the benefit of all." Then draw several CR symbols and activate each of them with the mantra for intensifying the Reiki flow of power.*

*

255

Assume the Mudrâ *Ongyô in*.

Visualize yourself as *Dai Marishi Ten*, as described in Practice 1.

Visualize one energy column each to the right and left of the central energy column[80]. They begin at the tip of the nose, travel over the brain, and then down the back to the perineum.

Visualize these energy columns as hollow channels. In the left one, the *Siddham a*[81] appears. In the right one, the Siddham *ka*[82] appears.

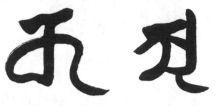

ILL. 100 – SIDDHAM KA AND A

Visualize the outlines of the *Siddham*[83] as fine as a hair in a red color. While exhaling, leave your Crown Chakra with one *Siddham* after the other and return again while inhaling. Once you have mastered the visualization of the individual *Siddham*, concentrate on the series of the *Siddham*. They form a chain like a *Mâlâ* and light up one after the other like a fairy fire.

This practice opens the energy channels so that the *ki* can flow through them in a controlled way.

*

[80] The right energy column is called *Pingalâ nâdi* and the left is *Idâ-nâdi* in Sanskrit.

[81] When an advanced level is reached, the *Siddham* symbols *a, â, i, î, u, û, ri, rî, li, lî, e, eî, o, oû, ang* and *å* are added.

[82] When an advanced level is reached, the *Siddham* symbols *kha, ga, gha, nga, cha, chha, ja, jha, nya, ta, tha, da, dha, na (hard sounds); ta, tha, da, dha, na (soft sounds), pa, pha, ba, bha, ma; ya, ra, la, va; sha, ksha, sa, ha* and *kshya* are added.

[83] According to the Hindu tradition, the *Siddham* sounds and syllables of Brahma, the Creator, were given to Ganesha, the God of Learning, and Ganesha passed them on to human beings. When pronounced and written correctly, these words that have been transmitted by the gods have direct psychic influences like "gift waves" of loving-kindness. Adding up all of the *Siddham* results in the number 50, which is symbolized by 50 skulls of the Great Shakti, the divine mother *Vajra-Yogini*.

Take leave from the distant contact in the usual way.

Practice 5: Yabyum Meditation

Establish the connection with the Great Sun Buddha **Dainichi Nyorai** *through the distant contact. Also establish the connection with* **Kongôsatta** *through the distant contact.*[84] *Greet both of them with the words: "Dear* **Dainichi Nyorai** *and* **Kongôsatta,** *I come to you as a sick person and request healing. I come to you as an ignorant person and request teaching. I come to you as someone who does not know the way and ask for protection and guidance. I come to you as someone who is helpless and ask you for power in order to better serve. As compensation, I send you Reiki. Please use it as you wish for the benefit of all." Then draw several CR symbols and activate each of them with the mantra for intensifying the Reiki flow of power.*

*

Assume the mudrâ *Chiken in* (Mudrâ of Spiritual Wisdom).

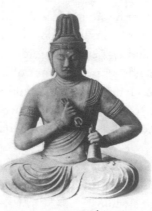

ILL. 101 – KONGÔSATTA

---

[84] *Vajra Dhara* (Tib. *Dorje Chang*) is a special form of *Vajrasattva* (Tib. *Dorje Sempa*, Jap. *Kongô Satta*). He represents the Tantric aspect of *Vairocana* in the *Yabyum* position. They are the Buddhist equivalent of Brahmâ (Jap. *Bonten*). In Japan, he usually rides a white elephant.

257

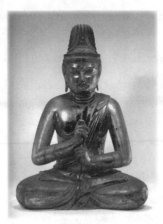

ILL. 102 – DAINICHI NYORAI WITH THE MUDRA CHIKEN IN

Visualize *Dainichi Nyorai* in your Heart Chakra. He sits in a lotus posi-tion and wears a crown. His hands are held in the mudrâ *Chiken in*. His body glows in a golden light.

Kongôsatta floats above his head. He is also adorned with a crown and is a luminous blue color as he sits in the lotus position. His Shakti sits on his lap with her arms and legs embracing him. As he embraces Shakti, *Kongôsatta* holds his hands crossed in front of his Heart Chakra. In his left hand, he holds a *Vajra* bell and a *Vajra* in the right hand.

Alternately devote your attention to the two of them.

As you do this, recite the mantra *Om abira unken* 108 times or a multiple of it.

Dainichi Nyorai and *Kongôsatta* now merge with each other and dis-solve in light, which is now distributed throughout your entire body. Remain in this state for a while.

*

Take leave of the distant contact in the usual way.

Practice 6: Dai Marishi Ten Goddesses Meditation for Awakening the Inner Fire

The proper posture: Sit upright with a straight spinal column and imagine that your spinal column consists of coins stacked on top of each other. While inhaling, press the diaphragm as far forward as possible. Lower the chin in the direction of the chest and place your tongue on your palate. Assume the Mudrâ of Meditation (*Zemui in*). Place your hands beneath the navel on the thighs. Always look in the same direction and concentrate on your mind.

Calm Breathing: Move your head slowly from right to left while inhaling and from left to right while exhaling (3 times). Slowly breathe in and out (3 times) while looking to the front. Repeat the total of six breaths to the sides and to the front more strongly. Breathe slowly up to this point. Do the same thing one more time, but more intensely. And once again, even more intensely for a total of nine times.

Making Contact and Visualization: Establish a connection with the Goddess *Dai Marishi Ten* through the distant contact. Greet her with the words: "Dear Goddess *Dai Marishi Ten*, I come to you as a sick person and request healing. I come to you as an ignorant person and request teaching. I come to you as someone who does not know the way and ask for protection and guidance. I come to you as someone who is helpless and ask you for power in order to better serve. As compensation, I send you Reiki. Please use it as you wish for the benefit of all." Then draw several CR symbols and activate each of them with the mantra for intensifying the Reiki flow of power.

Assume the mudrâ *Ongyô in* (Mudrâ of the Great Goddess *Dai Marishi Ten*). Visualize yourself as *Dai Marishi Ten* in a red color and empty on the inside.

Perception of the Energy System through Visualization: Meditate on the first four major chakras. Visualize the chakras like round flowers in the hollow inside. They now all have the color red, which represents the delights of life here. Each chakra is translucent and brilliant. Positioned on top of each other, they symbolize the trunk of the Tree of Life. The trunk extends from the Root Chakra to the Crown Chakra. To the right and left of it run additional energy channels. They begin at the First Chakra, run across the back to above the brain, and end at the face at the level of the nose. Many more energy channels radiate from the individual chakras.

Awakening Dai Marishi Ten's Secret Power: In your Hara, create the *Siddham a* with lines as thin as a hair, floating, and about as high as half a finger. It is reddish brown and burning hot. From the syllable *a*, the seething sound of *phem* is heard rings out. *Phem* is like the crackling of a burning candlewick.

The syllable *ham* in a white color now appears in the Crown Chakra. The syllable *ham* looks like sweet nectar wants to drip from it. While inhaling, imagine how the life energy penetrates into you through the crown into the middle, right, and left energy column. The life energy immediately shoots downward and meets the syllable *a* in the Hara. Touched by the life energy, the syllable *a* lights up even redder, just like blowing on coal makes it glow. Every time you inhale, the life energy is drawn in through the energy channels, upon which the chakras are located. During exhalation, it is distributed throughout the entire body.

As soon as you can do this without too much effort, continue on to the next step. Otherwise, end the practice by taking leave from the distant contact in your usual way.

ILL. 103 – SIDDHAM A

Visualize how a little flame in the length of half a finger is flickering upward from the syllable *a*. The flame is vertical, translucent and luminous, red, and empty. At the same time, the flame looks like a turning spiral.

With every breath, the flame now grows a little bit upward. With the eighth breath, the flame reaches the Second Chakra. With ten more breaths, all of the lotus petals of the Second Chakra are filled with the flame. With the next ten breaths, the entire lower body fills with flames down to the tips of the toes. During the following ten breaths, the body fills with the flames up to the height of the Fourth Chakra. With the next ten breaths, the flames rise up in the body into the Fifth Chakra. With the next ten breaths, the flames finally reach the Crown Chakra.

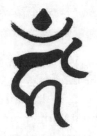

ILL. 104 – SIDDHAM HAM

With the next ten breaths, the syllable *ham* melts into the Crown Chakra and transforms into the moon energy (the power of the Goddess) that completely fills up the Crown Chakra.

With the next ten breaths, the moon energy now fills up the Fifth Chakra. With the next ten breaths, it fills the Fourth Chakra. With the next ten, it fills the Third Chakra. With the next ten, it fills the Second Chakra and with the next ten, the First Chakra. And with the next ten breaths, the moon energy now fills the entire body down to the fingertips and tips of the toes.

Remain a while in the state of the flames.

End the meditation by taking leave of *Dai Marishi Ten* is your usual way.

Note: For done on a daily and regular basis, the number of breaths can gradually be decreased since the volume of the lungs expands over time.

Benefit: Increases physical and mental vitality; supports the perception of subtle energies, reduces sensations of coldness in individual body parts, and awakens the inner fires.

Practice 7: Gasshô Flame Meditation

*Establish a connection with the Goddess **Dai Marishi Ten** through the distant contact. Greet her with the words: "Dear Goddess **Dai Marishi Ten,** I come to you as a sick person and request healing. I come to you as an ignorant person and request teaching. I come to you as someone who does not know the way* *and ask for protection and guidance. I come to you as someone who is help-less and ask you for power in order to better serve. As compensation, I send you Reiki. Please use it as you wish for the benefit of all."* Then draw several CR symbols and activate each of them with the mantra for intensifying the Reiki flow of power.

*

Assume the mudrâ *Ongyô in*. Visualize yourself as *Dai Marishi Ten* in a red color and hollow, with the three energy columns, the chakras, and the syllable *a* in the Second Chakra, as described in the previous practice.

Now visualize a radiant sun in the Hara and the Hand Chakras and Foot Chakras. Sit on the floor, draw up the legs so that you can place the feet together—which is practically doing *Gasshô* with the feet. Place your palms in *Gasshô* in front of your heart.[85] By rubbing the hands and feet, flames raise up from the sun that touch the sun in the Hara. From there, another flame rises upward and meets the syllable *a*. From the syllable *a*, the fire spreads throughout the entire body. Then a bright light radiates from the body in all directions, as if the body was a big sun. The entire world is filled by this light. In closing, perform the *Mahâ-Mudrâ* physical practice of *Dainichi Nyorai Kidô* for 21 times. Sit with extended legs on the floor. Place the right foot with its sole on the left lower leg. Inhale deeply. When exhaling, move the forehead as far as possible in the direction of the knees. Place the hands forward next to the feet. Relax, contract the anal sphincter, inhale deeply, and lower the chin to the chest. Remain in this position until it becomes unpleasant, while continuing to hold the breath. Repeat the exercise on the other side.

*

*Conclude the meditation by taking leave of **Dai Marishi Ten** in your usual way.*

---

[85] This meditation position corresponds with the Rainbow Reiki *Gasshô* Medi-tation as it is described in detail in *The Complete Reiki Handbook* by Walter Lübeck, Lotus Press. See pages 131-139.

Practice 8: "Flame and Drop" Meditation

*Establish the connection with the Imperturbable Buddha **Ashuku Nyorai** through the distant contact. Greet him with the words: "Dear **Ashuku Nyorai**, I come to you as a sick person and request healing. I come to you as an ignorant person and request teaching. I come to you as someone who does not know the way and ask for protection and guidance. I come to you as someone who is helpless and ask you for power in order to better serve. As compensation, I send you Reiki. Please use it as you wish for the benefit of all." Then draw several CR symbols and activate each of them with the mantra for intensifying the Reiki flow of power*

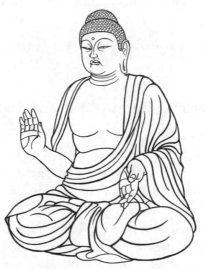

ILL. 105 – ASHUKU NYORAI

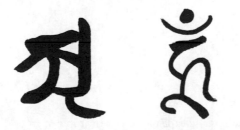

ILL. 106 – THE SIDDHAM SYMBOLS A AND HÛM

263

Visualize yourself as *Ashuku Nyorai* in a masculine form and a sky-blue color. Your body contains the three energy columns and chakras. The syllable *a* is in the Hara and the syllable *hûm* is in the Crown Chakra. With a crackling, a flame quickly slips downward. This stirs the fire and reaches the Second Chakra. Because of the rising heat, the syllable *hûm* now begins to melt. Hot drops fall down from the *hûm*. Wherever they touch the flames, these become even stronger and climb up along the chakras to the Fifth Chakra. Finally, the last bit of the melted *hûm* drips into the flames of the Fifth Chakra. Stay for a while in this state. From here, the melted *hûm* glides into the Heart Chakra. Also stay in this state for a while. This also continues on to the Third, Second, and First Chakra.

*

Conclude the meditation by taking leave of Ashuku in your usual way.

Grounding Exercise After Each Meditation

In closing, do the following physical exercise after the meditation: Place your the hands on your knees and swing your hip from right to left. Remain in the same position and circle your head, then move it forward and backward. Now kneel down. The hands remain on your knees. From there, move your upper body from side to side. If you are sitting on the floor, support yourself with your hands behind you and shake your legs in the air. Lift up the legs and move the upper body from side to side. Exhale powerfully and rub or massage your entire body.[86]

---

[86] Further suggestions and explanations on the topic of grounding can be found in the chapter on the meaningful integration of spiritual experiences

CHAPTER 13

Mount Kurama

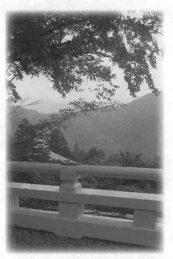

ILL. 107 – THE VIEW FROM MOUNT KURAMA

After Dr. Usui had attempted for a long time to discover the meaning and applications of the symbols that he had found in the old texts, he spent three weeks on Mount Kurama in order to meditate there. This mountain, which is about 1870 feet high, lies in the north of the Kyoto Prefecture, about 12 kilometers from the palace of the Tennô in the city of Kyoto. Today it is possible to go to the base of Kurama by the train. From there, it is a leisurely walk up the mountain itself. However, in Dr. Usui's day it was anything but easy to get there. There are many mountains in Japan, including many sacred mountains that Dr. Usui could have climbed. So why exactly did he choose the very remote Mount Kurama?

In the *Sarashina Nikki*, a diary from the early 11th Century, it says: "Kurama is so overgrown that even if you decide to go there on a pilgrimage, you will not set off because of your fear." Since time immemorial, Mount Kurama had the reputation of teeming with nasty demons that terrorize the approaching visitors. In addition to the demons, there are still other obstacles that should not be underestimated. However, if you

265

do not speak Japanese, you will not have to worry about them. As you may know: Ignorance is bliss. To be precise, there are signs in the Japanese language on the path to the top that urgently warn against going deeper into the forest—unless you would like to become more closely acquainted with one or more Japanese bears. About once a year, there is a newspaper article on how someone wanted to feed honey to the bears. In such cases, it is not rare for the bear to be so enthusiastic that it also polishes off an arm or some other limb of the honey-provider. Incidentally, anyone fleeing from a bear should be careful not to step on a *Mamushi*. This is a poisonous Japanese snake with a very pretty yellow-black pattern. Anyone who gets bitten by such a snake does not have much time left to go to Kyoto and be written up in the newspaper. If, despite all of this, you still feel the desire to climb Mount Kurama, then just let me (Mark) know. I would be happy to guide you there—and naturally, back again as well. Since I spent some weeks of my life in the Japanese forests, I know my way around there quite well.

In terms of nature, Mount Kurama is forested. The air is very pure and refreshing. In the town at the foot of the mountain, there is also a hot spring by the name of *Kurama Onsen*. I highly recommend a detour there in either the summer or the winter. Since this is a so-called *Rotenburo*, a hot spring in the open, there is a wonderful view of Mount Kuruma while century-old cedars surround you. If you are not accustomed to boiling water, it is best to avoid the volcanic spring that has hot water rising from deep inside Mother Earth. The temperature can vary greatly as a result. In order to cool off later, you can also jump into a waterfall on the way to the temple. There is a spot to meditate under the waterfall. This is also one of the places where Dr. Usui meditated.

The Kurama Temple

In addition to the minor obstacles and the enchanting natural surroundings, Mount Kurama is known in Japanese history and literature as a very sacred mountain where more than one person had an enlightening experience (Jap: *Satori*).

The monk *Kantei*, the best student of *Ganjin*, was led to Mount Kurama in the year 770 A.D. by a white horse. Like Dr. Usui, he had a vision during which he received a transmission of spiritual energy from *Maôson* and was enlightened by *Bishamonten*. This was the reason for him to establish a temple on Mount Kurama.

A few years later, in the year 796, the head representative for the building of the *Tôji* Temple, *Fujiwara Isendo* (759-827), had a similar experience on Mount Kurama with the 1000-Armed Goddess *Senju Kannon*. As a result, he added some buildings and a pagoda to the temple. It is quite probable that Dr. Usui knew of this and selected Mount Kurama for his plans because of this.

As a result of the mystical experiences had by some people in the Eighth Century, *Maôson, Bishamonten,* and *Senju Kannon* are the light beings who are worshipped in the *Kuramadera* Temple as a trinity by the name of *Sonten*. They symbolically represent the soul inhabiting the universe, the glorious light, and the activity of the mind. In simple terms, this is power, light, and love.

Throughout the centuries, the temple has served to protect the capital city of *Heian kyô* (today: Kyoto) from the north. The temple lies half way up to the summit. The original structure was destroyed by a fire in 1126. In the following year, sculptures of the gods *Bishamonten* and *Kichijôten* were created and these are still intact. In 1133, the temple was repaired and newly consecrated by order of the resigned *Gotoba Tennô*. In the year 1236, the temple burned down again. However, it was possible to rebuild it by 1248. From then on, the temple remained intact up into the 20ᵗʰ Century. At the annual fire festival (*Hi matsuri*) in the year 1945, some sparks from a big torch (a torch is so large that it must be carried by several people) fell onto the old building and it burned to the ground as a result. The current main hall was built in 1971. This means that Dr. Usui experienced a completely different temple structure in 1922 than present-day visitors. Accordingly, the energy of the building is also not as strong as it probably was at that time. But Mount Kurama has obviously remained a power place. Anyone who goes there can experience the mystical presence of this power place.

In the course of the centuries, the Buddhist School of the temple changed a number of times. When the temple was founded in the year 770, Esoteric Buddhism did not yet officially exist in Japan and so there was no School of Esoteric Buddhism. Since the founder *Kantei* was one of *Ganjin's* best students, it is likely that the first Buddhist School of the *Kurama* Temple dates back to him. It was probably the *Ritsu* School of *Mahâyâna* Buddhism. Between 889 and 1113, the temple belonged to the *Shingon* School that was established by the monk *Kûkai*. From then on, the temple reportedly belonged to the *Tendai* School. Both schools belong to Esoteric Buddhism in Japan. Two years after the big fire, the *Kurama Kôkyô* School was founded. It took over the temple in 1949 and consecrated it as its main temple.

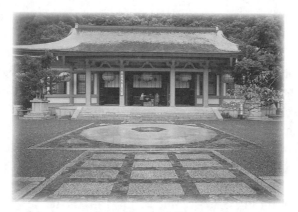

ILL. 108 – MAIN HALL OF THE KURAMA TEMPLE

The Kurama Kôkyô School

The *Kurama Kôkyô* School was established in the year 1947 as a branch of the esoteric *Tendai* School especially on the basis of the enlightening experiences of many pilgrims from legends, history, and the present. One of these pilgrims was Dr. Usui.

The teaching of the *Kurama Kôkyô* School says that the arduous climb up Mount Kurama is like the striving for enlightenment. Enlightenment can also mean achieving a goal through the help of the light beings. Enlightenment can be attained precisely there on the mountain. However, the descent is like a Bodhisattva who comes down into the world to help all sentient beings. This is because heaven, earth, and beings in between are emanations of the Great Sun Buddha *Dainichi Nyorai*, who preaches all of the sutras and from whom the spiritual life energy of Reiki comes.[87] Does this remind us of Dr. Usui? While searching for the solution to the mystery, he climbed Mount Kurama, attained enlightenment after a three-week meditation, and returned to bring the whole world much good. Seen in this way, anyone who practices Reiki is also on the path of the Bodhisattva in a certain sense because they all begin with Dr. Usui or *Dainichi Nyorai* and make a contribution toward the dawning of a new Golden Age on earth as soon as possible.

The energy that awakens every living being to life comes from the three light beings of the *Kurama* Temple. They are the 1000-armed *Senju Kannon, Bishamonten,* and *Maôson.* The three light beings are called *Sonten* as a trinity. It is important for each of us to find this trinity within ourselves. They are love, light, and the life force. In order to achieve them, there are three life principles that are called *Shinkô no sankajô.* They remind us of Dr. Usui's life principles.

1. It is necessary to work on ourselves and our karma by avoiding bad deeds and malicious gossip. Therefore, in order to actualize a modest self, we should be kind to our fellow human beings and work on ourselves and our own karma.

2. We should strive to be someone who walks through the world with a pure heart.

3. We should receive the noble power of the three light beings *Sonten* and develop a strong belief.

The three light beings *Sonten* express love, light, and the life force. The love is represented by the 1000-armed *Senju Kannon.* She is also seen as the light being of the moon. Her symbol is the SHK. *Bishamonten,* who carries the light with his pagoda of *Dainichi Nyorai,* stands for the sun (spiritual father—God) here. Incidentally, the two characters of sun 日 and moon 月 together result in the third character of the Reiki Master Symbol (*myô* 明). Finally, *Maôson* brings the life force and represents the earth (spiritual earth—the Great Goddess) and the creative force here.[88]

[87] Usui, Shiro. *A Pilgrim's Guide to Forty-Six Temples,* Weatherhill, Tokyo, New York, 1990, page 80.

[88] *Nihon no bukkyô zenshû ha.* Daihôrinkaku: Tokyo, 1994.

The Mythology of Kurama

More than 6 million years ago, *Maôson* supposedly came from Venus to the earth. As a king who is responsible for overthrowing evil and as a light being of the earth, it is his task to lead all sentient beings to happiness. One method of doing this consists of showing a path through initiation to those who are sincerely seekers and come to Mount Kurama to meditate. During his three-week stay on Mount Kurama, Dr. Usui did the Morning-Star Meditation. The Morning Star means Venus, from where the light that is frequently described came to him.

In *Maôson's* time, the Japanese Islands did not yet exist. Then an underwater volcano used the power of Mother Earth to create Mount Kurama and filled it with life energy consisting of love, light, and the life force (in the sense of activity). Since then, many people have been able to receive *Reiki* on Mount Kurama. But only the people who have been mentioned in its history are known. Dr. Usui was certainly aware of this.

If we follow the path deep into the forest, we come to the Inner Shrine (*Oku no in*) where *Iwakura*, the Demon King of the Six Higher Worlds of Wishes is worshipped because this is exactly the place where he is said to have descended to earth. In Japan, there are several mountains where gods descended to earth. This also always means that their energy can be felt in these power places. The *Kurama Engi,* a text about the origins of the *Kurama* Temple, tells how many good omens are connected with the Demon King *Iwakura.*

Folk Hero Yoshitsune

There are countless wondrous stories about well-known personalities such as monks, *Samurai,* and Tennôs, but also about a great many light beings in relation to Mount Kurama. I would like to briefly include what is probably the best-known story:

In the 12th Century, there were many conflicts between the newly emerging warrior families of the *Samurai*. The two strongest were called *Taira* and *Minamoto*. The *Taira* family had at some point wiped out the most important people of the *Minamoto*, but left the women and children alive. One of the children by the name of *Yoshitsune* was concealed in the Kurama Temple. The intention was for him to become a monk far away from the political events. His background was also kept secret from him. Driven by his great need for freedom, he slipped away every day from the monastery into the forests and learned the Japanese sword fight *Kenjutsu* from a sylvan with a long nose (Jap.: *Tengu*).

The *Tengu* of Mount Kurama are actually known for their fondness of hanging monks and ascetics with their heads down from the trees and then eating them alive. This does not sound very nice. But it appears that they made an exception for Yoshitsune. In reality, it was not the *Tengu* that taught *Yoshitsune* but the Ninja. The writers of Japanese history try to avoid mentioning something like this because the Ninja are accused of all types of evil in order to depict the Samurai as honorable (cf. chapter on *Kuji kiri*). In turn, the Ninja have a close connection to the mountain ascetics *Yamabushi* who practice the Japanese magic of *Shugendô*. The place in the forest where *Yoshitsune* trained can still be seen today. Many roots grow above the earth here so that it is easy to stumble. It is an ideal place for perfecting footwork in the martial arts. Today there is a *Yoshitsune* shrine in his honor on Mount Kurama close to the many roots.

When *Yoshitsune* went to Kyoto many years later, he played the flute while coming to a bridge where the warrior monk *Benkei,* who was greatly feared at that's time, waited. He had actually sworn to himself to conquer 100 men in order to collect their swords and to let no man cross the bridge who did not fight against him. But he wanted to let the little *Yoshitsune* pass because of his young age. Yet, *Yoshitsune* annoyed the big *Benkei* so much that a fight finally did occur. However, instead of going into the offensive, he pranced and weaved back and forth like he had learned to do between the roots so that *Benkei* finally fell exhausted to the ground after much effort and admitted defeat. From that time on, *Benkei* became *Yoshitsune's* bodyguard and accompanied him for the rest of his life.

One day, *Yoshitsune* learned of his true origin and swore that he would bring fame back to his family. There were many battles until *Yoshitsune* finally conquered the *Taira* family on 4/25/1185 (my, Mark's date of birth, except for the year) in the battle of *Dan no Ura*. *Yoshitsune* was then celebrated as the greatest hero in the entire country. *Yoshitsune's* older half-brother *Yoritomo*, who had built up a large seat of power in Kamakura in the meantime and soon also became the first Shôgun, was violently angry and envious of his greatly celebrated little brother *Yoshitsune* and therefore had him pursued by his troops through all of Japan. Because of a betrayal, *Yoshitsune* was discovered in Northern Japan in Hiraizumi. One legend says that he was killed by the troops, another alleges that he committed ritual suicide (Jap.: *seppuku*), and another claims that he fled to the mainland from there and later turned out to be Djingis Khan.

Be that as it may, his story did much to contribute to the fame of Mount Kurama and the temple. In addition, it shows how close the healing arts and martial arts are.

Dr. Usui and His Spiritual Experience on Mount Kurama

Dr. Usui searched for many years to find a method with which he could make the spiritual life energy of Reiki available in a lasting way. While doing this, he came across old writings in which some of the symbols appeared that he later integrated into Reiki. Although the symbols are explained in terms of their effect and function, he did not know how to use them in a concrete manner. No matter whom he asked, no one could show him how to make the knowledge of these writings useful in a practical way. Although it may be possible that there was someone in Japan during Dr. Usui's lifetime who could have imparted this to him, Dr. Usui could not find anyone who could do it or wanted to do it. The secret of learning regarding these types of topics does not just lie in the imparting of knowledge. As previously discussed in many sections of this book, it also involves connecting an individual with the spiritual power by means of initiation. Dr. Usui was certainly aware of this since it is explained in many writings and he would otherwise have hardly climbed up Mount Kurama in order to meditate there; after all, it was his intention to make Reiki available in a lasting way through meditation. So he set out to find a suitable place. Since Mount Kurama has been praised in literature for centuries as a location for visions and experiences of enlightenment, this was the appropriate power place for him.

Dr. Usui meditated for three weeks on Mount Kurama. In order to count the days, he piled up 21 stones and threw one of them away each morning. Then, during the last night as he already believed that he would go home the next morning without any success, he suddenly saw a light in the distance that was approaching him. As this light reached him, he fell into a trance, during which he was personally initiated into Reiki by *Dainichi Nyorai*. This was the fulfillment of his longstanding dream. Now he could both give Reiki and also initiate other people into it.

The question now arises as to the details of what Dr. Usui did on Mount Kurama. There are many types of meditations. Did he simply practice Zen meditation or a meditation from Esoteric Buddhism? The latter is quite probable since the symbols appeared in Esoteric Buddhism and *Dainichi Nyorai* is its main figure. The third point is that in the long history of Japan there is a special meditation with which spiritual seekers have repeatedly had experiences such as those that Dr. Usui had on Mount Kurama. One of them is the Morning-Star Meditation (Jap.: *Gumonji hô*)—which, incidentally, is the same meditation also practiced by the monk Kûkai in Japan 1,200 years before Dr. Usui. Even today, he is still considered the most famous monk of Japan, among other things because of his healing power. The other meditation is the visualization of the *Siddham* seed syllables (Jap.: *Ajikan*).

The Morning-Star Meditation is explained in detail in the next section. The instructions for meditating with the *Siddham* was already included in the chapter on *Dainichi Nyorai Kidô* as "Practice 4: Opening the Energy Channels for Letting the *Ki* Flow in a Controlled Way" (page 255).

The Morning-Star[89] Meditation

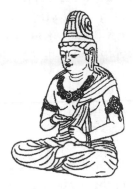

ILL. 109 – KOKÛZÔ BOSATSU

The Morning-Star Meditation is very complex and requires some aids such as water, incense, and prayer beads. This is the form of practice that is traditionally done in Shingon Buddhism. A simplified variation will be included at the end of this section with a sequence that is less complicated for Reiki initiates.

The main practice in the Morning-Star Meditation lies in reciting the mantras of the Bodhisattva *Kokûzô*. The number of repetitions is not exactly small—one million of them 108 times. As a multiple of nine, the number 108 is a sacred number in Buddhism. It is the number of the small beads in a large Buddhist prayer-bead chain (Jap.: *Juzu, nenju*, Skr.: *mâlâ*). Through the enormous amount of manta repetitions, the adept merges with the Bodhisattva *Kokûzô*, which makes a direct experience with *Dainichi Nyorai* possible. This is exactly what happened to Dr. Usui during his meditation practice on Mount Kurama. Dr. Usui was initiated into Reiki in this way.

In terms of its sequence, the Morning-Star Meditation is a shortened part of the four-part preparation practices (Jap.: *Shido kekgyô*) as the groundwork for achieving enlightenment in this life. Its Japanese name *Gumonji hô* means "Method for Keeping What Has Been Heard." So those who do this meditation from beginning to end can always remember everything that they have seen, heard, read, etc. This is why this meditation

---

[89] The Morning Star refers to Venus.

has been a popular method for training the memory in Japan since the Nara period. But this is actually more of a side effect. The actual esoteric goal lies in experiencing the nature of the esoteric teachings through the practice. In the ritual handbook of this meditation[90], the correlation with the Morning Star is explained. The Morning Star (Venus) is related to the content of the meditation instead of its name. While the mantra is recited, you simultaneously imagine the Bodhisattva *Kokûzô* in form of the planet Venus (Morning Star).

After the Indian monk *Subhâkarasimha*[91] translated the Morning-Star Meditation into Chinese in the year 717, many versions of this text came to Japan. The meditation continued to be developed there. Among other things, this was necessary because the meditations could otherwise not have been done with all of the rituals in Japan and because it is traditionally in the nature of the Japanese to adapt and optimize what they have adopted from foreign cultures. So Dr. Usui was also able to use the form of the meditation that had been adapted to his needs in order to realize his great dream and make Reiki available to all people at any time through initiation and training. However, this does not mean that the Morning-Star Meditation can be changed at will. Just like the symbols, certain rules must be followed so that the effect is reliably retained to its full extent.

Explanations on the Sequence of the Morning-Star Meditation

The following section describes how the Morning-Star Meditation is still performed in the Shingon School in Japan. Find a location that is calm and secluded from civilization for the Morning-Star Meditation. This may be in nature, as chosen by Dr. Usui, or a meditation hall set aside especially for this purpose. Build an altar with the appropriate symbols and offerings to establish contact with the light beings and request that they come to this place.

There are special opening and closing rituals that you should perform on the first and last day. The number of days that the meditation

---

[90] Name of the Handbook: *Kokûzô bosatsu nôman shogan saishô shin darani gumonji hô.* 虚空蔵菩薩能満諸願最勝心陀羅尼求聞持法
[91] One of the eight Shingon patriarchs.

is done depends upon how many times the mantras are repeated. If the meditation lasts 21 days, the mantra must be respectively repeated about 50,000 times every day. This explains why Dr. Usui meditated day and night. The mantras are counted with special prayer beads made of wood or crystal quartz with two times 54 beads (108) and two large ones as separation in the middle.

In no case should you interrupt the meditation. If you become ill or are forced to stop for some other reasons, you must start over again at a later point in time. In the ideal case, the time plan should be established in such a way that the last day of the meditation coincides with a lunar and/or solar eclipse.

The sequence of the meditation largely corresponds with the practices described above. However, considerably more symbols and light beings are visualized here. The right hand forms the Mudrâ of the Wish-Fulfilling Gem and the left hand holds the Mudrâ of the *Vajra* Fist on the hip. The mantra to be recited is the *Kokûzô*. The words are: *Nô bô akyasha kyarabaya on arikya mari bori sowaka.* Seat yourself in such a way that you are facing the east during the meditation.

All of the vital needs of the body such as eating, drinking, sleeping, and answering nature's call are also ritualized. Overall, the intake of food during the ritual is like a Japanese method of fasting.

Sequence of the Everyday Practice of the Morning-Star Meditation

Use the ritual to connect with the Morning star. Get two buckets of water from a clean well or spring. Cleanse yourself by drawing water from the bucket with your left hand, transferring it to your right hand, and then rinsing out your mouth. Then wash your hands, face, and body. While washing, recite the mantra and visualize how you are becoming pure both inside and outside.

Now prepare the offerings and enter the place of meditation. Show the light beings your respect and sit down to meditate.

In order to protect existence, recite the mantra and form the mudrâ above the five parts of the body. As you do this, visualize how *Kokûzô* and all of the Buddhas remove the veils from your eyes and how your mind becomes pure.

276

Activate the water with a mudrâ and recite the mantra as you do this. Then sprinkle the water upon the altar, the offerings, and the ground.

Now carry out the ritual for pulverizing the incense and use it to empower the altar and the offerings. As you do this, request the protection of the light beings and perform the ritual for purifying the body, speech, and mind.

Visualize the place of the practice and unite it with *Kokûzô*. Now invite the light beings to come to the altar.

Then take the activated water and use ritual movements to cleanse the feet of *Kokûzô*. Now greet the light being on a flower by ringing the little bell and making the five offerings.

Using this as the basis, build up the reciprocal spiritual transmission *kaji* with *Kokûzô* by forming mudrâs above the appropriate areas of the body, reciting mantras, using *Bîjas (Siddham*-symbols*)*, and merging with *Kokûzô*.

Now begin reciting the mantras with the special prayer beads. Visualize a moon disk in *Kokûzô's* chest upon which the *Siddham* of the mantra appear one after the other. From the mantra, golden light radiates into your Crown Chakra. It fills you up completely, circulates through your body, and finally flows out of your mouth. Now the golden light once again enters *Kokûzô* through the feet. Maintain this image until you have completed your daily 50,000 repetitions of the mantra.

Now enter into the realm of the Buddhas by raising your mudrâ to the level of the chest. Visualize how the *Siddham* expand with the moon disk until they fill up the entire universe. Then the *Siddham* grow smaller with the moon disk back to the normal size. Repeat the reciprocal spiritual transmission *(kaji)* with *Kokûzô* by forming the mudrâs above the appropriate body areas, reciting mantras, using the *Bîjas*, and merging with *Kokûzô*.

Then perform the same practice several hundred times with *Dainichi Nyorai* and his four emanations.

Finally, make the closing offerings, show your respect and gratitude to the light beings, and perform the reciprocal spiritual transmission for the three cosmic forces and the five great promises. Now express the wish for all the good that has been created through the meditation to be for the highest good of all beings.

Now dissolve the protective circle around the place of meditation and take leave of all the light beings. Do this practice once more for the protection of all existence. Recite the mantra for this and form the mudrâ above the five parts of the body. As you do this, visualize how *Kokûzô* and all of the Buddhas remove the veils from your eyes and how your mind becomes pure.

Massage your body and leave the place.

Applications of the Morning-Star Meditation for Reiki Initiates

Now that you have read the instructions for the meditation practice, you may be thinking that it would be rather difficult for you to do the Morning-Star Meditation on your own. However, if you are initiated into the 2nd Degree, you can use the Reiki symbols as tools for doing a variation of this meditation that is quite simple. But if you would like to do the meditation in exactly the same way as Dr. Usui, then follow the guidelines described above. The question could now come up as to why Dr. Usui did not do the meditation according to the following description. The answer is actually very simple. When Dr. Usui climbed up Mount Kurama in order to meditate there, he had not yet been initiated into Reiki and the symbols. This only happened after years of training and a course of studies, as well as the three-week intensive meditation.

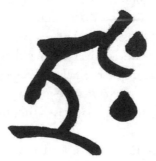

ILL. 110 – SIDDHAM SYMBOL TRAM OF KOKÛZÔ BOSATSU

Here are the applications for the Morning-Star Meditation:

Connect you with **Kokûzô Bosatsu** *through the distant contact. Greet him with the words: "I come to you as a sick person and request healing. I come* *to you as an ignorant person and request teaching. I come to you as someone who does not know the way and ask for protection and guidance. I come to you as someone who is helpless and ask you for power in order to better serve. As compensation, I send you Reiki. Please use it as you wish for the benefit of all."*

*

Hold your hands with the palms facing away from and intensify the contact with several CR Symbols. Now let the light beings receive Reiki for 10-15 minutes. Simply assume that *Kokûzô Bosatsu* is in front of you and are receiving Reiki. This part replaces the preparatory rituals for the light beings.

Then explain to *Kokûzô Bosatsu* that you would like to do the Morning-Star Meditation and request his cooperation. Assume the mudrâ *Kanjô in* (Mudrâ of Initiation). Visualize *Kokûzô Bosatsu* diagonally in front of you and above you. Visualize a moon disk lying flat on his chest. When you see this clearly, draw the *Siddham* symbol *tram* of *Kokûzô Bosatsu* as if it was standing on the moon disk and activate it by saying the mantra *tram* three times. Then also use a CR with its mantra. Now a spiral begins at the foot of the *Siddham* with the mantra of *Kokûzô Bosatsu*. The mantra is: *Nô bô akyasha kyarabaya on arikya mari bori sowaka*. Begin reciting the mantras.

A golden light emanates from the mantra spiral and flows into your Crown Chakra. It fills you up completely and circulates through your body. Finally, the golden light radiates from your mouth back into *Kokûzô Bosatsu* through his feet.

If you cannot imagine all of this at the same time, then direct your attention for a while to *Kokûzô Bosatsu* and then to the moon disk, to the symbol and mantra and then to the circulating golden light. Sometimes it is helpful to imagine that the golden light streams into you when you inhale and back to *Kokûzô Bosatsu* when you exhale. Repeat the mantra 108 times or a multiple of this.

ILL. 111 – STROKE SEQUENCE FOR TRAM OF KOKÛZÔ BOSATSU

When you have completed the recitation, raise your mudrâ to the level of the chest. Now imagine that you are becoming *Kokûzô Bosatsu*. The moon disk, *Siddham,* and mantra spiral are now within your own chest. Keep your attention there for a moment. Now imagine how the moon disk, *Siddham,* and mantra spiral are expanding until they are as large as you. Then they are as large as a house, a mountain, the entire earth, and finally the entire universe. Next, reduce the moon disk, *Siddham,* and mantra spiral back to their normal size.

Now the golden light returns back to the mantra spiral and the mantra spiral merges into the *Siddham* symbol *tram*, which also unites with the moon disk. The form of *Kokûzô Bosatsu* also falls into the moon disk, which then becomes increasingly smaller and finally completely dissolves. Pause for several minutes.

*

Now express the wish that all of the good that was just created through the meditation may work for the highest good of all beings. Then give thanks to **Kokûzô Bosatsu,** *wish him all the best and that the blessing of the creative force may be with him on his path. Request that you may soon be allowed to come to him again. Blow strongly through your hands and rub them together.*

If necessary, ground yourself for several minutes by giving Reiki to the soles of your feet and your toes.

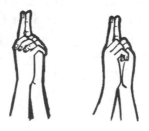

ILL. 112 – MUDRA OF INITIATION

PART III –

ORIGIN, MEANINGS, AND MYTHOLOGICAL BACKGROUND OF THE TRADITIONAL REIKI SYMBOLS

CHAPTER 14

The SHK Symbol

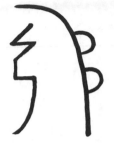

ILL. 113 – THE SHK SYMBOL

The Siddham Script: The Basis of the SHK Symbol

As the Buddhist teachings were written down in the classic Indian language of Sanskrit after hundreds of years of being an oral tradition, the ancient Indian *Siddham* script was used as the alphabet. The sacred texts of Buddhism created in this way are called sutras.

In addition to the function as script, the form and sound of the individual *Siddham* signs have a spiritual and symbolic meaning with concrete effects when they are used correctly. In this case, they are called seed syllables (Skr.: *Siddham* or *Bîja*). The SHK Symbol[92] is one of these seed syllables. However, they were changed somewhat—probably by Dr. Usui—and then integrated into the Reiki System of Healing. This is somewhat different than changing the Reiki symbols in retrospect, as frequently occurs today, because the effect can be lost if later formal changes that are not compatible with the spiritual qualities of the Reiki tradition deviate too much from the original. Through his decades of spiritual studies, Dr. Usui possessed the ability of making symbols useable for practical energy work in a very specific way and of connecting them

[92] The SHK Symbol at the top of this page shows the way it was written by Hawayo Takata.

with deities. Anyone who does not possess this ability will achieve a lesser effect or none at all by changing the Reiki symbols. In Rainbow Reiki, this method is taught in the 3rd Dan (the highest degree of Mastership).

The syllable *om*, which is familiar to people throughout the entire world, is also one of the *Siddham* seed syllables. Several or more *Siddham* form a *mantra*, which is used as the highly effective recitation in rituals and meditations. In *dhâranîs*, which have a function similar to that of mantras but simultaneously also have a meaning in terms of their content, the *Siddham* are used as the alphabet together with the *Bîjas* as seed syllables. When the sutras were translated into Chinese, the mantras and *dhâranîs* related to the rituals were not translated into Chinese. *Siddham* or *Bîjas* were just transcribed into *Kanji* for clarifying the pronunciation. Other than the originals of the sutras in Sanskrit, the Chinese translations have been completely preserved to this day with the *Siddham* that they contain. Accordingly, the *Siddham* are also extensively explained in the Buddhist reference books from China, Japan, and Korea.

Many words that are used in Buddhism, in esotericism, in this book, and also in everyday usage like normal words come from Sanskrit. The best-known are probably Buddha, chakra, sûtra, mantra, and mudrâ. All of these terms, which are now written in the West with Latin letters, are actually just written in *Siddham* in Buddhism. Since the current customary spelling in the West involves Latin words and not the symbols that are in close resonance with the spiritual powers, the words written in Latin script also do not have the same effect as a *Siddham* symbol. As a symbol, the SHK Symbol also does not just have the qualities of "normal," worldly script that solely serves as the bearer of meaning for the spoken language in individual or compounded or successive signs.

The History of the Siddham

During the second millennia B.C., the Aryans, a warring nomadic tribe from Turkestan, invaded India and soon mixed with the original inhabitants who lived there as they became settled. The Vedic religion with the literature collection called the *Vedas* arose among these Indo-Aryan people of the Indian subcontinent. The *Vedas* were written about 1200-600 B.C. and include four collections, consisting of the hymns to the gods

283

(*Rigveda*), ceremonial chants (*Sâmaveda*), rites, and ceremonial mantras (*Yajurveda*) and spells, as well as the incantations (*Atharvaveda*). A special meaning was given to the magical formulas, which, among other things, were used to heal diseases, prolong life, be strong against the enemies, or influence the weather, for instance.

The *Vedas* include ritual texts with explanations about applications and the effect of the offering (*Brâhmana*) and the philosophical treatises on the liberation of human beings (*Upanishads*).

ILL. 114 – EXCERPT FROM THE RIGVEDA

The *Vedas* are said to not have been invented by human beings but "heard" by seers and spiritual mediums. In addition, the God *Brahmâ* is known to be the author who supposedly wrote the *Vedas* in Sanskrit on golden leaves. However, the people of that time also believed that the live recitation of the texts was more correct because this would transfer their power and effect. So it still took a long time for it to be written down. During this time, trained memory experts learned the *Vedas* by heart from mouth to ear in special schools and then preached them to the people by memory. One of these schools exists in India today and the *Vedas* are occasionally recited from memory at spiritual events.

Until Buddhism (since about 500 B.C.), *Brâhmi-lipi* was used as the sacred script and understood by just a few scholars. Buddha (about 565-486 B.C.) insisted that his teachings should be transmitted to all people in their own language. King *Ashoka* took Buddha at his word and ordered that pillars with the words of Buddha be erected throughout the country in order to spread Buddhism. The edicts on the pillars were written in all of the languages of India's various regions.

284

Brâhmi-lipi is the precursor of many Indian, Tibetan, and South-East Asian scripts. From the Northern Indian variation, various types of script such as the *Gupta, Siddham, Devanâgarî* developed, as well as *Tibetan* and *Khotanisch*.

Siddham and *Devanâgarî* are both successors of the Western *Gupta* script. In the *Gupta* period (320-674), many Buddhist monasteries flourished and many literary works were also created. In the early phase of Buddhism, the teachings were transmitted orally since very few monks could write. Then, as the *sutras* were gradually written down, it became indispensable for the monks to learn the script.

The Buddhist training in the *Gupta* region began with a primer in twelve chapters, in which the characters and 10,000 combinations of the vowels and consonants were taught. The script system initially did not have a name of its own. This arose through the training in the script itself. At the beginning of the lesson, the students had to practice the two characters for the term *Siddham*. The root of this word is *siddh*, which means something like "realized, successful, or perfect" in a sacred sense.

ILL. 115 – PILLAR WITH THE WORDS OF BUDDHA

285

On the primer, or as the title of character lists, *siddhir-astu* (May it be perfect!) or *namah sarvajnâya Siddham* (Hail the Omniscient Perfection) is written. As a result, the term *Siddham* became a synonym for the characters and the primer itself. The primer had to be mastered within six months. This was followed by the *Sutras* of *Pânini*, the book of *Dhâtu*, and the three *Khilas*.

Manuscripts were usually written with a wooden writing brush and red paint on palm leaves (Skr.: *tâla*) and sometimes also on birch bark. Holes were bored through the leaves and they were tied together with a piece of string.

The *Siddham* in their original form as symbols were seen as perfect in themselves in the spiritual sense since they were created by *Brahmâ*. Buddhism teaches that the *Siddham* were created from the void *sûnyatâ*. *Shâkyamuni*, who is a manifestation of *Dainichi Nyorai* 大日如来, taught the *Siddham* as symbols within the scope of Esoteric Buddhism (*Vajrayâna*, *Mantrayâna*, *Tantrayâna*). Up until the time of *Nâgârjuna*[93], the first human patriarch and founder of Esoteric Buddhism, they were kept secret.

The Buddhist *sutras* that were exported to China were mostly written in *Siddham* script. The texts were translated into Chinese. However, there was little interest in the correct pronunciation or *Sanskrit* grammar. Because of the many dialects in China, more attention was placed upon the script than the language in order to make it understandable. As a result, there was more concentration on the form of the *Siddham*. At the same time, special value was placed upon the effectiveness of mantras, *dhâranîs*, and *Bîjas* in *Siddham*. The *Siddham* in China, and later also in Korea and Japan, were therefore exclusively seen and used as a sacred script. In addition, the inventors of other script systems, such as *Hangul* in Korea and the syllable script systems of *Hiragana* and *Katakana* in Japan, who were enthused about Buddhism, let themselves be inspired by the system of the *Siddham* in the creation of their new script.

---

[93] *Nâgârjuna* (exact biographical data is not known; Jap.: *Ryûju* 龍樹 or *Ryûmyô* 竜猛) was the founder of the *Mâdhyamika* School. From the perspective of *Mahâyâna* and *Vajrayana* Buddhism, as well as many studies, he was born in the 3rd Century into a Brahmanic family. He first studied *Hînayâna* and later *Mahâyâna* in the Himalayas. When he returned to Southern India, he wrote some texts on the teaching of emptiness *sûnyatâ*. In China and Japan, he is known as the founder of the Eight Schools; for Esoteric Buddhism, he is the third patriarch of the *Shingon* School and lived in the 7th Century.

The Siddham in Japan—Symbols for Rituals and Healing

Until quite recently, it was assumed that the *Siddham* came to Japan with the introduction of the secret teachings of Esoteric Buddhism at the beginning of the 9th Century through the monks *Kûkai* and *Saichô*. Although a wave of introduction of documents and their general spread began with these two monks, the secret teachings (*mikkyô*) of Esoteric Buddhism came at least one-hundred years earlier and the *Siddham* had already arrived in the 6th Century. This is at the same time that Buddhism officially came to Japan.

In the year 538 or 552, the Japanese Tennô was gifted sculptures, *sutras* with *Siddham,* and ritual implements from Korea. We can conclude from this that the rituals for worshipping the sculptures were also sent along to Japan since such gifts could hardly have been intended as souvenirs. Although the *Siddham* are a special characteristic of the secret teachings of Esoteric Buddhism, the recitation of mantras was also customary in *Mahâyâna* Buddhism, which was first spread in Japan. These mantras are written in *Siddham* and *Kanji*. These can still be admired today on the old scrolls in the *Hôryûji* Temple (the oldest wooden house in the world).

In various literary sources, exciting stories describe time and again how the *Siddham* are used in rituals. For example, the Korean monk *Nichira*[94] (?-583) allegedly performed a secret ritual by the name of *Shôgun jizô bosatsu hô* in Japan. We know that this involved the invocation of the Bodhisattva *Jizô* as the protective God of War by using *dhâranîs* and *mantras,* as well as symbols in Siddham.

As a ritual for averting disaster, it was later adopted in the 7th Century by the founder of the *Shugendô*[95], *En no Ozuno*[96] and performed on a regular basis on Mount Atago in Kyoto.

---

[94] *Nichira*: Nobleman from *South Kyûshû* who went to Korea as an envoy.

[95] *Shugendô* is a religious school that unites elements from Esoteric Buddhism and Japanese mountain-belief concepts with each other. The members (*yamabushi*) perform various ascetic practices in the mountains. See the corresponding chapter in this book.

[96] *En no Ozuno* (exact biographical data is not known; late 7th Century) is the legendary founder of *Shugendô*, which is also known under the name of *En no Gyôja*.

In the process, the Bodhisattva *Jizô,* flanked by the Wisdom King *Fudô Myôô* (不動明王; Skr. *Acala*), and the Deva *Bishamonten* (毘沙門天; Skr. *Vaisravana*) were depicted on talismans in *Siddham.*

In the year 607, the Japanese envoy *Ono no Imoko*[97] brought *sutra*s in *Siddham* written on palm leaves to Japan. Even today, they are still preserved in the *Hôryûji* temple. Afterward, the Indian monk *Hôdô*[98] brought the belief in the eleven-headed *Jûichimen Kannon* (十一面観音; Skr. *Ekadasamukha avalokitesvara bodhisattva*) to Japan. By means of the secret *dhâranîs* and symbols in *Siddham,* he performed rituals for the healing of diseases. A bit later, in the year 722, the mountain ascetic *Taichô*[99] (683-767) healed the *Genshô* Tennô[100] (680-748) with the help of rituals using a three-pronged thunderbolt (Jap. *sankosho*; Skr. *vajra*) and a thunderbolt ritual bell upon which the *Siddham* were engraved (Jap. *sankorei,* Skr. *vajra ganthâ*). At the same time, the scholarly monk *Dôji*[101] (?-744) went to *Tang*-China (618-907) and received a Buddhist ritual meditation, the *Gumonji hô* 求聞持法, there from *Subhâkarasimha*[102], the Fifth Patriarch of the *Shingon* School. The *mantra* of the Bodhisattva *Kokûzô* and the symbols in *Siddham* are indispensable for this meditation. Incidentally, this is also the same meditation (Morning-Star Meditation) that Dr. Usui practiced on Mount Kurama. The fundamental goal of this meditation is, as the Japanese name also suggests, "to keep what has been heard."[103] The monk *Kûkai* also practiced this meditation in his youth long before his journey to China.

[97]   *Ono no Imoko* was a Japanese envoy who was commissioned by *Shôtoku Taishi* in 607 to travel to *Sui*-China to study the Chinese culture and institutions there. His knowledge, which also influenced the *Taika* Reform of 645, shaped the Japanese culture to a large degree.

[98]   *Hôdô* (exact biographical data unknown; 7th Century).

[99]   *Taichô,* mountain ascetic of the *Nara* period (710-794).

[100]   Tennô of the early *Nara* period.

[101]   *Dôji*: an especially gifted monk who was selected from 100 high-ranking monks during his stay in *Tang*-China to teach the *Ninnô hannya kyô* 仁王般若経 (Skr.: *Prajnâpâramitâ sûtra*). After his return, he taught the teachings of the *Sanron* School 三論宗 in *Daianji.*

[102]   *Subhâkarasimha* (637-735; Jap.: *Zenmui* 善無畏): Buddhist monk from Southern India who translated the *Danichikyô* (Skr.: *Mahâvairocana sûtra*) into Chinese and spread Esoteric Buddhism in China during his stay in Chang'an, together with *Vajrabodhi* (671-741; Jap.: *Kongôchi* 金剛智).

[103]   Details on this are in the chapter about Mount Kurama.

The two *Siddham* scholars *Daoxuan*[104] (702-760) (Jap. *Dôsen*) from China and *Bodhisena*[105] (704-760) from India went to Japan together and played a leading role there in the year 752 as ritual masters in the eye-opening ceremony of the Great Buddha (*Daibutsu* 大仏) of *Tôdaiji*[106]. This ritual is the consecration of a Buddha statue. It is used to awaken the power of this Buddha within it. Apart from the ceremonial "painting of the eyes," it is similar to a Reiki initiation in its broader aspects.

Afterward, *Bodhisena* taught *Siddham* in the *Daianji*[107] temple for about 15 years. The Vietnamese monk *Buttetsu*[108], who had followed *Bodhisena* to Japan, reportedly brought the *Siddham* collection (*Shittanzô* 悉曇蔵) to Japan. It has since been lost. He also taught *Siddham* and the ritual dance music *Gagaku*. And we also know that *Ganjin*[109] (688-763), who finally reached Japan in 753 used the *Siddham* for the initiation rituals with monks on an ordination platform.

In the 9th Century, many monks and officials were sent as envoys to *Tang*-China to study Esoteric Buddhism. Eight especially well-known monks, including *Kûkai*, all of whom were focused on the *Siddham*, were given the nickname of the "Eight *Siddha* Monks" (*Shittan hakke* 悉曇八家). There were repeated reports on how they were introduced to the secret teachings of Esoteric Buddhism (*mikkyô* 灌頂) through the initiation rituals (*kanjô* 密教, Skr. *abhisheka*) because the *Siddham* in

---

[104] *Daoxuan* (Jap.: *Dôsen*) taught Buddhism in Japan since 736 and influenced *Saichô* (767-822), the founder of the *Tendai* School in Japan.

[105] *Bodhisena* (702-760) (Jap. *Bodaisenna* 菩提僊那): Buddhist monk from India who received the honorary title of *Baramon Sôjô* 婆羅門僧正 after his arrival in Japan. When *Bodhisena* still lived in India, he heard that a reincarnation of *Manjusrî* lived in China on Mount *Wutai*. As a result, he traveled to China through Indonesia. However, when he arrived in 733 he learned that there was no reincarnation of *Manjusrî* on Mount *Wutai* but that, according to other rumors, this incarnation lived in Japan. So he arrived in Japan in 736. He taught Sanskrit there in Nara beginning in 750.

[106] *Tôdaiji*: Buddhist temple in Nara that was established in 752.

[107] *Daianji*: Buddhist temple in Nara that was established in 617 by *Shôtoku Taishi* (574-622).

[108] *Buttetsu* (exact biographical data not known; 8th Century): studied in Southern India under *Bodhisena*; followed Bodhisena to China and Japan.

[109] *Ganjin*: Buddhist monk from China who established the *Ritsu*-school 律宗 in 753 and the *Tôshôdaiji* 唐招提寺 in 759.

particular have an important meaning in the correct transmission of the Buddhas' power.

Kûkai brought not only abundant material with him from China but also laid the foundations for the *Siddham* as an organized teaching and wrote several treatises about it. The content of these treatises was familiar to Dr. Usui since the basis for the symbols was set down in them.

Kûkai explained in his writings on the *Siddham* that both the meaning of their appearance and that of their form are significant and that they have special functions and effects as symbols. In teaching the *Siddham*, *Kûkai* placed great value on the proper spelling since the effect would otherwise be lost. This obviously also means that intentional or even unintentional changes of the Reiki symbols in a form that is not in keeping with the spiritual rules of the tradition can weaken or even negate the effect. In practice, this means that there may very well be various proper spellings for the Reiki symbols, but that it is absolutely necessary to create the symbols according to the rules that apply to them in order to guarantee their full and reliable effectiveness.

In the initiations, the Mandalas of the Two Worlds[110] (*Ryôkai mandara*) and their *Siddham* played an especially important role for *Kûkai*. They are the essence of the *Shingon* teaching and depict *Dainichi Nyorai* as the Great God and the Great Goddess. Since Reiki's spiritual power has its source in *Dainichi Nyorai* and he equally embodies the feminine and the masculine spiritual principle, Reiki is a *non-polar* energy form.

Within this context, *Kûkai* composed many calligraphic works in *Siddham*. These include the "Mantra of Light" (*Kômyô shingon* 光明真言), which was written with wooden brushes and has especially increased in significance since the 12th Century for the spiritual power transmission in initiations, healing rituals, and meditations. This *Siddham* mantra is closely related to the symbols DKM and SHK.

The wave of introducing the *Siddham* in the 9th Century was followed by a phase of researching the available materials. This is related to the fact that the contact with China was abruptly broken off in the year 894. In the various temples of Esoteric Buddhism, the *Siddham* were studied and

---

[110] Combination of the Mandalas of the Diamond World *kongôkai* 金剛界 (Skr.: *vajra dhâtu*) and the Womb World *taizôkai* 胎蔵界 (Skr.: *garbha dhâtu*).

explanatory texts were written. Since they have an important function for the rituals of Esoteric Buddhism, they spread together with the secret teachings (*mikkyô*).

Because *Kûkai* placed great value on calligraphy, eight *Shingon* monks up until the 14th Century followed his example by producing the calligraphies and providing explanations about the *Siddham*. One thing they all have in common is that they used the *Siddham* as symbols for purposes such as meditations and rituals for the healing of diseases, the dissolution of karma, and death rituals. Another factor is that they learned the *Siddham* through meditation and wrote new texts on this topic as a result. For example, the monk *Seigen* (1162-1231) wrote many books on fire rituals[111] (*Goma hô* 護摩法) and initiation rituals.

Up until the 20th Century, there was hardly any interest in studying the grammar of *Sanskrit*. The enthusiasm for the *Siddham* was limited to the expressive calligraphies in *Siddham* and the effective esoteric rituals and meditations. Only in recent years has a slow change taken place in Japan in terms of people studying the grammar and language of Sanskrit. Within this context, I also became acquainted with my calligraphy master, a Chinese-Japanese Zen monk. He made a special trip to Germany in order to learn Sanskrit since this is simply not possible in Japan.

While searching for Reiki, Dr. Usui became familiar with the *Siddham* in the course of his research and integrated the SHK Symbol for the healing of the mind into his method. I consider it possible and probable that Dr. Usui would have incorporated even more *Siddham* into Reiki if he had had more time to teach Reiki. Unfortunately, he only taught his system for four years before his death.

Siddham—Symbols of the Light Beings

There are many different ways to describe a light being. They are usually just called by their names. Some names have a meaning and can be translated into various languages. For example, the *Great Sun Buddha* is a translation of *Dainichi Nyorai*. This is the Japanese pronunciation. In Chinese, it is pronounced as *Dari Rurai* and written with the same char-

---

[111] *Goma hô:* Fire ritual in which *Fudô myôô* (不動明王, Skr.: *Acala*) is usually worshipped as a protection-bringing figure of liberation.

acter of 大日如来. But both of these are translations from the Sanskrit. Here he is actually called *Mahâ Vairocana Buddha*, which is written in different characters of the *Siddham*.

Those who have never heard about *Dainichi Nyorai* also cannot say what type of light being he is. This is comparable with the chakras in the energy system of a human being. In India, each chakra is associated with a god and not with a color. When they hear the name of the god, people in India can immediately recognize the meaning of this chakra. People in the West normally cannot do this because they do not come from this culture and are hardly familiar—if at all—with the gods there and their characteristics. In order to simplify the chakra system and make it understandable for Western individuals, the individual chakras had colors assigned to them. This probably occurred at the beginning of the 1980s in the Northern Scottish spiritual community of Findhorn.[112]

In the same way, each light being—including those in the chakras—has a *Siddham* symbol associated with it. Whenever they appear as seed syllables, the *Siddham* are always the equivalent of the light being itself. The special thing about this is that these symbols speak for themselves. It is said that the knowledge and wisdom of the entire cosmos is contained in just one symbol.[113] This knowledge can practically be "tapped into" through meditations with the *Siddham*. If the *Siddham* are correctly used in rituals or healing, they retain their effect even if the practitioner does not know what they mean or is incorrectly informed about them. This also applies to all of the Reiki symbols, the origins of which have been largely unknown up until the writing of this book.

Mental or spiritual healing is performed with the SHK symbol in Reiki. The fact that this is possible is related to the light beings that are expressed by the *Siddham*. The SHK Symbol is one of the few *Siddham* that simultaneously represent more than one light being. These are the

[112] Cf. Walter Lübeck: *The Aura Healing Handbook*, Lotus Press.

[113] This view is also found in the spiritual philosophy of ancient China. The following has been said about the famous *I Ching*, the ancient Chinese book of oracles and wisdom: "The saints and sages established the images (of the *I Ching*) in order to completely express their thoughts." The master spoke: "The script cannot completely express the words. The words cannot completely express the thoughts." (Attributed to Confucius but the origin is probably much older.)

Paradise Buddha *Amida Nyorai* and the 1000-Armed Goddess *Senju Kannon*. Both light beings have special functions in rituals and meditations. As the Paradise Buddha, *Amida Nyorai* tends to be responsible for death rituals and the Goddess *Senju Kannon* is the helping Bodhisattva for spiritual healing. Both work hand in hand since rebirth in a paradise is especially possible when the soul of the deceased has a very pure mind. In the depictions of this in works of art, we frequently see how *Kannon* brings the soul on a lotus blossom to *Amida* in Paradise.

ILL. 116 –	ILL. 117 –	ILL. 118 –
AMIDA NYORA	SIDDHAM HRIH	SENJU KANNON

Incidentally, spiritual healing and the related personality development already make it possible to be happy in this life because the individual reaches a state in which the world is experienced in the way desired from the depths of the heart, from the soul, which perceives the unique spiritual vision for the person's life. In this way, both light beings work in this one symbol.

Pronunciation and Meaning of the SHK Symbol

Although the SHK Symbol is a *Siddham*, the mantra uses the Japanese pronunciation of *Sei heki* instead of the Indian. "Japanese pronunciation" means that there must also be characters for the pronunciation. But if we take the Japanese pronunciation *Sei heki* and translate it into characters, the result is the *Kanji* 正癖. This *Kanji* means "correcting habits," which is equivalent in its meaning to the function of mental healing in Usui Reiki. Expressed simply, the original Indian SHK Symbol—a so-called *Siddham*—was given a Japanese pronunciation through which the general function of the SHK Symbol in Reiki can easily be recognized.

293

It is not possible to determine the pronunciation on the basis of the symbol or use the symbol to figure out the pronunciation. The pronunciation of the SHK Symbol does not correspond with the pronunciation of the original *Siddham* seed syllable. In Sanskrit, this actually sounds like *hrih*.

We could presume that the pronunciation is a translation of *hrih* into Japanese. However, this also is not the case here. When the *Siddham* came to China, the Chinese already had difficulties in correctly pronouncing the Siddham. It was even more difficult to write them in the Chinese translations of the sutras because the appearance of the *Siddham* does not reveal the pronunciation in China. So the Chinese used a trick to deal with this problem. Each *Siddham* had a Chinese character assigned to it. In the process, only the pronunciation was important but not the meaning. The Chinese characters were intended as an aid in pronunciation so that an individual did not have to make an extra effort to learn Sanskrit and *Siddham*. The SHK Symbol had the character 紇利 assigned to it.

When the *Siddham*—as well as the SHK Symbol that was included with them—came to Japan, the Chinese-Indian pronunciation was additionally adapted to Japanese. This ultimately led to the Indian pronunciation of *hrih* becoming the pronunciation *kiriku* in Japanese. When they are compared, we discover that they only have the middle letters *ri* in common. Both of the *h*s have become a *k*. The remaining letters *i* and *u* are Japanese adaptations that can be ascribed to the Japanese way of writing syllables. In Japanese script and pronunciation, it is hardly possible to have several consonants following each other. In addition, a word is also not permitted to end with a consonant (the only exception is *n*). This means that either an *i* or an *u* are added between all of the consonants. Both of these rules come into play here. The following example is intended to clarify this phenomenon even more: When someone in Japan speaks about Christmas, it is called *kurisumasu*. This is the Japanese pronunciation for the English word "Christmas."

The pronunciation *kiriku* and the character 紇利 are in no way related to the pronunciation of *Sei heki* for the SHK Symbol and the character 正癖 for the pronunciation of the SHK Symbol. Without the appropriate explanation, it is therefore neither possible to draw a conclusion about the pronunciation of *Sei heki* nor can we draw conclusions about the symbol from *Sei heki*. Yet, mental healing with the SHK Symbol functions excellently, as long as it is done according to the rules of the art. As already mentioned by way of introduction, changing the form or completely modifying the pronunciation of a symbol **at a later point** in time leads to the symbol no longer functioning. Although Dr. Usui slightly changed the form and considerably modified the pronunciation, he did this before he integrated the SHK Symbol into Reiki. As part of this process, he used an ancient Taoist method of creating talisman symbols that had already been accepted into *Shingon* Buddhism at an early time in Japan. This guaranteed that the effect and function of the symbol remained the same and his students could use the symbol in very simple ways. When he decided to do this, it is very likely that he did not know what path Reiki would take after him, even though he had wished for the wisdom of the Reiki System to spread throughout the world to all people who are open to it, as we can read on his tombstone.

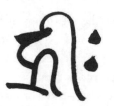

ILL. 119 – SIDDHAM HRIH

The Function and Effect of the SHK Symbol

In Reiki, the *main function* of the SHK Symbol is mental healing. In order to perform such a treatment effectively, not just any symbol can be used. It is necessary to use this specific *one*, which has been stored over the course of time on the mental level. It has the power to dissolve habitual patterns that have an unpleasant effect on people and can initiate a meaningful re-orientation that is based upon the here and now.

We can discover why the SHK Symbol in particular is especially well-suited for this if we analyze the original *Siddham* as it is described in the sutras. The SHK Symbol was originally the *Siddham* symbol *hrih*. Similar to the other *Siddham*, the SHK Symbol is composed of a number of individual *Siddham*. This can be compared with numbers, for instance: several individual numbers represent various individual qualities such as 1, 2, and 3. If we put these three together, we have a new number (123) with a completely different quality than those of the individual numbers from which the new figure has been created.

The SHK Symbol (*hrih*) can be broken down into the *Siddham ha, ra, i,* and *a.* Each individual *Siddham* has both a meaning of its very own and an individual, practical spiritual function. Taken together, the above-mentioned *Siddham* have the effect of dissolving attachments of the mind through so-called disruptive feelings such as envy, rage, jealousy, greed, and illusions. Related to the SHK, this means that the habits obstructing happiness, health, and contentment are healed.

Sign Analysis of the SHK Symbol (Hrih)

In the sûtra *Kongô chô kyô*, the meanings of the *Siddham* are explained. The monk *Kûkai* wrote additional explanatory commentaries on it. This indicates that it is necessary to break down the *Siddham* into their individual components and consider them separately from the compound form in order to gain a deeper understanding. The following section provides an analysis using the example of the SHK.

The Siddham Symbol Ha in the SHK Symbol

The syllable *ha* means "cause," but this is actually independent of cause and effect; correspondingly, this is an "unconditional" cause arising from the divine Free Will. As such, it is not subject to the law of karma in any way. At the same time, it is the spiritual basic characteristic of each individual being, which ultimately enters into existence through all of its unique characteristics in an act of the Creative Force's free will. The syllable *ha* corresponds with the element of air. In Sanskrit, the cause is explained by the opportunity and fate with the term *hetavah*. There are six forms of the cause. Five of them

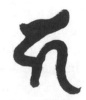

ILL. 120 – SIDDHAM HA

are conditional causes and can be explained as fate and/or effect. These are side effects, analogies, equivalents, movements of a complete unit, and outside. The sixth form of the cause describes the actual, divine cause of the creation, which is linked with the individual responsibility that is related to the free will of every human being. If the latter is recognized and integrated, this is a good precondition (cause) for a happy life. If we meditate on the syllable *ha*, the inner perception arises that all phenomena of the material world is based upon cause and effect.

The syllable *ha* is also a gateway to the perception that the final cause of things manifested is not visible because each cause resulted out of an additional cause and the chain ultimately "ends" in the unfathomable source of the creative force. This process is obviously infinite when we take a closer look at it. Expressed in different terms, nothing is created from an ultimate material cause in the temporal sense, but perhaps a cause that comes from the divine and cannot be located in time but outside of it. In keeping with its nature, life is an infinite process—without a beginning and without an end—that is just as infinite as it appropriately reflects the abstract potential of the divine in its state of oneness. This makes it understandable that only the use of the free will—which means unconditional decision in this sense of the word– is what connects a human being with the infinite flow of divine power. Consequently, fears, lust for power, envy, jealousy, and the like must be dissolved, which is done through meditation in most spiritual traditions in order to liberate the true self of the human being and make his divine legacy available to him. This obviously also means that a person must rise above the narrow boundaries of cultural values and standards in order to follow the divine law of life. In turn, this non-conditional state must be balanced through the relativization that consists of allocating it a place in the world, just like the conditionality. Unconditionally and conditionality are the yang and yin that are organized in their eternal changes through divine meaning in such a way that life comes into being, is maintained, and can develop.

In addition, *Kûkai* pointed out that the innumerable phenomena in the material world that have existed since time immemorial only arise from consciousness.[114] This consciousness is a knowledge in which the seeds of every form of existence are contained, meaning the infinite potential of the creative force in the state of oneness. The only thing that does not exist there is that can be considered to be the cause. This becomes clear through the meditation in the syllable circle of the *Siddham*. If we visualize the entire *Siddham* alphabet in succession, beginning with *a*, we eventually reach *ha* since this is the last sign. So we approach the absolute truth, the meaning of which is the lack of a beginning. The syllable *a* was born from the original unborn of all conditions. It is the spiritual potential that appears in the material world as an individual creation, which has not yet been influenced by any type of karmic resonance. Consequently, both syllables indicate the same thing. Although they are the farthest removed from each other, they are still very close to each other.

The Siddham Symbol Ra in the SHK Symbol

ILL. 121 – SIDDHAM RA

The syllable *ra* expresses purity and not being able to be touched by dirt and dust. In Esoteric Buddhism, *ra* represents the great heavenly fire (Jap.: *kadai*) from which everything is created.[115] This is differentiated into three types: the fire of anger, the fire of the will, and the fire of purification. All three are equally important for the healing of the mind. The Fire of Anger is the aggressive energy of the 1st Chakra that secures the will to exist in the material world. The Fire of the Will is not just limited to

[114] This is a fact that is also known to the modern science of quantum mechanics. More than a half a century ago, the physicist Schrödinger discovered that subatomic particles such as electrons only appear through the process of observation. This discovery became famous through the story of Schrödinger's cat. In the meantime, it has been frequently confirmed by the corresponding experiments. If you would like to find out more about this topic, please look in the chapter on "Spiritual Cosmology" and the Commentated Bibliography in the Appendix.

[115] There are interesting parallels in the Nordic mythology, which originates from the same cultural area as the *Vedas*. The rune teachings describe how the primordial ice was melted through the Divine Fire and the water that was created in this way was the precondition for the formation of things in the material world. In Chinese Qi Gong, this would be the essential Qi of the kidneys that then becomes the archetypal Water-Qi of the kidneys in the Hara (*Dan Tien*). Disseminated through the Small Energy Cycle (Server Vessel and Governor Vessel), it provides fresh life energy to all the other meridians.

the drive for survival. Other chakras are also resonating here, dependent upon which life theme is involved, but particularly the 3rd Chakra. In addition, this is about the self-responsible decision to change something and having enough power of endurance so that the new quality can also be manifested. Ultimately, this is the precondition for the fire of purification that transforms all of the energies detrimental to well-being by burning them or transforming them into something meaningful. The energy center that resonates with this is the 5th Chakra, the chakra of self-expression. Through the purification of the fire, these energies can go to where there is a greater need for them.

The Siddham Symbol Î in the SHK Symbol

The *Siddham î* consists of three circles that form a triangle together. As a trinity in a triangular form, they are the strongest. This is why they are inseparable from each other here. At the same time, this inseparability is the meaning of the syllable *î*. In Buddhism, this means the three

ILL. 122 – SIDDHAM Î

virtues of *hosshin, hannya,* and *gedatsu* from the sûtra *Nehan kyô* (Nirvana-Sûtra*).* They also simultaneously represent the Great Goddess, the Great God, and the Creative Force in their state of oneness.

Hosshin is the infinite abundance and scope of *Dainichi Nyorai's* teachings. It corresponds with the Creative Force.

Hannya has various levels of meaning and represents the qualities of the Great Goddess. *Hannya* originally stands for the intuitive wisdom through which all types of suffering, created by the delusions of the mind caught up in the ego, can be dissolved. In addition, it causes resonance with the life net of the Great Goddess[116]. On a deeper level, *hannya* is therefore also called the spiritual mother and teacher of all Buddhas. *Dainichi Nyorai* is the teacher of all Buddhas because the great radiant light *Daikômyô* shines from him as the Cosmic Buddha into the world in the form of the original, spiritual teaching. Both the masculine and the feminine aspects of *Dainichi Nyorai* are at work here On the one hand, he

---

[116] The life net of the Great Goddess is extensively explained in the chapter on Spiritual Cosmology.

gives birth (in his feminine aspect) to the wisdom of his spiritual mother Dai *Marishi Ten*, who encircles him with protection. On the other hand, he directs the absolute truth of wisdom into the right channels (in his masculine aspect) by means of the divine light.

Gedatsu is another word for meditation and corresponds with the Great God, the masculine aspect, since things are set in motion through meditation. Meditation is the means for freeing ourselves from the shackles of illusions and suffering by charging ourselves and orienting ourselves on the divine yang forces. These yang forces get the rigid material yin structure of human beings to flow again and give it the possibility of once again tuning into the divine order. As a result of meditation, we become conscious of things. Only then can they be autonomously processed and integrated with love, a deeply feminine quality.

The Siddham Symbol A in the SHK Symbol

The *a* is also contained in the above-described *ha*. *A* is the mother of all sounds and has three levels of meaning: being unborn, being empty/unlimited, and existing. When we meditate on the syllable *a*, we recognize the non-existence of everything that is conditioned by laws, meaning all manifestations in the material, individual existence.

ILL. 123 – SIDDHAM A

The syllable *a* is a gateway to all laws; it transcends them. This also corresponds with the Buddha consciousness, which contains the non-duality, the result of all laws and the law-regulated nature of all existence in the sense of the divine order that is manifested in the material creation.

Non-duality should not be equated with the unity of all things. Non-duality is the Primal Mother, the invisible goddess who creates the preconditions of manifestation from the Creative Force in the state of oneness. As a result, the syllable *a* is the most direct connection to the Creative Force. As a mantra, the syllable *a* is the key to every other spiritual form of power that appears in the manifested world. It is the root and the power source of every mantra. The famous *Gayatri* Mantra, which is taught in the higher training levels of Rainbow Reiki by means of initiation, refers to this mantra and its goddess, *Gayatri*. After the Primal Mother, whose worship since the beginning of time has been verified, the Great God and the Great Goddess assume the ultimate manifestation of the Creation. The Primal Mother is identical with the Cosmic or Divine Heart (*Dai-Kokoro*), which accepts the creation of the world and its beings from its endless love so that they may enjoy their existence in love and become acquainted with each other. In the chakra teachings, the mantra *a* is associated with the Heart Chakra as the focusing point of all the yin chakras (2nd, 4th, and 6th major chakras). Through the power of the 5th chakra, it creates a meaningful manifestation of a spiritual idea in the material form that corresponds with the Divine Order.

In other words, the syllable *a* is expressed in the unborn state of all laws and is therefore like the earth from which everything else develops. The cosmic order is therefore never apparent in nature. It is unfathomable, in the true sense of the word and can only be recognized indirectly on the basis of its effects.

The Effect of the SHK Symbol

In the *Shingon* School, there are special rituals of energy transmission, which are called *kaji*. They can be used to ward off misfortune and disease as described in the chapter on the DKM Symbol. This was also the method with which *Kûkai* was able to spread *Shingon* Buddhism for the protection of the state, initially at the court of the Tennô and then throughout all of Japan for the benefit of the people. Depending on what the attention of the mind is focused upon in this ritual, the effect is also the strongest in the place to which the most energy flows. This principle can be applied for many things in a meaningful and beneficial way without hurting others in the process. This is why there is an entire series of various *kaji*. Among others, these include the general energy transmission of *kaji kitô* and the energy transmission for healing the sick *byônin kaji*. In addition, the power of the light beings can also be transmitted to objects[117]. A popular method is energy transmission to sand *dosa kaji*. In Japan, this method is especially used in death rituals in order to make the path to the light easier for the deceased. It consists of transferring the power inherent to *Dainichi*

---

[117] Dr. Mikao Usui did this by, for example, charging quartz crystals with Reiki and giving them to certain patients so that they could support their healing at home by placing the stones on their bodies.

Nyorai's Dhâranî of the Great Light (*kômyô shingon*) to the sand, which is then sprinkled on the deceased before the cremation for an optimal effect. Among other things, the SHK Symbol is always necessary for this ritual. The book *The Best Reiki Techniques* by Walter Lübeck and Frank Arjava Petter describes a beautiful ritual for wish-fulfillment with sand that uses the principles explained in the above section.

It is also especially interesting to note that *kaji* can also be used on objects of everyday use such as the *mâlâ* for reciting mantras, incense sticks, or sacred water for strengthening their effects. The simplest method consists of just simply giving Reiki to these things. However, the symbols can also be used for doing a great many other useful things.

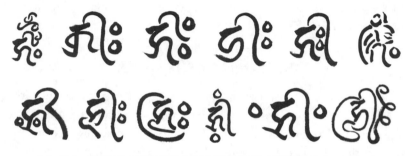

ILL. 124 – WRITING VARIATIONS FOR THE SHK SYMBOL (HRIH)

The SHK Symbol and HS Symbol in the Heart Sûtra

The Heart Sûtra in Transcription

Bussetsu Maka Hannya Haramita Shingyô

Kanjizai bosatsu, gyô jin hannya haramitta ji, shôken go´un kai ku, do issai kuyaku, sharishi, shiki fu i kû, kû fu i shiki, shiki soku ze kû, kû soku ze shiki, ju sô gyô shiki yakubu nyoze, sharishi, ze shôhô kûsô, fushô fumetsu, fuku fujô, fuzô fugen, zeko kû chû mu shiki mu ju sô gyô shiki, mu gen ni bi zesshin i, mu shiki shô kô mi soku hô, mu genkai, naishi mu ishikikai, mu mumyô, yaku mu mumyô jin naishi mu rôshi, yaku mu rôshi jin, mu ku shû metsu dô, mu chi yaku, mu toku, imu shotoku ko, bodai satta, e hannya hara mitta ko, shin mu kei ge, mu kei ge ko, mu u kufu, onri issai, ten dô mu sô, kûgyô nehan, sanze shobutsu, e hannya hara mitta ko, toku ano ku tara sanmyaku sanbodai, kochi hannya hara mitta, ze daijinshu, ze daimyôshu, ze mujôshu, ze mutôdôshu, nôjo issai ku, shinjitsu fu ko, ko setsu hannya hara mitta shu, soku sesshu wa´.

Gyatei, gyatei, hara gyatei, hara sô gyatei, boji sowaka.

Hannya hara mitta shingyô.

The Heart Sûtra in Chinese

ILL. 125 – THE HEART SÛTRA IN KÛKAI'S HANDWRITING

303

The Translation of the Heart Sûtra

Buddha's word, the Heart Sûtra of the great, perfected wisdom

If the Bodhisattva *Kannon* devotes himself to the deep practice of perfected wisdom, his Seeing will enlighten the five foundations of being to emptiness in this time and leads away from every type of suffering and evil.

O *Sharishi*. Form is nothing other than emptiness and emptiness is nothing other than form.[118] Form is the same as emptiness and emptiness is the same as form. It is the same with regard to perception, imagination, action, and thought.

O *Sharishi*. All teachings are forms of emptiness. They are not created and not obliterated. They are neither dirty nor are they pure. They do not increase nor do they dwindle. This is why there is no form, no perception, no imagination, no actions, and no thinking in the emptiness[119]; neither eyes, ears, nose, body, mind, nor sensual pleasures, sound, scent, taste, touch, and thought; no world of seeing and also no world of consciousness; there is no delusion and no end to the delusion, and also no aging and dying. But there is also no end to aging and dying—there is neither suffering nor the cause of suffering—no obliteration and also no path—there is no knowledge and attainment because there is nothing to attain.

The Bodhisattva rests in the wisdom that has been perfected. Because his heart is free of attachments, he has no fear. Free of all illusions, he enters into Nirvana for once and for all. All Buddhas of the past, the present, and the future who trust in the perfected wisdom achieve absolute enlightenment. This brings us to the insight that *Hannya hara mitta* embodies the magic formula of the Great Goddess—it is the magic formula of the Great Light—and is incomparable with other magic formulas. Since it is the pure truth, it has the power to take away all suffering. The magic formula for the perfected wisdom should be spoken like this:

Gyatei, gyatei, hara gyatei, hara sô gyatei, boji sowaka.

This is the Heart Sûtra of the perfected wisdom.

---

[118]   Compare this to the comments about the double nature of existence in the chapter on Spiritual Cosmology.

[119]   The Creative Force in the state of unity.

The HS and SHK and the Esoteric Meaning
of the Heart Sûtra

The Heart Sûtra is probably the shortest of all Buddhist sacred texts. It is among those that simultaneously make a statement and have a high degree of effectiveness. During my (Mark's) pilgrimages and many visits to temples in Japan, I frequently heard groups of Japanese reciting this sûtra. Something stirred within my Heart Chakra every time I heard it and it was always in the same part of the text. It is the essence of the Goddess of Great Compassion *Kannon*, who, as previously mentioned, is represented by the SHK Symbol.

How could it be otherwise since the Heart Sûtra plays an especially important role in Esoteric Buddhism and the monk *Kûkai* left the world a valuable commentary called *Hannya shingyô hiken* on this sûtra (Secret Key to the Heart Sûtra of the Perfected Wisdom). On the one hand, this was intended to make the sûtra easier to understand; and on the other hand, the secret keys—symbols—are revealed. In *Kûkai's* text, a type of interview also appears in which Kûkai answers various questions. I find the asking of questions and especially the responses given by *Kûkai* to be particularly interesting because I frequently hear the same questions today: "Why are the symbols, which are actually secret, now published in a book despite this fact? Isn't that a desecration of the symbols themselves?" *Kûkai's* response is very complex. Astonishingly enough, it is also appropriate for our current age. This is why both the question and the answer appear to be timeless while the contents of the books have slightly varied through the centuries. *Kûkai* responded: "In the teachings of Buddha, there were both the exoteric as well as the esoteric. For those who have opened themselves to the exoteric teachings, Buddha has spoken many explanatory words. For the people who have an understanding of the esoteric teachings, he provided symbols such as the *A* and the *Om*. The symbols had already been explained and published much earlier by the Indian monks and *Shingon* patriarchs *Nâgârjuna, Subhâkarasimha,* and *Amoghavajra*. Which manner of teaching a person prefers depends completely upon the type and extent of the individual student's resonance. Speaking and silence both belong to the intention of the historical *Buddha Shâkyamuni*."

Even in his preface to this text, Kûkai wrote that enlightenment rests in the heart of every person and just needs to be awakened with the right means. He points to the spiritual principle of personal responsibility within this context. It is up to each of us whether we turn toward the light or the darkness. With trust and practice, each of us can attain the light of truth.

Through the repeated reading, explaining, and revering of this sutra, we can attain joy. If we also meditate with this sûtra, we can attain enlightenment[120] and supernatural powers. In the same way as the *I Ching*, the Heart Sûtra contains the wealth of inexhaustible manifestations within it. The individual aspects of wisdom come to light at the right point in time.

---

[120] In Esoteric Buddhism, the types of enlightenment are differentiated. The last of these is spiritual awakening, as explained in the chapter on "What Is Enlightenment?" The first type of enlightenment (*Rigo-Jubutsu* = embodiment of reality) consists of recognizing that one's own Self and the Buddha (*Dainichi Nyorai*) have always been ONE in a perfect way and always will be. The ego exists here, but it is largely powerless. The second type (*Kaji-Jobutsu* = transmission of strength and response in the sense of the strength of the divine and the response of the only truth) is characterized by the complete destruction of the ego, and a mind that is totally peaceful and conscious in the sense of the divine perspective. The third type (*Kentoku-Jobutsu* = manifestation of what has been achieved) shows the respective person the great errors in the world, the false viewpoints and ways of life, the evil attitudes and behavior patterns. Through the infinite compassion with beings trapped in this cage of delusions, the spiritually awakened individual decides to participate in this world and help the others who are not awakened to attain his state of being. This state is the highest. It is the nature of the Bodhisattva and the foundation of the Bodhisattva vow that is unlimited in terms of its time and is effective in every incarnation once it has been taken. In Zen, the spiritually awakened is only considered to be perfect when he behaves in a completely natural way as a human being. If his behavior shows conspicuous features in which he lets others see that he has attained enlightenment, this is called *Goseki*, the Trace of Enlightenment. In colloquial speech, the Zen monks then say that he stinks of enlightenment. So this enlightenment is not integrated. It is not true enlightenment. Only when the enlightened person no longer makes a fuss about of his state and has integrated it into normal everyday life, and is capable of living a normal life, the integration is complete. However, in the practice the enlightened person is faced with challenges time and again in order to further integrate the enlightenment…

Depending upon how receptive we are each of us receives the wisdom that is appropriate for us at this moment.

The Heart Sûtra is not just a text with meanings and metaphors of everyday language but also a mandala of *Siddham* symbols with a gateway to mantric absorption. As in the HS Symbol, each sign is a symbol that bears the seeds of absolute truth within itself.

In the Heart Sûtra, the Goddess *Kannon* (SHK) represents everyone who becomes involved with the sûtra. *Kannon* helps the practitioner return to his or her natural origin. The actual light being who transmits the power here is the Boddhisattva *Hannya haramitta*. He embodies the absolute wisdom of the Buddhas, which is why she also bears the names "Mother of Wisdom" and "Mother of the Buddhas." The term "Wisdom Heart" (Jap.: *hannya shin*) in the title of the Heart Sûtra means that there are mantras for the body and also for the heart (the mind). So the Heart Sûtra is a great, powerful magic formula for the heart.

The Heart Sûtra can be divided into five parts. The five sections indicate a connection with the five-syllable HS Symbol that, like the Heart Sûtra itself, depicts a symbol mandala.[121]

The **first part** describes the teaching contents for the practitioner, which are expressed through the Goddess *Kannon* (SHK) here. It contains the five main points of cause, practice, enlightenment, Nirvana, and time. These five points result in the HS Symbol. The Goddess *Kannon*, who stands for the practitioner here, has always carried enlightenment within her heart—just as the practitioners do. With the mental healing and meditations with the SHK Symbol, which express the spirit of the practice in concrete terns, we can—as Dr. Usui mentioned time and again—return to the natural original state, which is enlightenment. Through this return to true being, the ability is developed to see things as they really are. This "seeing" is the knowledge of enlightenment. It leads beyond every type of suffering and evil. In other words, *Kannon* practices the wisdom and recognizes the emptiness of the five realms of existence: the physical appearance of all things in the world is sensed. Sensation leads to perception—perception leads to ideas—ideas lead to will—will leads to action—and action ultimately leads to consciousness.

[121] Cf. the chapter on the HS Symbol.

The **second part** discusses the essence of the teaching. As in the HS Symbol, this also consists of five aspects: establishment, separation, form, two, and one. The establishment means the teachings about the meditative absorption of truths related to the body (mudrâ), speech (mantra), and mind (*Samâdhi*) with which we create the fertile soil for enlightenment. The essence of the establishment is the all-wise Bodhisattva *Fugen*. He symbolizes both the teaching and the meditation practice in one. *Separation* corresponds with Wisdom Bodhisattva *Monju*, who rides on a lion and whose sharp flame sword frees the mind from the insight-inhibiting thoughts.[122] *Form* means the teaching of meditative absorption of the future Buddha, who at this time is still the Bodhisattva *Miroku*. Through him, the secret is revealed that all phenomenon and laws only exist in consciousness. *Miroku* is the provider of great joy. Time and again, he revokes the laws of cause and effect, as well as the differences between the form and the beings concealed behind it. He shows the pure areas of consciousness in their most natural state and separates it from the forms, the outer forms of manifestation. This dissolves the belief in the second self that has been created through the illusion of material existence—the ego. *Two* points to the two opinions: the first says that there is only phenomena, meaning nothing that truly exists in the psychosomatic realm. Of course, this completely negates the ego with its greed, fears, and worldly judgmental patterns; the second is the questioning of the patriarchal path to enlightenment that is hostile to the body and sensuality. *Kûkai* emphasizes at this point the importance of physical existence and sensuality as a path to true joy that represents a central cause of enlightenment and the subsequent spiritual awakening. *One* means the fruit of meditative absorption by the Goddess *Kannon*. *Kannon*, who is symbolic of the practitioners, shows human beings a path of purity that resembles a lotus blossom. The lotus blossom is pure and beautiful. It grows out of a dirty swamp. The swamp is the feeding ground for the pure and beautiful. The swamp is the world of suffering and the lotus blossom is great joy. As it grows out of the swamp, it leaves the dirt behind. In other words, this mean that as people move toward happiness, they let go of their suffering.

---

[122] In Western mysticism, this is done by the Archangel Michael with his sword of flames.

We can perceive the purity of the mind by looking at the lotus blossom in its purity. By looking at its fruit, we can also recognize the power of the heart that grows out of spiritual purity.[123]

The **third part** of the Heart Sûtra explains what the practitioner can achieve with the power of the Goddess *Kannon* (SHK). On the one hand, this is the path to be recognized and also the truth of cause, practice, Buddha-consciousness, and Nirvana to be recognized. Wisdom is the cause that leads to the ability to practice. Through practice, it is possible to purify the mind and let go of all obstacles. In turn, this awakens the Buddha-consciousness, which opens the gateway to Nirvana, the Creative Force in the state of oneness.

The **fourth part** provides an additional summary of the previous content. The mantras contain symbols that awaken insight and supernatural powers. This leads to the **fifth part**—the esoteric treasure—the mantra itself: *Gyatei gyatei hara-gyatei hara-sogyatei boji sowaka*[124]. As part of this, the five parts of the mantra are decoded. The first *gyatei* stands for the result of the practice and the second *gyatei* represents the Buddhas who have achieved enlightenment by themselves. *Hara-gyatei* indicates the highest goal (Beingness), *hara-sogyatei* describes the success of the completely realized *Shingon Mandala,* and *boji sowaka* is the access to highest enlightenment. The mantra removes the darkness of the mind. One single word has a thousand-fold meaning. To achieve inner peace, it helps to return to the natural origin. In truth, all beings are a whole, creative power, and infinity.

---

[123] There is also a beautiful parallel here in Western mysticism: The unicorn that places his head in the lap of the virgin of his own free will. In this sense, the virgin is not a woman who is sexually untouched or disinterested but a woman who is pure of heart because of her naturalness and freedom from prejudice. She does not use her sensuality because of fear or greed but is naturally completely in unity with this divine power that leads to oneness.

[124] This is the Japanese version. The one that is much more familiar in the Western world is the Indian: *Gate Gate Paragate Parasamgate Bodhi Svaha.* A rough translation of this is: "Gone, gone, gone across, gone across together. Oh, great awakening! Hail!" It is not difficult to recognize that the meaning of this mantras points to the Bodhisattva vow.

Practices with the SHK Symbol

The Hands in Esoteric Buddhism

Mudrâs, spiritual hand positions, play a central role in Esoteric Buddhism. But how did people actually come up with the individual gestures? For a better understanding of this approach, a type of esoteric map of both hands is provided below. They contain many types of zones that are on top of each other with various functions and meanings.

The diagrams and tables show that each hand is a mandala on its own, and both together represent perfection. The world mandala means "circle" and is intended to depict the cosmos in an abstract, simplified form with which magical rituals and healing can be performed. In order to use these hand-mandalas—how could it be otherwise—initiation and special symbols are necessary.

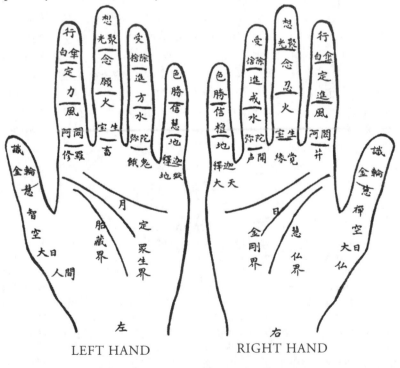

LEFT HAND   RIGHT HAND

ILL. 126 – CLASSIFICATION WITH THE HANDS

Area	Left Hand	Right hand
Thumb	識 Consciousness dependent upon VAKOG[125] 金輪 Golden world beneath the earth in the cosmology of Buddhism; the three karmas of body, speech, and mind 慧 Trust that strengthens the ability to make decisions and extinguishes doubt 智 Wisdom 空 Element of air 大日 *Dainichi Nyorai* 人間 Human realm	識 Consciousness dependent upon VAKOG 金輪 Golden world beneath the earth in the cosmology of Buddhism; the three karmas of body, speech, and mind 慧 Trust that strengthens the ability to make decisions and extinguishes doubt 禅 Meditation 空 Element of air 大日 *Dainichi Nyorai* 仏 Buddha
Index finger	行 Action: activity of the hears through practice 白傘 Wise aura of the moon 定力 Powers that can be attained through meditative absorption (practice) 風 Element of wind 阿 *Ashuku Nyorai* 修羅 Demon realm	行 Action: activity of the heart through practice 白傘 Wise aura of the sun 定進 Development and progress through meditative absorption (practice) 風 Element of wind 阿 *Ashuku Nyorai* 牟 Silent meditation
Middle finger	想 Visualization with VAK-OG, manifesting something in the mind 光聚 The light to be gathered 念願 Wish from the heart 火 Element of fire 宝生 *Hôshô Nyorai* 畜 Animal realm	想 Visualization with VAK-OG, manifesting something in the mind 光聚 The light to be gathered 念忍 Patience from the heart 火 Element of fire 宝生 *Hôshô Nyorai* 縁覚 Enlightenment by one's own efforts

[125]   V = visual, seeing; A = auditive, hearing; K = kinesthetic, the bodily sensation; O = olfactory, taste; G = smell.

311

Ring finger	受 Perception 捨除 To reject 進方 Methods and form 水 Element of water 阿弥陀 *Amida Nyorai* 餓鬼 Realm of the hungry ghosts	受 Perception 捨除 To reject 進戒 Rules and principles 水 Element of water 阿弥陀 *Amida Nyorai* 声聞 Enlightenment through listening to Buddha's teachings
Little Finger	色 Form 勝 Victory 信慧 Trust in wisdom 地 Element of earth 釈迦 *Shaka Nyorai* 地獄 Hell realms	色 Form 勝 Victory 信檀 Supporting the trust 地 Element of Earth 釈迦 *Shaka Nyorai* 大天 Gods and goddesses
Palm	月 Moon 定 Meditative absorption 胎蔵界 Womb World 衆生界 Human realm	日 Sun 慧 Understanding *Prajna*, trust, wisdom that strengthens the ability to make decisions and extinguishes doubt 金剛界 Diamond World 仏界 Buddha realm

Mandala Hand Ritual with Dai Marishi Ten, the Goddess of Light and Glory

The left hand forms a mandala of three circle-shaped zones. The fingers are the outermost circle. Here are the goddesses with the elements:

Finger	Element	Goddess
Thumb	Earth	Patani
Index finger	Water	Marani
Middle finger	Fire	Akarsani
Ring finger	Air	Narttesvari
Little finger	Ether	Padmajalini

The fingernails form the middle circle and represent the Buddhas to be invoked:

Finger	Buddha	Color	Symbols
Thumb	Amoghasiddhi	White	Om hah namah
Index finger	Dainichi Nyorai	Yellow	Hi swâhâ
Middle finger	Amida Nyorai	Red	Hum vausat
Ring finger	Ashuku Nyorai	Black	He hum hum hoh
Little Finger	Hôshô Nyorai	Green	Phat ham

Finally, the palm is the inner circle—a red lotus with the five petals of the goddesses:

Direction	Goddess	Color	Symbols
East	Yaminî	Black	Ham yom
North	Mohanî	White	Hrim mom
West	Sancalinî	Yellow	Hrem hrim
South	Santrasinî	Green	Ngam ngam
	Chandika	Gray	Phat phat

In the end, the Red Goddess Dai *Marishi Ten* with the two symbols *Om* and *Vam* is in the center of the lotus blossom.

Kannon also has various powers for granting protection. The best-known example on the *Saikoku* pilgrimage route is *Kannon* in *Okadera*. This mainly involves protection against harm in especially critical phrases of life (*yakudoshi*). In *Okadera*, a talisman (*fuda*) is preserved that was written by the *Kôken* Tennô (around 749-758) and the *Shôtoku* Tennô (764-770) as they prayed for lifetime protection against evil and harm.

Making a Talisman 1 (Dosa Kaji 土砂加持)
Transferring the Light of a Mantra to a Talisman

Select an object or material as a storage medium for making a talisman. Particularly suitable for this purpose are crystal quartz and healing stones that contain crystal quartz, as well as water, sand, and sugar. Here is a detailed description of the practice using the example of a crystal quartz.

*Connect with the Great Sun Buddha (Dainichi Nyorai) through the distant contact (HS Symbol plus its mantra three times, then the CR Symbol plus its mantra three times, and three times Dainichi Nyorai). Greet him with the words: "Dear Great Sun Buddha **Dainichi Nyorai,** I come to you as a sick person and request healing. I come to you as an ignorant person and request teaching. I come to you as someone who does not know the way and ask for protection and guidance. I come to you as someone who is helpless and ask you for power in order to better serve. As compensation, I send you Reiki. Please use it as you wish for the benefit of all." Then draw several CR symbols and activate each of them with the mantra for intensifying the Reiki flow of power.*

*

Take the crystal quartz in one hand and draw the SKH Symbol on it with the other hand. Activate it with its mantra and then a CR Symbol, which you must also activate. Now say: this crystal quartz – this crystal quartz – this crystal quartz.

Recite the Light Mantra (*Kômyô Shingon* 光明真言) 108 times while you hold the crystal quartz between your hands: *Om a bo kya bei ro sha na ma ka bo dara man i han doma jinba ra hara ba rita ya hûm.*

*

Give thanks and take leave from distant contact in the usual way. If necessary, ground[126] yourself for a few minutes by giving Reiki to the soles of your feet.

Translation of the Light Mantra: "*Om*—The great seal of the eternally shining perfect light is the symbol *Daikômyô* of *Dainichi Nyorai*. The virtue of all treasures, of the lotus, and of the bright shining light contains

---

[126] More detailed information on the topic of grounding can be found in the chapter on The Integration of Spiritual Experiences.

wisdom and talents within itself. We request that you, *Dainichi Nyorai*, realize the Buddha consciousness—the spirit of enlightenment within us."

Effect: The Light Mantra promotes the purification and development of the heart, even on the level of the light body. It cleanses traumatic experiences and dissolves karma. This leads to healing the causes of karmic diseases that could develop in this or the following lifetime. In addition, it promotes wisdom, love, and inner abundance, as well as a long, happy life.

Duration: The effect of the talismans made in this way is lost again after approx. 2 weeks. However, if you repeat this ritual for a total of three times at intervals of one each week, the Light Mantra will stay stored in it. Then it becomes a quality of this crystal and also cannot be erased anymore.

Making a Talisman 2 (Dosa Kaji 土砂加持) Power Transmission to Sand

Preparation: Take some clean crystal sand. This is normal sand like that at the beach or in a sandbox (ground crystal quartz). However, it should be very pure for the ritual. Large amounts can be purchased in building-supply stores and smaller amounts as bird sand in drug stores. The sand can remain in a container or bag during the rituals. Cleanse and activate the sand and container with Reiki, a Reiki Shower, the Rainbow Reiki Power Song *Hey loa kei loa*[127], or with the *Goddess Crystal Radionic Tool*.

Procedure: *Connect with the Great Sun Buddha (**Dainichi Nyorai**) through the distant contact (HS Symbol plus its mantra three times, CR Symbol plus its mantra three times, three times Dainichi Nyorai). Greet him with the words: "Dear Great Sun Buddha **Dainichi Nyorai**, I come to you as a sick person and request healing. I come to you as an ignorant person and request teaching. I come to you as someone who does not know the way and ask for protection and guidance. I come to you as someone who is helpless and ask you for power in order to better serve. As compensation, I send you Reiki. Please use it as you wish for the benefit of all." Then draw several CR symbols and activate each of them with the mantra for intensifying the Reiki flow of power.*

*

---

[127] See pg. 459.

Take the sand in one hand and draw a SHK Symbol with the other hand in the sand, activate it with its mantra, and then draw a CR Symbol, which you also need to active. Now say: this sand – this sand – this sand.

Recite the Light Mantra (*Kômyô Shingon* 光明真言) 108 times while you hold the sand between your hands: *Om a bo kya bei ro sha na ma ka bo dara man i han doma jinba ra hara ba rita ya hûm.*

*

Give thanks and take leave of the distant contact in your usual way. If necessary, ground yourself for several minutes by giving Reiki to the soles of your feet.

Application: Now you can do all kinds of useful things with this Light Mantra Sand: In Japan, it is scattered on the deceased before the cremation in order to ensure a good rebirth. However, it is also possible to scatter the sand in the open countryside or fill it into a container or brooch that you can wear on your chest for rituals at power places.

Effect: With the Light Mantra Sand, you bring *Dainichi Nyorai's* wish into the material world. The Light Mantra promotes the purification and development of the heart, even on the level of the Light Body. It helps resolve traumatic experiences and dissolve karma. The result is healing the causes of karmic diseases that could come in this lifetime or the following. In addition, it promotes wisdom, love, and inner abundance, as well as a long, happy life.

Duration: The effect of the talismans sand made in this way is lost again after approx. 2 weeks. However, if you repeat this ritual for a total of three times at intervals of one each week, the Light Mantra will stay stored in it. Then it becomes a quality of this crystal sand and also cannot be erased anymore.

SHK Meditation (1)
for the Purification and Healing of the Heart

Connect with the 1000-Armed Goddess of Great Compassion (Senju Kannon) through the distant contact (HS Symbol plus its mantra three times, the CR Symbol plus its mantra three times, three times Senju Kannon). Greet her with *the words: "Dear Goddess of Great Compassion **Senju Kannon,** I come to you as a sick person and request healing. I come to you as an ignorant person and request teaching. I come to you as someone who does not know the way and ask for protection and guidance. I come to you as someone who is helpless and ask you for power in order to better serve. As compensation, I send you Reiki. Please use it as you wish for the benefit of all." Then draw several CR symbols and activate each of them with the mantra for intensifying the Reiki flow of power.*

*

Hold your hands with the palms placed together, but with a distance of about 15 cm (5 inches) in front of the heart (as in the *Gasshô* meditation but at the distance of 15 cm (5 inches). Mentally draw a SHK Symbol between the hands and activate it by repeating its mantra three times. Maintain the visualization of the SHK Symbol the entire time. Imagine that bright radiant light from the SHK Symbol is streaming into your heart as you inhale. This light purifies your heart, dissolves knots, and fills your chest with increasingly more love with each breath you take. As you exhale, imagine how Reiki is flowing through your hands to the SHK and nourishes it, causing it to light up even more intensively with each exhalation.

While you slowly inhale and exhale in this way, recite the mantra *Om bazara tarama kiriku* 108 times or a multiple thereof.

Now imagine how the SHK Symbol dissolves in the light, which then flows into your heart. Leave your hands together (*Gasshô*) and continue to feel the spiritual power within you and around you for a few more minutes.

*

Give thanks and take leave from the distant contact in the usual way. If necessary, ground yourself for a few more minutes by giving Reiki to the soles of your feet.

SHK Meditation (2)

*Connect with the 1000-armed Goddess of Great Compassion (Senju Kannon) through the distant contact. Greet her with the words: "Dear Goddess of the Great Compassion **Senju Kannon,** I come to you as a sick person and request* *healing. I come to you as an ignorant person and request teaching. I come to you as someone who does not know the way and ask for protection and guidance. I come to you as someone who is helpless and ask you for power in order to better serve. As compensation, I send you Reiki. Please use it as you wish for the benefit of all." Then draw several CR symbols and activate each of them with the mantra for intensifying the Reiki power.*

*

Draw one SHK Symbol on the right hand and one on the left, and then activate each of them with the mantra. Place your hands on your heart and recite the mantra *Om bazara tarama kiriku* 108 times or a multiple thereof.

*

Continue to feel this for a while. Give thanks and take leave in the usual way from the distant contact.

Distant Healing with the Power of the 1000-Armed Goddess Senju Kannon

Connect with the 1000-armed[128] *Goddess of Great Compassion (Senju Kannon) through the distant contact. Greet her with the words: "Dear Goddess of the Great Compassion **Senju Kannon,** I come to you as a sick person and request healing. I come to you as an ignorant person and request teaching. I come to you as someone who does not know the way and ask for protection and guidance. I come to you as someone who is helpless and ask you for power in order to better serve. As compensation, I send you Reiki. Please use it as you wish for the benefit of all." Then draw several CR symbols and activate each of them with the mantra for intensifying the Reiki power.*

*

Place your hands in *Gasshô* (palms of your hands together) in front of your heart and visualize yourself as *Senju Kannon*. Imagine that you are a wonderful woman with 1000 arms. You hold one pair of hands in *Gasshô* in front of your heart. Another pair forms the Mudrâ of Meditation. To

---

[128] The 1000 arms represent her infinite power to help those who are suffering.

do this, place your hands in your lap beneath the navel. The right hand rests in the left, meaning that the fingers of the right hand are laid on top of the fingers of the left hand. The tips of the thumbs touch each other so that the front view is a triangle formed between the fingers. The other hands hold all of the symbols of purification that come to mind for you (for example: a broom, a sword, or a water pitcher). There are 10 additional heads on top of your head that look in all directions. Your body is empty on the inside.

Visualize how the SHK Symbol is created within your heart and activate it with its mantra. At the foot of the SHK Symbol, a CR Symbol now appears. Also activate this with its mantra.

Now use the distant contact to connect with the being that you would like to heal. Imagine how your 1000 arms are giving Reiki to this being. The SHK Symbol in your heart radiates purifying light through your 1000 arms into the being to be healed. As you do this, recite the mantra *Om bazara tarama kiriku* 108 times or a multiple thereof.

In closing, ground the being with two hands by giving Reiki to the soles of his or her feet. Take leave of the being from the distant contact in the usual way. Then imagine how your form of the 1000-armed *Kannon* dissolves in the light. This light now flows into the SHK Symbol in your heart. This is followed by the CR Symbol.

The SHK Symbol finally dissolves in the light and radiates into the entire cosmos. Continue to feel the spiritual power for a while.

*

Then give thanks and take leave from the distant contact in the usual way.

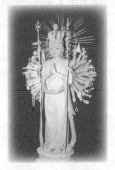

ILL. 127 – SENJU KANNON

319

Healing with the Power of Senju Kannon

*Connect with the 1000-armed Goddess of Great Compassion (Senju Kannon) through the distant contact. Greet her with the words: "Dear Goddess of Great Compassion **Senju Kannon,** I come to you as a sick person and request healing. I come to you as an ignorant person and request teaching. I come to you as someone who does not know the way and ask for protection and guidance. I come to you as someone who is helpless and ask you for power in order to better serve. As compensation, I send you Reiki. Please use it as you wish for the benefit of all." Then draw several CR symbols and activate each of them with the mantra for intensifying the Reiki power.*

*

Draw a SHK Symbol on your right hand and one on your left, and then activate each of them by saying its mantra three times. Place your hands in front of your heart with the palms together and recite the mantra *Om bazara tarama kiriku* seven times. Now ask the Goddess of Great Compassion for the healing of this being (add the name of client) on all levels. In addition, ask her to guide your hands.

Now give Reiki wherever your hands are led (this can be on the body and in the aura). As you do this, recite the mantra *Om bazara tarama kiriku.*

*

In conclusion, give thanks and take leave from the distant contact in the usual way.

Balancing and Purifying the Chakras with the SHK Symbol

*Connect with the 1000-armed Goddess of Great Compassion (**Senju Kannon**) through the distant contact. Greet her with the words: "Dear Goddess of Great Compassion **Senju Kannon,** I come to you as a sick person and request healing. I come to you as an ignorant person and request teaching. I come to you as someone who does not know the way and ask for protection and guidance. I come to you as someone who is helpless and ask you for power in order to better serve. As compensation, I send you Reiki. Please use it as you wish for the benefit of all." Then draw several CR symbols and activate each of them with the mantra for intensifying the Reiki power.*

Draw a SHK Symbol on the right hand and one on the left hand, and then activate each of them with its mantra. Hold your hands at a slight distance above the 1st and 6th Chakra. Draw a SHK Symbol above each of these chakras, and then activate each of them with its mantra. In addition, draw one CR Symbol above each of the chakras in order to strengthen the flow of power. Recite the mantra *Om bazara tarama kiriku* 108 times.

Hold your hands at a slight distance above the 2nd and 5th Chakra. Draw a SHK Symbol above each of these chakras, and then activate each of them with its mantra. In addition, draw one CR Symbol above each of the chakras in order to strengthen the flow of the power. Recite the mantra *Om bazara tarama kiriku* 108 times.

Hold your hands at a slight distance above the 3rd and 4th Chakra. Draw a SHK Symbol above each of these chakras, and then activate each of them with its mantra. In addition, draw one CR Symbol above each of the chakras in order to strengthen the flow of the power. Recite the mantra *Om bazara tarama kiriku* 108 times.

*

Do the aura cleansing technique. In conclusion, give thanks and take leave from the distant contact in the usual way.

Moon Meditation with the SHK Symbol

When the moon is full, go to a place where you can easily see it.

*

Connect with the 1000-armed Goddess of Great Compassion (Senju Kannon) through the distant contact. Greet her with the words: "Dear Goddess of Great Compassion **Senju Kannon,** *I come to you as a sick person and request healing. I come to you as an ignorant person and request teaching. I come to you as someone who does not know the way and ask for protection and guidance. I come to you as someone who is helpless and ask you for power in order to better serve. As compensation, I send you Reiki. Please use it as you wish for the benefit of all." Then draw several CR symbols and activate each of them with the mantra for intensifying the Reiki power.*

*

In your mind's eye, draw a SHK Symbol on the moon until it completely fills it, and then activate it with its mantra. While you continue to look at the moon, constantly visualize the SHK Symbol and recite the mantra *Om bazara tarama kiriku* 108 times or a multiple thereof.

Hold your hands upward in a receptive position. As you inhale, imagine that the moon energy is radiating into you through your hands and your Crown Chakra from the SHK in the moon. As you exhale, you give the SHK in the moon your healing energy by allowing a ray of light from your heart to shine to the SHK in the moon. This is a form of *Kaji* (energy transmission).

*

Now give thanks and take leave from the distant contact in the usual way. If necessary, ground yourself for a few minutes by giving Reiki to the soles of your feet.

CHAPTER 15

The HS Symbol

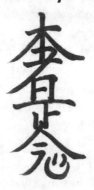

ILL. 128 – THE HS SYMBOL

The Pronunciation of the HS Symbol

With its traditional Japanese spelling, the HS Symbol is probably the most complex of all four Reiki symbols[129]. In more precise terms, this is a conglomerate of five compounded Chinese characters. Japan originally had no script of its own. Since the introduction to Buddhism in the year 538 and the following centuries, Japan assumed the Chinese script with its many thousands of signs and applied it to its own Japanese language. These Chinese signs are called *Kanji* (漢字) in Japanese, which means something like the "signs of the *Han*." *Han* was actually the name for China during the *Han* period (206 B.C. to 220 A.D.), but this means China in general. *Kanji* is the Sino-Japanese (Chinese-Japanese) pronunciation for the Chinese word *hanzi* (漢字), which has the same meaning and is written in the same way.

The introduction of the script soon made it possible for the Japanese to write their own Chinese texts and read the imported literature from China. However, a great deal of additional effort was required in order to integrate the *Kanji* into the Japanese language. Other than in the Western

[129] The SH Symbol illustrated above corresponds with the way that Hawayo Takata wrote it.

323

alphabet, each *Kanji* is already a word, and combinations of this sign continually result in new words. Since the Japanese had their own language and words with the same meanings in the form of characters (*Kanji*) were introduced from China, the *Kanji* were assigned a pure Japanese reading (i.e. pronunciation) in addition to the Chinese. Since the Chinese pronunciation has changed in the course of the centuries and the *Kanji* were frequently also imported again to Japan in a number of batches, there were soon *Kanji* with several different Chinese readings. Not only is the pronunciation different from time to time but there are also variations dependent on the topic. This means, for example, that identical *Kanji* are read differently in the Buddhist context than in the Confucian.

This is also apparent in the Reiki Principles of Dr. Usui. One of these rules reads as follows in Japanese: 今日だけは業に励め. Dr. Usui was also kind enough to leave us the pronunciation of this sign. In transcription, this sentence is: *Kyô dake wa gô ni hageme*. Because the *Kanji* 業 is read here as *gô* and not as *gyô*, as in modern Japanese, it is a Buddhist reading and also has a Buddhist meaning. This is why it is possible to see the principle of "Just for today, work hard" within the Buddhist context. Here, 業 actually means "karma" (the law of cause and effect) instead of work: Just for today, work hard on your karma[130].

---

[130] Karma is defined as the spiritual law of causes and effect. For the most part, this should be understood in a very practical sense. For example, when I want to build a house I may partially finance it with a mortgage. In order to do this, I may pay interest and reimbursement fees. This means that I have a—karmic—obligation for many years that binds me on the one hand but opens up beautiful, useful opportunities on the other hand that would not be available without the house. Since, in accordance with the spiritual law of "As above, so below. As within, so without." every action is reflected both inside and outside of the person taking the action, good acts in the sense of the divine order create meaningful, healthy, useful, and high-frequency structures within and outside of a human being—negative acts in the sense of the divine order obviously create structures that have disharmonious and negative effects. Karma is not inescapable. It can also be influenced, transformed, and dissolved by the spiritual practices such as Dr. Usui's *Gassho* Meditation, Zen, or the Three-Ray Meditation in combination with the respective actions and insights that contribute to a constructive reorientation of thinking. A mortgage, for example, can be prematurely terminated when the house is sold or if the person inherits a large sum of money or wins the lottery. Then the related obligations do no longer apply.

Related to the HS Symbol, this means that we can draw many conclusions about the meaning of the sign on the basis of its pronunciation. The HS Symbol is made of five *Kanji* and is read as *Hon sha ze shô nen*. The little roof above the *ô* of *shô* means that this *Kanji* is read with a long *o* (as in "boat"). The other syllables are all pronounced short (as in "golf").

Although the third *Kanji* by the name of *ze* is written in the transcription with "z," it is pronounced like a soft "s." Incidentally, the same also applies to the word "Zen" meditation. The correct pronunciation is *sen* and not a hard "z." No Japanese person will understand it if someone speaks of *Sen* Buddhism.

Based on the pronunciation of the last two signs, which result in the word *shônen* when used together, it is recognizable as a Buddhist-influenced word here. The pronunciation of the overall symbol is also Buddhist because the signs are pronounced as in the mantras and sutras. This way of reading the signs is called "stick reading" (Jap.: *bô yomi* 棒読み) since the sign is read in one go as in Chinese but with a Sino-Japanese pronunciation. If the HS Symbol was read as if in a Japanese sentence, the pronunciation would be completely different. But the way it is read not only provides insights about the meaning but also the purpose and use, which will be explained in more detail below.

Each individual *Kanji* is just a sign with one or more meanings. If, in addition to the known readings, we look at the additional readings, the spectrum of possible meanings also expands correspondingly.

This sign becomes a mantra only in the order shown here and with the correct pronunciation. Through the systematic and ritual combinations of the signs, they become a talisman[131] or an amulet. Without initiation into the symbols and mantras, no one can achieve an effect by doing this as energy work. Then these are just a mixture of signs, ink on paper and any people think it's an artwork like the one of Nichiren.[132]

---

[131] In a magical way, a talisman attracts good effects of various qualities, depending upon the "attitude" of the talisman. An amulet protects against specific negative effects or experiences.

[132] Also see the chapter on Symbols and Mantras as Tools for Spiritual Energy Work.

The Characters Concealed in the HS Symbol and Their Meaning

On the basis of the pronunciation *Hon sha ze shô nen*, we can conclude that five *Kanji* are concealed in the HS Symbol. A more precise analysis and the help of a sign lexicon reveals the appropriate pronunciation of the five *Kanji* (本 *hon*, 者 *sha*, 是 *ze*, 正 *shô*, 念 *nen*).

I (Mark) know many people who study the Reiki symbols and have come across these five signs on their own with the help of reference works. This is obviously quite an achievement for someone who does not speak the Japanese language. So I congratulate anyone who has already done this detective work on his own from the bottom of my heart. However, this is precisely where a major trap occurs that has been a headache for me for a long time. Since the individual characters have more than one meaning, it is very difficult to come up with a meaningful translation without interpreting something into the symbol that is not there or does not pertain to the meaning. Here is a list of meanings that can be found in most dictionaries.

本 *hon*	book, basis, root, origin, true
者 *sha*	person, human being
是 *ze*	this, correct, being
正 *shô*	correct, improve
念 *nen*	sense, meaning, feeling, wish

How many possibilities are there when we attempt to combine the meanings of the words with each other in such a way that a sensible sentence is created? Can we really say that one of them is the right one? It becomes obvious that this approach is more difficult than it first appears to be. It is also completely correct; unfortunately, things are actually not that simple. Interpreting new meanings into the symbols and creating interpretations of them is like a lottery and tends to lead away from the original meaning of the HS Symbol.

The following interpretation is initially just based upon the existing material. To do this, it is absolutely necessary to examine whether the individual signs can also be translated as single words or whether these are word combinations. The last two signs— *shô* 正 and *nen* 念—are actually a sign combination, which means that they result in a word together.

In addition, it is important to see whether this is an entire sentence with a grammatical structure. If there is a sentence structure, then we must find out whether this sentence is actually Japanese or Chinese. Since all five signs are *Kanji*, which means it consists solely of Chinese characters, there is a high probability that this is a Chinese sentence. If the HS Symbol was Japanese, signs from the Japanese script systems *katakana* and *hiragana* would then also appear here.[133] Yet, this does not necessarily mean that the HS Symbol was created in China. This is what I initially assumed, especially on the basis of the Buddhist pronunciation. I also thought that the HS Symbol could be found in the Buddhist sutras, but have unfortunately been unable to find it there up to now. On the other hand, the DKM Symbol appears countless times in them. Of course, it is possible on a purely theoretical basis that the HS Symbol appears in another Chinese text such as those of Taoism or Confucianism. Yet, although these are good reasons it would still not be adequate evidence that the HS Symbol is Chinese.

But this has been suspenseful long enough: Although the HS Symbol is Chinese, it was created in Japan. The inventor of this symbol was Dr. Usui himself. He created this symbol according to special criteria in order to provide help to his students in freeing themselves from time and space in their Reiki energy work; in other words, to make distant healing considerably easier for them and to make it more reliable, safe, effective, and simple to use.

Now that we know the background, the following section will explore the significance of the HS. This includes the various levels of its meaning since the HS Symbol contains a great deal of knowledge and wisdom in a condensed form. We will also explore its creation, which is the method by which Dr. Usui was able to invent such an effective symbol.

---

[133] Cf. the history of how script was developed in the chapter on Calligraphy.

The HS Symbol– a Chinese Sentence

The subject always comes before the predicate in Chinese and Japanese. However, the predicate can also be an adjective or noun instead of a verb. This is why it sometimes looks like the verb is missing or a series of nouns follow each other. In the HS Symbol, both of these situations seem to be the case. Anyone unfamiliar with the characters and the classic Chinese language will not find the verb in any of the positions. When the verb is formed by a noun, the auxiliary verb "to be" is not necessary. There is a very well-known example of this in the *Lunyu*, the Words of Confucius. One day, when Confucius was asked how he would rule a state, he responded: 君君臣臣父父子子 (literally: The nobleman is the nobleman, the subject is the subject, the father is the father, and the son is the son.) But this literal translation is only possible when we know that a verb is not required between the nouns. Otherwise, this sentence would say: "Nobleman nobleman subject subject father father son son," which has little meaning to it. Here is an example of a more elegant translation into English: "The nobleman acts in a way befitting to a nobleman, the subject acts in a way befitting to a subject, the father acts in a way befitting to a father, and the son in a way befitting to a son." So this is a sentence in which the verb is missing for the Western reader because only the nouns are strung together. However, the verb results on its own in classic Chinese. In the HS Symbol, exactly the same thing applies to the *Kanji* 本者是正念. Because of this alone, a meaningful and correct translation is not possible without the necessary knowledge.

Since about the 3rd Century, the third *Kanji* of the HS Symbols *ze* 是 has been used like the auxiliary verb "to be" under the influence of Japanese colloquial language. In Japanese, this is originally a demonstrative pronoun with the pronunciation of *kore* or *kono* and means "this." In many Japanese kitchens today, the following Chinese saying can be found as a calligraphy: 日日是好日. This literally means: "Day day this good day. We can translate it accordingly as: "Every day is a good day." The sign for day, which appears here three times, is the same as in *Dainichi Nyorai* 大日如来 and can also mean "sun." But here it means "day" because this is how this sentence has been interpreted in Japan for many centuries:

that every day we should be content with what we have. In simple terms, this is an essential summary of the Reiki Principles.

Since the third character of *ze* 是 also corresponds with the HS Symbol's verb "to be," the following construction can be assumed from it: "*Honsha* is *shônen.*" On the basis of the Buddhist pronunciation of the HS Symbol, the last two signs *shô* and *nen* mean a word that is summarized to mean the "Buddha consciousness." I use the word "summarized" because there are entire treatises on just the meaning of the spiritual term *shônen.*

A possible and meaningful translation would then be: "The true (in the sense of spiritual) human being is not separated from Buddha consciousness."

Within this context, the Buddhist concept of the "ten-thousand things in the universe" (*banyû* 万有) is also mentioned. This expresses that space—the universe—connects the beings instead of separating them, as is frequently assumed. The realized mind (in Japanese, this is the heart—*kokoro*) knows this state, as well as the origin of all things. In this case, *Honsha* (the true human being) can also be translated with the "origin of the human being" in this case on the basis of the *Kanji* and how they are combined. The translation would then be: "The origin of the human being is not far removed from Buddha consciousness." This is very reminiscent of a sentence that was used by Dr. Usui and Dr. Hayashi within the scope of the Reiki mental healing: "Human being, Crown of Creation, stop ... (the name of the problems) and return to your natural, normal state." This means that this sentence used by Dr. Usui offers an explanation of the HS Symbol. At the same time, this is an exhortation with which Dr. Usui wanted to aid his students in attaining the awareness that illumination lies directly at their feet. The Crown of Creation is not mentioned directly in the *Kanji* of the HS Symbol. This is probably an allusion to the Buddhist way of thinking that only beings reborn as humans can achieve enlightenment in this existence.[134] Animals, for example, cannot do this because they do not have the possibility of dealing with the mind and acting out

---

[134]   There are six realms of existence in Buddhism: the hell realms, the realms of the hungry ghosts, the animals, the human beings, the demigods, and the gods.

of individual responsibility—key word: free will—and consciously with wisdom and lovingly with compassion.

However, based on the shamanic perspective and my personal experience, this situation is completely different because there are animals that are known to act in a very spiritual, conscious manner. For example, they may accompany special people as familiars, support them on their path, and have healing powers, great compassion, as well as the capacity to impart deep wisdom. Anyone who does this and uses strong means such as the esoteric teachings (*mikkyô*), can be released from *Samsâra*, the eternal cycle of death and rebirth and attain complete enlightenment. This is not possible in the purgatory realms because the beings there are so caught up in suffering that they no longer think of anything else. This situation is similar for the hunger ghosts since they are never satisfied because of their overly large bellies and very thin throats and are always greedily searching for something edible. If they should find something, it immediately turns into fire or something else that cannot be consumed. According to Buddhist teaching, the animals tend to be ruled by their instincts. The demigods are much too caught up in their competitive mentality and think only of themselves. The gods[135] are so occupied with the joys that it does not occur to them to be concerned with the mind, let alone do something good for others. However, this also does not correspond with my experience in dealing with light beings. The statements about the purgatory realms and the hungry ghosts should be understood symbolically—as the levels of a being's consciousness. They do not exist in the literal sense.

In the figurative sense, all of the levels listed here can also be observed on the earth. This reflects the law of cause and effect (karma). Dr. Usui wanted to illustrate this correlation for his students with the sentence "Human being, Crown of Creation, return to your natural state" and with the HS Symbol.

---

[135]   In more precise terms, the type of gods described here are not subtle beings (light beings) with divine qualities but incarnations in another level of existence (dimension) that is also limited in its properties. At some point, their lifetime also comes to an end and then they are reborn—for example, on the earth—when the good karma has been used up.

The Origin of the Kanji in the HS Symbol and Its Mystical Background

When each of the five characters of the HS Symbol are decoded, its meaning can be grasped on even deeper levels. To make this easier to understand, the following is an explanation of where each individual sign came from—how they were created. In this process, the individual signs are not *arbitrarily* divided into individual components but analyzed according to the explanations of the signs *in relation to their creation and meaning* in very comprehensive Japanese and Chinese reference works that have been written for such purposes. Some of these have been renowned in their use by experts for centuries. This is important to mention because it sometimes seems that the individual signs could also be deciphered in other ways, but this could deviate from the actual history of the sign's origin based on the information in the reference works.

The Chinese Character Hon 本

The *hon* 本 is a combination between the sign for tree 木 and the number One 一.

ILL. 129 – KANJI— ORIGIN FOR TREE 朿 ˙ 朿	The upper part corresponds with the crown, the middle with the trunk, and the lower part with the roots. In the present-day sign, the horizontal stroke is the ground. Beneath it we see the roots and above the earth just the trunk.	ILL. 130 – KANJI— ORIGIN FOR THE NUMBER ONE ― ˙ ―	There is not much to say about the emergence of the number One. It solely corresponds to a horizontal stroke. In the number Two (二), there are then two strokes and the number Three (三) has three.

Adding the number One to the roots of the tree makes them strong and thick. Solid roots are the basis for a tree so it does not fall over during the next gust of wind. The same applies to other areas as well. Without a strong foundation, whatever we build upon it will not last. This is why *hon* 本 is also translated as "basis" or "foundation" and used in corresponding word combinations. The tree is associated with the *element of wood*.

Meanings of the Kanji Hon 本

In addition to the derivation of *hon* 本, this *Kanji* has an entire series of other meanings that cannot always be expressed with one word:

The focal point of all things

Beginning, origin, and basis

Original, fundamental

Unique, the thing in itself, the essence

True

Writings such as books

Word for a unit used in counting long objects

Readings of the Kanji 本

Sino-Japanese[136]: *hon, bon*

Japanese[137]: *moto, hajime*

Japanese names[138]: *nari, hajime, moto*

I Ching Classification ䷳

The corresponding hexagram of the ancient Chinese oracle and wisdom book I Ching is No. 52, Gen 艮, Keeping Still, Mountain.

Word Combinations

Depending upon in which combination the sign *hon* 本 appears, the quality of its content also changes. For example, Japan is known as the "Land of the Rising Sun." This is based upon the old name of *Hi izuru kuni* 日

---

[136] This is the Sino-Japanese pronunciation, which means the Chinese pronunciation in Japan. In the classic or modern Chinese, the *Kanji* are pronounced differently.

[137] The pure Japanese pronunciation that is given to a *Kanji*.

[138] The *Kanji* may have a reading of their own in names.

出ずる国. However, Japan is now called *Nihon* or *Nippon* 日本, which combines the sign for "sun" and "basis." The sun rises very far in the east at the basis of the earth and this is where Japan is located.

As a comparison, here are also the explanations of the Reiki character: The sign *rei* 靈 gives the energy *ki* 氣 the special quality. This makes it difficult to decide which meaning an individual sign has that stands alone. Under the ideal circumstances, the sought-after sign combination can be found in a dictionary. Unfortunately, this is frequently—as also here in the case of the *hon* 本 of the HS Symbol—not possible. As in the character for *Reiki,* it is only through combinations of other signs with the sign *hon* that we can actually correctly grasp the intended meaning and the possible range of intended meanings.

Two important, revealing sign combinations for the spiritual understanding of the *hon* will be extensively explained.

本門 *Honmon* means "main gateway"

The gateway refers to a teaching or a teaching system as the access to true understanding and liberation. The *honmon* teaching explains the original state of a being, that all beings are actually Buddhas but they do not know it in most cases. This is also a reason why *Kûkai* was firmly convinced that every human being could attain enlightenment in this life and this body. The original state is equated with the "natural state," of which Dr. Usui spoke and to which we should return. This correlation is also explained in the second half of the Lotus Sûtra. In contrast to this, the first half of the *Shakumon,* which means something like "the Gateway of the Tracks" or unreal manifestations. *Shakumon* therefore generally teaches *Mahâyâna* Buddhism and *honmon* goes further and brings all beings to enlightenment.

本覚 *Hongaku* means "original perception"

The original understanding is related to the heart nature of all living things, which means the principle of true reality that is identical with the *Dharmakâya*[139] of the Buddha. This state is symbolically embodied by *Dainichi Nyorai.*

---

[139]   *Dharmakâya* is the absolute nature of the Buddha consciousness. It cannot be grasped in words or things. It is the highest spiritual wisdom that incorporates all perfection within itself.

Related to the HS Symbol, this means that the next character after *hon* 本 must be something natural to which we should return in order to liberate ourselves of time and space. The HS Symbol makes it possible for us to enter into this state during its use for a limited time with one part of our being. This is necessary until we no longer need the HS Symbol because the personal direct understanding and the ability to take action in terms of spiritual powers have developed in an appropriately extensive and detailed way. Dr. Usui personally created the HS Symbol in order to make it easy for his students to do distant healing—among many other fine things. But he probably did not use the symbol very often, at least not for distant healing, since he had already returned to his natural state, his Buddha nature, in his human body during his lifetime. So he also achieved what is actually the highest goal in Esoteric Buddhism according to *Kûkai*.

The Chinese Character Sha 者

Sha 者 primarily means "person." However, this is not the character for human being. There are other *Kanji* for this such as the two people 人 in the *rei* 靈 of Reiki. Instead, this is an active person who is doing or performing something,

Sha 者 is mostly used to emphasize something. An appropriate example for this is *konsha* 今者. In modern Japanese, this term is *ima wa* 今は and means "right now." This has a parallel to Dr. Usui's Principles, which always begin with the structure of doing something "just for today." In Japanese, *kyô dake wa* is called 今日だけは. Here as well, the last syllable *wa* corresponds in its meaning with the *sha* 者. Consequently, the *hon* 本 represents emphasizing the original state. In order to achieve this, we can take various paths. One of them is Reiki. Therefore, the Principles are a powerful tool for becoming increasingly aware on the path of the hearts—Reiki—of our own "natural state."

In the sign *sha* 者, the sign "earth" for the element of earth 土 is above and the sign "sun" 日 for the element of the heavenly fire is below.[140]

---

[140] If we speak of the five elements by themselves, other *kanji* are used. However, this is not about the character for an element but the element inherent to the character.

Since the earth and sun appear in one sign, this is an equivalent to the Mandalas of the Two Worlds, which describe the transcendental Buddha *Dainichi Nyorai*, the spiritual light beings, and the entire Creation from the spiritual perspective. As in *hon* 本, the *sha* 者 is not a composite sign. This becomes clear in the development of the *sha* 者.

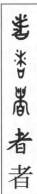

The origins of *sha* 者 can be traced back to the burning of firewood on a hearth, which means that this sign is associated with the element of fire. In order to kindle the heavenly fire here on earth, the power of the sun and of the earth are necessary. This is also the reason why both the earth and the sun appear in *sha* 者. Depending on the spelling, a comma-like slash can be added above the 日, as in the illustration.

ILL. 131 – ORIGIN FOR THE KANJI SHA

Meanings of the Sha 者
A person, a being, a group of people
Someone who does something
This
At the end of a sentence to express something in a commanding tone

Readings of Sha 者
Sino-Japanese: *sha*
Japanese: *mono, koto*
Japanese names: *hisa, hito*

Word Combinations with Sha 者
There are very few word combinations with *sha* 者 that are not related in any way to the HS Symbol.

I Ching Classification ䷝
The corresponding hexagram of the ancient Chinese oracle and wisdom book I Ching is No. 30, Li 離, The Clinging/Fire.

The Chinese Character Ze 是

This sign primarily means "this" in Japanese. First of all, "this" means exactly what is closest to a person. The *ze* 是 has many similarities with the character for foot (*ashi* 足). Since our feet are closest to the earth, this sign is associated with the element of earth.[141]

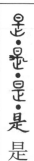 The explanation of this sign may sound a bit unusual, but according to the clarifications found in various sign dictionaries this involves a spoon that has been straightened. With the foot, we can move the earth in an upward direction. The human foot (in Eastern Asia, the foot and the leg are the same) is bent—it is something like a shovel or spoon. A foot that has been straightened to be a tool is the equivalent of a spoon with which we can pick up something that is close—soil.

ILL. 132 – ORIGIN FOR THE KANJI ZE

Meanings of Ze 是

Is used to indicate something that has a connection in the sense of: this
Is used to emphasize something
Expression of agreement, confirmation, affirmation
Proper goal, right course.

Readings of Ze 是

Sino-Japanese: *ze*
Japanese: *kore, kono, ko*
Japanese names: *kore, sunao, tadashi, tsuna, yuki, yoshi*

I Ching Classification ䷼

The corresponding hexagram of the ancient Chinese oracle and wisdom book I Ching is No. 61, *Chung Fu* 中孚, The Inner truth.

---

[141]   In case this appears to be a bit far-fetched, please remember that in Eastern Asia the attention is frequently focused upon areas that are considered less important by people in the West. For example, the color white—the areas left empty—plays a very important role in the painting of Eastern Asia and gives pictures a very special atmosphere. This is why it sometimes appears that we have to think around the corner. This is a case of other countries, other perspectives, other customs, and different ways of thinking...

For a Deeper Understanding of Important Word Combinations with Ze 是

是正 *Zesei* To Set Something Straight

The sign combination of *ze sei* 是正 within the HS Symbol leads to a different interpretation than the translation of the entire symbol: "The Buddha consciousness is attained through the correction of the wishes/ideas." This interpretation is not possible in the Takata lineage because its pronunciation of the symbol is *Hon sha ze sho nen* and not *Hon sha ze sei nen*. In the Japanese pronunciation, this pronunciation may be changed when, for example, several consonants follow each other (*hon sha* becomes *honja*). In this case, the meaning remains the same. However, if the individual *Kanji* are combined differently, this changes not only the pronunciation but also the translation.

是非 *Zehi* Absolutely

This is a joining of the affirmation and the negation. Originally, it meant something like "no matter whether it is right or wrong, this is how it was meant to be," which then was shortened into "absolutely."

The Chinese Character Shô 正

Shô 正 primarily means "correct." As a verb, it means "to correct" or "to bend straighten" or "adapt."

Shô 正 is composed of the sign for the number One 一 (*ichi*) and the verb stop 止. "Stop" means this verb, at least for today. This was originally also a sign for "foot" and shows that someone is moving straight forward on a line, described by the *Kanji* for the number One. This is why there is also a trace of sincerity contained in the meaning.

ILL. 133 – ORIGIN FOR THE KANJI SHÔ

Walking "straight" on the path in the "right" way means acting for the highest good of everyone involved—taking the golden path. In this sense, the *shô* 正 is connected with the element of metal. Incidentally, the terms for "metal" and "gold" have the same character. In addition, *shô* 正 has a close relationship with the third *Kanji* in the HS Symbol, the *Ze* 是. The sun 日 in the upper part of the sign, which represents *Dainichi Nyorai*, melts the metal of the earth, which makes it possible to bend it straight. This resembles the principle of personality development, which is influenced in an especially beneficial way through Reiki.

In Japan, it is also customary to use *shô* 正 for counting (for example: when including things in a list) from one to five. While in the West four vertical strokes that are crossed by a horizontal line amount to five, in Japan it is the *Kanji shô* 正. This makes the number five complete as a unit. If a stroke is missing, the sign is not complete and also not correct.

Readings of Sho 正

Sino-Japanese: *shô, sei*

Japanese: *tadashii, tadasu, mato, masa ni, masashiku, kami*

Japanese names: *akira, osa, kami, kimi, sada, taka, tada, tadashi, tadasu, tsura, nao, nobu, masa, masashi, yoshi*

I Ching Classification ䷹
The corresponding hexagram of the ancient Chinese oracle and wisdom book I Ching is No. 58, *Tui* 兌, The Joyous/Lake.

The Chinese Character Nen 念

Nen 念 has an entire series of meanings. It primarily involves the perception of a "feeling" or "mood." Other meanings are "attention" or "wish" and "desire." Depending upon the context in which *nen* 念 is used, the meaning also changes.

The *Kanji nen* 念 is composed of an upper and a lower part. Both can also be used as individual signs independent of each other. Because this is a combination of words, there is no graphic depiction for the origin of *nen* 念 alone.

The upper part 今 means "now." The explanation of the sign is that an object is pressed until it is as flat as the *Kanji* for the number One, which represents a horizontal stroke (一). A type of stamp that narrows toward the top is used for pressing. Through the pressing, the power is concentrated into one point in the moment "now."

ILL. 134 – KANJI ORIGIN FOR NOW

The lower part 心 means "heart." The *Kanji* is a simplified depiction of the heart as an organ. However, at the same time it also means that a mood or a substance spreads throughout the entire available space. In terms of the organ, this is related to how the lifeblood is distributed from the heart throughout the entire organism. For distant healing with the HS Symbol, this means that Reiki is distributed from the heart of *Dainichi Nyorai* throughout the entire cosmos.

ILL. 135 – KANJI ORIGIN FOR HEART

If a seal is used in Asia, its color is always red like blood.[142] When the stamp is pressed onto the paper, this red color distributes itself as an imprint of the seal itself. Of course, only the protruding (previously determined) areas of the seal show on the paper. This corresponds with the explicit characteristic of the Reiki recipients in a distant treatment.

According to an explanation from a Japanese dictionary[143], this phenomenon is also compared with reciting a *sûtra* or mantra, whereby the mouth is not wide open and one does not need to shout, and yet the effect is distributed through the entire room. This is why the general term for

---

[142] There is also an interesting parallel to this in Europe: Runes, the Nordic sacred alphabet, were always colored red when people want to work with their spiritual power. Only then is the magical power effective in the material world.

[143] *Gakken* 学研. *Super Nihongo Daijiten* スパー日本語大辞典. Tokyo, 1998.

invoking the Buddha (*nenbutsu* 念仏) is described with the *nen* 念. With an invocation such as *Namu Amida Butsu* (南無阿弥陀仏), which means something like "Praised be the Amida Buddha," he is reached through the developing power. Similar invocations are also practiced with the names of other Buddhas.

In Buddhism, *nen* 念 has a meaning of its own that is a closely related to the above sign explanation and is decisive for understanding the HS Symbol. In Buddhism, it is namely the translation of the Sanskrit term *smriti*, which means something like "there where the heart is" or "memory of the heart." Someone who is completely merged with his heart, continually moving closer to it or, in other words, lets himself fall increasingly deeper into the heart energy, comes to where there is only love, which is comparable with the state of *Dainichi Nyorai*. The *nen* 念 therefore once again describes *Kûkai's* thesis that every human being can attain enlightenment in this lifetime. The art of this is solely directing the attention to the love that is stored in the hearts of all beings. Assuming that the energy flows where the attention is, the love of *Dainichi Nyorai*, which is simultaneously expressed by both the God and the Goddess, is transmitted to other beings. With the HS Symbol, which depicts the source of the spiritual power of love (= Reiki), attention is focused upon a goal. In the process, the Reiki practitioner detaches with the HS Symbol from time and space in order to let the Reiki power flow in the distance (both the spatial and the temporal). The Reiki channel (the person using Reiki) receives this energy in the same way from a non-tangible distance, which is then transmitted through him from the hands or via the HS Symbol to a recipient.

Word Combinations with Nen 念

The last two *Kanji* of the HS Symbol—*shô* 正 and *nen* 念—result in one word when they are combined. But before this is described in more detail, here are some additional sign/word combinations to promote a better understanding of *nen* 念 beforehand.

念力 Nenriki

This is a Buddhist term with which the concentrated power in the heart is described without any type of doubt.

念珠 **Nenju**
Prayer beads of pearls for reciting mantras, dhâranîs, and sutras (*mâlâ*).

念旧 **Nenkyû**
The constant memory of a true friendship.

念呪 **Nenju**
The recitation of magical formulas.

念念 **Nennen**
An extremely short period of time in Buddhism.

念じ入る **Nenjiiru**
Doing or expressing something whole-heartedly.

念ず **Nenzu**
Without speaking it aloud, wishing for something in the depths of the heart and asking the various light beings for protection and guidance.

Readings of Nen 念

Sino-Japanese: *nen, den*

Japanese: *omou, yomu*

Japanese names: *mune*

I Ching Classification ䷜

The corresponding hexagram of the ancient Chinese oracle and wisdom book I Ching is No. 29, *K'an* 坎, Water.

The Meaning of the Shônen Terms within the HS Symbol

Although Japan took over the Chinese sign with its meanings, the definitions for some of the terms have changed over time. In Japanese—and only in Japanese—*shônen* 正念 means "mentally healthy." However, this was originally a Buddhist expression that is described as follows in the current dictionaries: Right thought—genuine idea—one of the Eight Paths—recognizing (the teaching of Buddha) that has always already been there and keeping it in the heart—not letting oneself be distracted from the heart energy, calling upon Buddha from the whole heart, and taking refuge in him.

Since I have been involved with the symbols, I have repeatedly asked Chinese, Japanese, and Koreans what the five *Kanji* of the HS Symbol mean and if they know where or in which written sources this expression could be found. No one was able to answer this question for me. However, educated Asians were particularly drawn to the last two *Kanji* of *shô* 正 and *nen* 念. They said that although *shônen* 正念 is translated as "right idea" or "right thought," it is simultaneously a Buddhist term and it would be important to more closely explore this aspect.

The Buddhist encyclopedias give very extensive descriptions of the word *shônen* 正念, which are briefly summarized in the following section.

Shônen 正念 in Buddhism

Shônen 正念 is a specialized Buddhist term about which several books could be written in order to precisely explain its meaning. In brief, *shônen* 正念 stands for the "Buddha Consciousness," which is very close. How many people travel to distant countries seeking enlightenment and then at some point discover (or maybe not) that they have already carried enlightenment, the "Buddha Consciousness," with them the whole time!

The *Avatamsaka Sûtra* explains that the Buddha Consciousness is related to *Dainichi Nyorai*. It provides an extensive description of the Lotus-Blossom Treasure World in which *Dainichi Nyorai* dwells as the cosmological Buddha at the center of the universe. From here, light radiates from his pores into all areas of the entire cosmos and illuminates them. But this is not just light. Under the microscope, this would look like an infinite amount of little Buddhas. This is also an explanation of why so many little Buddhas are depicted in the mandorla of Buddhist sculptures. In keeping with this, all other Buddhas of the past, present, and future are also emanations of *Dainichi Nyorai*. These also include the historical Buddha *Shâkyamuni*.

With regard to our HS Symbol, this means that the HS Symbol is useful as a Reiki energy source and for making contact in distant healing. According to this sutra, the Reiki channel acts as a light-bearer for the spiritual life energy Reiki of *Dainichi Nyorai*. At the same time, anyone who gives Reiki is an emanation of *Dainichi Nyorai*. This means that all human beings carry the enlightenment of the cosmological Buddha *Dainichi Nyorai* within themselves and only need to recognize it.

As described above, the last two *Kanji* of the HS Symbol result in the word *shônen* 正念. 正 *shô* means "proper, correct" and is composed of the signs 一 *ichi* = One and 止 *tomeru* = stopping or pausing. 念 *nen* means "sense, meaning, feeling, wish" and is composed of the sign 今 *ima* = now and 心 *kokoro* = heart in the sense of "mind; the totality of wisdom, feeling, and sense; focal point."

On the basis of this, the translation of *shônen* 正念 results in the following sentence: "By pausing at the right moment, the mind is in the here and now." In Zen Buddhism, the ability to be (to live) in the "here and now" is an important goal. This is namely the moment of fusion with the Buddha Consciousness. This lends an even more comprehensible meaning to the translation of the five signs of the HS Symbol (The true human being is not far away from Buddha Consciousness) because the "true human being" means every person who entrusts himself with all his being to the Reiki power flowing through him during a treatment. This state is certainly familiar to anyone who gives Reiki. It happens almost on a regular basis when someone gives Reiki and over time becomes increasingly absorbed in the flow of power—no longer thinking about anything, no longer questioning, no longer observing, but just resting at the center of his being.

I Ching Classification ☷

The corresponding hexagram of the ancient Chinese oracle and wisdom book I Ching is No. 64, *Wei Chi* 未済, Before Completion.

The Form of the HS Symbol

Since Dr. Usui integrated characters as bearer of meaning into the symbols, this will be explained in great detail in the following section. I (Mark) have been practicing calligraphy for about as long as I have done Reiki. Over the course of many years, it has always remained exciting to write the symbols in calligraphy with a writing brush.[144] This is also a method of allowing the meaning of the symbols to decipher itself.

Since calligraphy is one of the meditative arts, it is no surprise that it has been especially popular among Buddhist monks for many centuries. It is also important to note that since copying or transcribing the sutras for the propagation of the Buddhist teachings creates good karma, the sutras were only copied in handwriting at that time and the transcribing of sutras developed into a form of meditation.

Based on my own experience, I know that it is possible to attain deep perceptions through meditative writing or drawing of the symbols. While I wrote the HS Symbol countless times some years ago, it suddenly occurred to me that its form is very similar to that of a pagoda. A pagoda is the further development of a *Stupa*—the tomb of Buddha. In Eastern Asia, this is a type of tower with several stories and the same amount of upturned roofs.

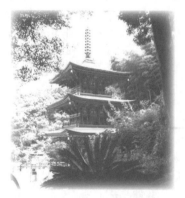

ILL. 136 – PAGODA ON THE ISLAND OF SHIKOKU

Each story has its own upturned roof. In the HS Symbol, there are correspondingly three upturned lines on the left side and two on the right side. A pagoda has a central middle pillar (Jap. *shinbashira* 心柱) that is visible as it protrudes from the tip at the top. The same can also be seen in the HS Symbol. The middle pillar can be literally translated as the "heart pillar" (心 *shin* = heart and 柱 *hashira* = pillar). The last three strokes of

144   Cf. chapter on Calligraphy.

the HS Symbol are an abbreviation for the character 心 *shin* = heart. The heart in this character does not refer to the heart as an inner organ since different characters would have been used in this case. The most important ritual object of the pagoda rests beneath the heart column. These are the relics of the historical Buddha, as well as other sacred cult objects that, simply expressed, make sure that the Buddha and his energy—meaning the "Buddha Consciousness"—are present.

The pagodas of Esoteric Buddhism depict a three-dimensional mandala with *Dainichi Nyorai* at the center. Consequently, *Dainichi Nyorai* is present at the center of the pagoda in the heart pillar. It is surrounded by a number of Buddhas and Bodhisattvas. Here as well, this means that *Dainichi Nyorai* illuminates the entire universe as the cosmological Buddha and the other Buddhas arise from him. If this is applied to the HS Symbol, the Room-cleansing of Rainbow Reiki[145] creates a mandala in the same way as the one that represents *Dainichi Nyorai* in the HS Symbol as a source of power. In order to transmit Reiki, we only need to additionally use some CR Symbols, which then signify the emanations of *Dainichi Nyorai*. Something very similar actually occurs in the applications of the HS Symbol to the distant treatment. Since the cosmos is infinitely large and *Dainichi Nyorai* is everywhere as the transcendental Buddha, its central point can also be practically anywhere. Through the visualization of the recipient and calling his name three times, the respective person is incorporated into the state described by the HS. Time and space are not boundaries for the Buddha Consciousness—it exists in every being as a potential and can be awakened to life through the right means. And this also shows the soundness of the translation for the character *Honsha ze shônen* as "The true human being is not far removed from Buddha Consciousness." The true human being is someone who consciously uses Reiki and devotes himself to this power. The more a person opens up, the more he lives Reiki as a state of being in everyday life, the closer he comes to individual enlightenment, the divine consciousness of life.

In applying the symbols, they are both drawn and visualized. Visualizations are also used in the secret teachings (*mikkyô* 密教) in order

---

[145] This technique is precisely explained in *Reiki—The Best Practices* by F. A. Petter/W. Lübeck, Lotus Press. Translated by Christine M. Grimm.

to show that appearances and truth, as well as mind and matter, are inseparable from each other in reality. The symbols to be visualized are like energy-charged beings. More precisely, the energy arises out of these symbols since they are equivalent to the embodiment of the enlightened cosmos. So the symbol as the means to realization cannot be separated from realization itself. The sûtra *Dainichi kyô*—in which *Dainichi Nyorai* plays the main role—says that the enlightened mind is originally inherent in all beings. This means that the HS Symbol is an allusion to the *Dainichi kyô* and reflects the essence of this sûtra.

The HS Symbol not only gives us the possibility of sending Reiki into the spatial distance but also into the past or the future. The commentary on *Dainichi kyô* includes the following statement on this: "Wherever the Buddha appears, this pagoda is also there. He is unique and yet not separate from the three realms of the past, the present, and the future."

Like the other symbols, the HS Symbol also has a form but is still something that is formless. This may sound paradoxical, but it is immediately followed by the solution. The things of form first appear to be like material things and the formless like fleeting images without color and shape. Anything that cannot be directly perceived is formless. In the secret teachings, the truth is depicted with symbols. This means that each mantra, each mudrâ, and each syllable is an image of enlightenment, just like the HS Symbol itself.

In Zen, there is a corresponding, central teaching: "Form is emptiness, and emptiness is form." This is the spiritual double nature of existence.

Dr. Mikao Usui, who integrated this sign into his Reiki System of Natural Healing as an essential component, had a rich wealth of knowledge and experience in Buddhism, Taoism, and the Japanese religions of Shugendô and Shintô. In my opinion, his special achievement was to also make available the complex spiritual correlations and possibilities of these traditions to the laypeople in a definite and quick practical way. As a result, someone who today would like to learn how to help himself and his fellow human beings in a spiritual way can do so without necessarily becoming a monk or a nun and spending many years in seclusion and asceticism to find access to the divine powers of healing.

The next step to explore is the question of how Dr. Usui could have come up with the idea of creating the HS Symbol to be like a pagoda in one of its levels of meaning. The Japanese and Chinese to whom I have showed the HS Symbol for the first time usually thought that I was unfamiliar with traditional calligraphy and therefore did not know how that space should be left between the individual characters. However, similar to other cultures, there is also a major difference between everyday spoken and written language, especially in terms of how it is used and understood in specialized areas. Consequently, this way of putting together sacred symbols is also very evident in Buddhism, Taoism, Shugendô, and Shintô. Yet, few people are familiar with this art outside the walls of certain monasteries and special university faculties. For example, there have been some emperors in China and Japan whose names, as well as short sentences, have been combined into one character. The Japanese temple names have been frequently created in this way.[146] This way of playing with the Chinese characters for many centuries had its origin in Taoism. In Taoism, it is completely normal to combine various characters for ritual and magical purposes. At the same time, it is even possible to combine the characters of various languages and cultures.

ILL. 137 – TALISMAN IN SIDDHAM AND KANJI—HELPS DISSOLVE UNWANTED CONTACTS TO THE SOULS OF THE DECEASED

Consequently, Dr. Usui took up this ancient tradition and filled the Taoist combination technique with Buddhist contents. Through this creative connecting of various spiritual methods, it became possible for him to construct a custom-made symbol with an immense amount of related levels of meaning that is simultaneously a functioning tool for energy work in his system. Time and again, I am astonished how simply Dr. Usui

---

[146] Cf. Seckel, Dietrich. *Buddhistische Tempelnamen in Japan.* (Names of Buddhist Temples in Japan) In: *Münchener Ostasiatische Studien.* Bd. 37. (Munich East-Asian Studies. Vol. 37) Franz Steiner Verlag Wiesbaden: Stuttgart, 1985.

created the access to a vast and practically applicable spiritual system. It is my hope that as many Reiki friends as possible will learn how to use the great opportunities concealed in the wisdom of Dr. Usui's symbols in addition to the healing power contained in the ABCs of energy work with Reiki. Through the divine powers that they also make available, it will become much easier for all of us to use the opportunities of this era and once again make the earth into a paradise in which each individual can walk his path to the light in peace and love.

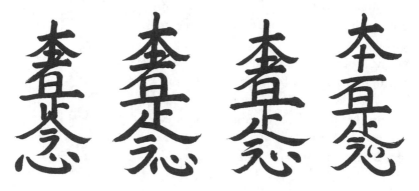

ILL. 138 – WRITING VARIATIONS FOR THE HS SYMBOL

The Siddham Symbols within the HS Symbol

When the Buddhist sutras were translated from Sanskrit into Chinese, the pronunciation in *Kanji* was transcribed but the content of the mantras and *Dhâranîs* was not translated. As a result, it is possible to use the *Kanji* of the HS Symbol to look up whether they are also associated with *Siddham*. Since there are many mantras that have a length of five characters, another approach was to see whether this could be a Buddhist mantra composed of Chinese characters.[147] Unfortunately, this direct path did not lead to any results. But this is no surprise, as I was allowed to learn one day, since Dr. Usui came up with the HS Symbol on his own. However, I was able to discover the nine levels of the HS Symbol, which are described in detail

---

[147] Although the original language of the mantras is Sanskrit, these were also translated into Chinese signs.

below. In addition, the HS Symbol corresponds in its esoteric meaning with the *Siddham hûm* of the Diamond Mind *Kongôsatta.*

When we send Reiki by means of distant contact, a type of consciousness-expansion takes place. This can be used in a great many ways. The simplest method consists of sending Reiki to others. If the time is not specifically programmed, Reiki comes to the recipient at the same time. However, it is just as possible to use the distant contact for many types of astral journeys—a special area of Rainbow Reiki. In Esoteric Buddhism, there are additional forms of consciousness-transmission that are integrated into special meditations and rituals. A general method is the transformation of the so-called Five Poisons into the Five Esoteric Wisdoms. When this is successful, we soon become a Buddha ourselves. The HS Symbol, which represents the power of the Diamond Mind *Kongôsatta* as the *Siddham* symbol *hûm*, is a strong means for this. The Five Wisdoms are expressed by the Five Transcendental Buddhas. This creates a mandala with *Dainichi Nyorai* (the Wisdom of the All-Penetrating Void) at the center and the four emanations that surround him: *Ashuku Nyorai* in the east (mirroring wisdom), *Hôju Nyorai* in the south (wisdom of equality), *Amida Nyorai* in the west (wisdom of magical perception), and *Fukujôju Nyorai* in the north (wisdom of perfection). The individual wisdoms continue to be symbolized by the Five Elements.

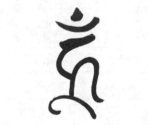

ILL. 139 – SIDDHAM HÛM

The Five Transcendental Buddhas and their powers are all contained in the *Siddham* symbol *hûm* (HS). They correspond with the Five Elements, which are depicted in a Five-Elements pagoda (Jap.: *gorintô*). The Great Brightly Shining Light (DKM) of the Great Sun Buddha *Dainichi Nyorai* radiates from him as the center into all corners of the cosmos. *Dainichi Nyorai* actively shows himself as the Diamond Mind *Kôngosatta* (HS)—the purifying power of all Buddhas. The elements are associated with colors, which help in transforming the five poisons of ignorance, rage, wrongful pride, egotistical urges, attachments, and jealousy into wisdom.

The upper point (circle)—a flame that extends into space—is *Dainichi Nyorai*. A literary translation of his name is "he who makes the forms visible." The trinity of the Great Goddess, Great God, and Creative Force inherent to him in its manifestation makes him into the source of all phenomena. He personifies the wisdom of the "World of Teaching" (Skr.: *Dharma dhâtu*). In the HS Symbol, this is the area of the Chinese character *shô* 正. Additional classifications are:

Field of the Partial Symbol Shô 正	Buddha
Buddha of the Diamond World	*Dainichi Nyorai* as God (potential; unrealized idea)
Buddha of the Womb World	*Dainichi Nyorai* as Goddess (an effect perceivable in the material world, also of an energetic nature; power)
Ritual implement	Pagoda
Associated finger and state	Ring finger – trust
Form of transformation	Highest form of skill
Color	White
Form	Circle
Direction in the mandala	Center
Element	Water
Body area	Belly

The second bowl-shaped line symbolizes *Ashuku Nyorai*—the personification of the mirroring wisdom. In the HS Symbol, this is the area of the Chinese character *nen* 念. Additional classifications are:

Field of the Partial Symbol *Nen* 念	*Vajra* (spiritually effective, masculine principle, comparable to the life- begetting masculine member)
Buddha of the Diamond World	Ashuku Nyorai
Buddha of the Womb World	*Hôdô Nyorai*
Ritual implement	*Vajra* with five points
Associated finger and state	Middle finger – progress
Form of transformation	Attaining enlightenment
Color	Red
Form	Triangle
Direction in the mandala	East
Element	Fire
Body area	Chest

The third line symbolizes *Hôshô Nyorai*—the personification of the wisdom of equality. In the HS Symbol, this is the area of the Chinese character *hon* 本. Additional classifications are:

Field of the Partial Symbol *Hon* 本	Treasure
Buddha of the Diamond World	*Hôshô Nyorai*
Buddha of the Womb World	*Kafuke ô Nyorai*
Ritual implement	Wish-fulfilling gem
Associated finger and state	Little Finger – concentration
Form of transformation	Practice
Color	Yellow
Form	Square
Direction in the mandala	South
Element	Earth
Body area	Hip

The fourth line symbolizes *Amida Nyorai*—the personification of the wisdom of magical perception. In the HS Symbol, this is the area of the Chinese character *ze* 是. Additional classifications are:

Field of the Partial Symbol *Ze* 是	Lotus
Buddha of the Diamond World	*Amida Nyorai*
Buddha of the Womb World	*Muryôju Nyorai*
Ritual implement	*Vajra* with one point
Associated finger and state	Thumb – absorption
Form of transformation	Realization
Color	Blue-green
Form	Drop – lotus petal
Direction in the mandala	West
Element	Emptiness
Body area	Crown

The fifth line symbolizes *Fukûjôju Nyorai*—who personifies the wisdom of perfection. In the HS Symbol, this is the area of the Chinese character *sha* 者. Additional classifications are:

Field of the Partial Symbol *Sha* 者	Karma
Buddha of the Diamond World	*Fukûjôju Nyorai*
Buddha of the Womb World	*Tenkuraion Nyorai*
Ritual implement	*Vajra* with three points
Associated finger and state	Index finger – compassion
Form of transformation	Nirvana
Color	Black
Form	Half-moon
Direction in the mandala	North
Element	Wind
Body area	Face and throat

The HS Symbol and the Five Elements

The individual *Kanji* of the HS Symbols are associated with the five elements of wood, fire, earth, metal, and water. The order of the elements, as arranged in the HS Symbol, corresponds exactly to that of the Chinese Five-Element teaching.

本 *hon* corresponds with the element of wood

者 *sha* corresponds with the element of fire

是 *ze* corresponds with the element of earth

正 *shô* corresponds with the element of metal

念 *nen* corresponds with the element of water.

The elements depict a cycle. The wood nourishes the fire, the fire nourishes the earth, the earth nourishes the metal, the metal nourishes the water, and the water ultimately nourishes the wood. If we begin with the element of water, the water conquers fire, the fire conquers the metal, the metal conquers the wood, the wood conquers the earth, and the earth conquers the water.

As a result, Dr. Usui appears to have done considerably more with the HS Symbol than just making contact with it for distant healing. The spiritual power of the Five Elements is virtually condensed within this symbol. The associations with the *I Ching* hexagrams provide additional insights into the esoteric qualities of the individual parts of the HS. Although it is apparent that the hexagrams of the *I Ching* do not always correspond with the element classifications according to the Five Elements, this is because there are Taoist and shamanic element associations with the hexagrams of the I Ching. Even if the Taoists and Confucians have been very successful in selling the perspective that the *I Ching* is "their" wisdom, this is definitely wrong. It was created during the time in which Wu Shamanism flourished in China. And Taoism and Confucianism did not even exist as concepts back then. In addition, the partial signs have different levels of meaning that complement each other.

In Asia, the Five-Elements teaching is used for classifying the entire Creation. In Traditional Chinese Medicine, as well as in the philosophy, the painting, music, and art of warfare—this very versatile system can be found everywhere.

The Attributes of the Five Elements

Each of the Five Elements has various associations with which the phenomena of life can be understood in both the practical and the theoretical sense.

Water 水: kidneys; bladder; colors of black/dark blue; salty; foul smell; north; winter. 1 Water Qi sinks downward. Curved, irregularly shaped horizontal forms. If the water is too weak, the fire blazes too strongly and burns too quickly (flash in the pan). If the water is too strong, the fire is extinguished. Feelings: fear and dread, fright, stress, gentleness, stillness, and calmness. Physical body: ears, brain, bones, and urogenital system. Organ clock: 3 p.m. to 5 p.m.—bladder; 5 p.m. to 7 p.m.—kidneys. Groaning. Too much fear harms the bladder.

Wood 木: liver; gallbladder; color of green; acidic; rancid smell; east; spring. 3 and 4 Wood Qi extends in all directions. Rectangular, rising forms. When the wood becomes weak, the earth is sluggish. If the wood is too strong, it disturbs the earth. Feelings: irritation, anger, aggression, friendliness, assertiveness, imagination, and openness. Physical body: eyes, muscles and tendons, diaphragm, and groins. Organ clock: 1 a.m. to 3 a.m.—liver; 11 p.m. to 12 a.m.—gallbladder. Screaming. Too much anger harms the liver.

Fire 火: heart, small intestine, (Triple Warmer); color of red; bitter; burned smell; summer; south. 9 Fire Qi shoots upward. Triangular forms. If the fire is too strong, the metal loses its form, durability, and strength. If the fire is too weak, the metal solidifies and becomes brittle. Feelings: joy, excitement, love, happiness, honor, respect, uprightness, creativity, enthusiasm, temperament, charisma, impatience, arrogance, a hectic pace, moodiness, cruelty, and violence. Physical body: tongue, armpits, and face. Organ clock: 11 a.m. to 1 p.m.—heart; 1 p.m. to 3 p.m.—small intestine; 7 p.m. to 9 p.m.—circulation and Triple Warmer. Laughing. Too much happiness harms the heart.

Earth 土: stomach; spleen; color of yellow; transitions between the seasons; sweet or neutral taste; fragrant smell; center. 2, 5, and 8 Earth Qi rotates around its own axis. Angular forms. When the earth is weak, the water sinks deeper. If the earth is too strong, it obstructs the natural movement of the water. Feelings: melancholy, worrying, brooding, sentimentality, openness, compassion, being centered, musicality, and equanimity. Physical body: mouth/lips, connective tissue, and pancreas. Organ clock: 7 a.m. to 9 a.m.—stomach; 9 a.m. to 11 a.m.—spleen. Singing. Too much rest harms the spleen.

Metal 金: lungs; large intestine; color of white; pungent; rotted smell (compost heap); west. 6 and 7 Metal Qi moves toward its own center and solidifies in the process. It contracts. Round, dome-shaped forms. If the metal is too weak, the wood expands too much. If the metal is too strong, the wood is damaged. Feelings: worry and sorrow, grief, depression, courage, honesty, ability to adapt, letting go, emptiness. Physical body: nose, mucous membranes, and skin. Organ clock: 3 a.m. to 5 a.m.—lungs; 5 a.m. to 7 a.m.—large intestine. Crying. Too much sorrow harms the lungs.

Each of the five different emotions can be produced by each of the five elements in turn. For example, there is anger (wood) that is created by fear (water), but also anger that is produced by unsatisfied arousal (fire).

The Constructive Cycle

Clockwise: Wood (thunder and wind) burns and therefore produces *fire*. The *fire* leaves ashes (earth). From the *earth* (earth and mountain), *metal* (sea and sky) is extracted. *Metal* gives power to the *water* and produces it because the constricting, inwardly directed movement toward the summit point turns into the downward motion of the *water*. The element of *water* is required in order for trees (*wood*) grow.

The Decomposing Cycle

Counterclockwise: Fire melts *metal.* The *metal* cuts *wood. Wood* takes vital powers of nourishment from the *earth.* The *earth* soils the *water. Water* can extinguish *fire.*

The Control Process

This type of interaction serves to avoid imbalances, so it is the process of self-regulation. Following a clockwise direction, it always controls (meaningfully organizes) the element that follows the next one.

Wood controls *earth. Earth* controls *water. Water* controls *fire. Fire* controls *metal. Metal* controls *wood.*

The Injury Process

This type of relationship causes the self-organization to become disharmonious. In this process, the element following the next one in the counterclockwise direction is influenced.

Wood harms *metal. Metal* harms *fire. Fire* harms *water. Water* harms *earth. Earth* harms *wood.*

The Mediation Process

If two hostile elements are too close together, a third can be used for mediation in order to eliminate the problem.

Wood mediates between water and fire.

Fire mediates between wood and earth.

Earth mediates between fire and metal.

Metal mediates between earth and water.

Water mediates between wood and metal.

The Five Practices of the Bodhisattvas

In addition to the Five Elements, the five *Kanji* of the HS Symbol also represent the so-called Five Practices of the Bodhisattvas.

布施 *fuse* Generosity

The focus of *fuse* is giving something out of abundance. This means wealth in the sense of material things, as well as teachings.

持戒 *jikai* Following the Path of the Heart

This focuses on following the path of the Buddha (the Path of the Heart), which means acting with compassion and wisdom for the greatest good of all involved and helping many beings achieve happiness in the process.

忍辱 *ninniku* Patience

This involves patience in the sense of appropriately responding to the way in which others behave, forgiving them, and wishing them all the best.

精進 *shôjin* Light Work

This means mentally following the teaching of the light and rejecting everything that harms the divine order.

止観 *shikan* Giving Up Illusions

This involves giving up illusions and experiencing the Buddha Consciousness.

The implications of all five practices result in a further level of meaning for the HS Symbol, which is very close to the translation of the HS Symbol: "Following the path of the heart with generosity and attaining the Buddha Consciousness through patience in our actions and light work in the mind."

Strictly speaking, this involves a special interpretation of Dr. Usui's Principles.

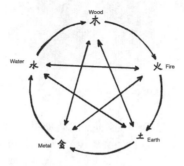

ILL. 140 – THE FIVE ELEMENTS

The Origins of Distant Healing in Japan

Anyone who climbs Mount Kurama, where Dr. Usui spent three weeks in meditation, will find the *Kuramadera* temple. This is where the spiritual light beings *Senju Kannon, Bishamonten,* and *Gohô Maôson* are worshipped[149]. Moreover, the *Kuramadera* temple is still a syncretistic monastery complex in which both Buddhism and Shintô are practiced.

It is necessary to explain more about *Bishamonten* within the context of the HS Symbol. He was originally one of the guardians of Buddhism. Since the early 10th Century, *Bishamonten* has also been mentioned as the Master of Distant Healing in written sources such as the *Shigisan engi monogatari*. This story is so famous that it was drawn in the 12th Century as a Japanese scroll painting. The story is about the three miracles of the monk *Myôren*. In the first part, *Myôren* made his begging bowl fly; in the second part, he healed the Tennô by means of distant healing; and the third part is about *Myôren's* older sister who was led to him in the *Tôdaiji* temple by the Great Buddha.

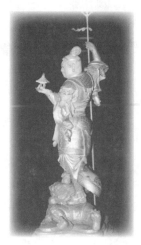

ILL. 141 – BISHAMONTEN—BEARER OF THE HS SYMBOL

Bishamonten is also the one who is responsible for distant healing. In sculptures, *Bishamonten* is customarily depicted with a staff of wisdom

---

[149] Cf. chapter on Light Beings and Mount Kurama

358

in his right hand and a pagoda in his left. Yes, you have read this cor-rectly—*Bishamonten* holds a little pagoda on his left hand (on the Palm Chakra) in shoulder height, as described in the section about the HS Symbol. This is how *Bishamonten* receives the energy of *Dainichi Nyorai* (Reiki) in distant healing, which enters directly through the pagoda in his Palm Chakra. In his right hand, *Bishamonten* holds a staff of wisdom, which shows the activity of *Bishamonten* with which he can fight, protect, and heal through the orientation of the power (action). The latter activity also corresponds with the function of the CR Symbol, whether in distant healing, mental healing, or the Reiki Shower. While the HS Symbol is the source of the power, the CR Symbol determines the direction in which Reiki flows and how it works. The wisdom is demonstrated in that *Bishamonten* acts for the greatest good of all involved. So the left hand is the receiving (*Yin*) and the right hand is the sending (*Yang*). There is also a relationship here with the Goddess and the God, as well as the Mandalas of the Womb and Diamond World. The womb or Goddess in the pagoda symbolize the receptive principle (HS), and the diamond and the God with the staff of wisdom symbolize the executing principle (CR). Originally, the staff of wisdom was a weapon consisting of a long staff with a blade at the end. Its form ensured the holding and drawing closer of a person or thing.

The above-mentioned scroll painting of *Shigisan engi* depicts how distant healing occurs. The light being walking on the clouds, *Bishamonten,* symbolically represents the HS Symbol here. The cloud express-es that *Bishamonten* moves very quickly. The Wheel of the Teachings (Skr.: *Dharma cakra*; Jap.: *rinbô*) rolls in front of him. On the material plane, the Wheel of the Teachings is the spiritual power that has a practical effect on the beings that exist there, which helps them once again become aware of their divinity and trust in their inner light. In my opinion, the CR Symbol is the equivalent of the Wheel of the Teachings within this context.

Bishamonten sends out *Fudô Myôô* as a powerful manifestation of *Dainichi Nyorai*. With the sword, he cuts away the things that are detri-mental to personality development and health, which are the causes of disease. With the lasso, he rescues the beings from the disease-causing things by drawing them closer to him.

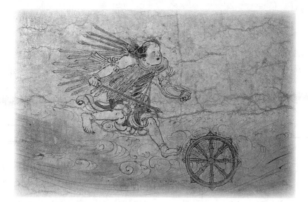

ILL. 142 – DISTANT HEALING IN THE SCROLL PAINTING SHIGISAN ENGI

The Wheel of the Teachings rushes ahead of the light being. The Wheel of the Teachings is one of the most important symbols in Buddhism. Because it rolls through the world, the teachings of Buddha are spread. It is therefore also said that Buddha himself turned the Wheel of the Teachings three times, which means the three sermons in which the Buddha taught the three Buddhist main schools of *Hinayana, Mahâyâna,* and *Vajrayâna.*[150] In addition, the eight-spoked wheel is an ancient symbol throughout the world for the shamans who work in the traditional ways. It shows the eight directions, the eight sacred festivals associated with the seasons that not only depict and explain the order of the year but also the entire life process. Furthermore, spiritual helper beings can be found within the eight-spoked wheel that support nature and human beings on their path through time so that everything occurs within the framework of support and is therefore coordinated with each other. The sacred medicine wheel of the Native Americans is an especially developed variation of this symbol, which was also introduced to Europe by the Native American master Sunbear and his life partner Wabun Wind. Anyone who has ever done ritual work and meditation in a medicine wheel and was allowed to experience the powerful, loving presence of the spiritual helper beings, knows the deep meaning of this universal symbol.

As in the SHK Symbol, there is a *Siddham* symbol for every light being in Buddhism. The comparison of the *Siddham* between *Fudô Myôô* in the

---

[150] Cf. the chapter on Esoteric Buddhism.

above-mentioned scroll painting and the *Siddham* of the light being *Gohô Maôson* in *Kuramadera* temple shows that this is the same sign, namely the syllable *hûm*. This relationship implies the connection between the two temples on the mountains of *Shigi* and *Kurama*. It is also interesting here to note the context of the three light beings' function in the temple *Kuramadera*. *Senju Kannon* represents love, *Bishamonten* stands for light, and *Gohô Maôson* depicts power. People also like to equate the latter with a *tengu*, a forest spirit with a long nose who has a special affinity with big trees. In my opinion, *Senju Kannon* is related to the SHK Reiki Symbol, *Bishamonten* with the HS Symbol and *Gohô Maôson* with the CR Symbol.

The Shigisan Engi Monogatari–
The Story About the Origin (of the Temple) on Mount Shigi

Part 1–The Flying Granary

A monk by the name of *Myôren*, who had not yet received the initiation as a monk, went to the *Tôdaiji* temple to have himself initiated. Afterward, he decided not to return to his hometown and prayed to the Great Buddha *Birushana*[151] in *Tôdaiji* to show him a place where he could devote himself to his Buddhist practices in peace. As he did this, he saw the outline of a mountain in the southwest to which he felt magically drawn. It was the mountain *Shigi*. Once he arrived there, he dedicated himself so diligently to his practices that he even made a Buddhist sculpture while in a trance. After its completion, he discovered that it was a sculpture of *Bishamonten*. He then built a hall for it.

The years passed and he performed some miracles, through which he unintentionally became very well known. At the foot of the mountain lived a very rich man. *Myôren* always let his alms bowl fly there and then return loaded with food. However, the rich man became aggravated at the bowl one day and said: "The usual bowl has come. It is so fresh and greedy!" Then he took it and threw it into the corner of his granary. This time he placed nothing in it. When the bowl was also locked into the granary after

---

[151] *Birushana*: *Vairocana* Buddha in *Mahâyâna* Buddhism. Comparable with *Dainichi Nyorai* (Skr.: *Mahâ Vairocana*) in *Vajrayana* Buddhism.

its work was done, the granary suddenly began to sway. The people were surprised and saw how the granary began to float. The bowl escaped from the warehouse, flew beneath it, and carried it away. The rich man and the others followed the bowl and the granary as it flew into the mountains where the monk *Myôren* lived. There it crashed down next to his hut.

This was obviously an extraordinarily embarrassing matter for the rich man. He went to *Myôren* and explained to him: "Oh, I was totally confused today and inadvertently put nothing in the bowl. Then I forgot it in the granary, which has now flown here with the bowl. Would you perhaps be so kind as to give me back the granary?" *Myôren* responded: "Since the granary has flown here and something like this has not been here before, it is sensible to put something in it. This is why I cannot give it back to you. But you can take the contents home with you." The rich man responded: "How should I just simply take it with me again? There are 180,000 kilograms of rice in the granary." *Myôren* explained to him that this would be very simple. If he placed a bale of rice on the bowl and let it fly away, the remaining rice bales would follow the bowl like wild geese. This made the rich man become fearful. Quite ashamed, he said that he wanted to leave him about one-third of it. But *Myôren* did not agree to this because he could not use this much by himself. Finally, the 180,000 kilograms of rice bales landed safely at the estate, right where the granary previously stood.

Part 2–The Healing of the Daigo Tennô

In the *Engi* period (901-923), during which *Myôren* distinguished himself through such miracles, the *Daigo Tennô* (885-930) became seriously ill. Although he had many prayers, mantras, and sutras said for himself, no one could ease his pain, let alone heal him. Then he heard: "In Yamato at a place by the name of *Shigi* lives a holy monk called *Myôren* who possesses extraordinary and venerable miraculous powers. He can even let his alms bowl fly so that he can meditate in the mountains in peace. If Your Majesty would let him come, he would be certain to heal you." As a result, the Tennô had an envoy sent to bring *Myôren* back to the court.

When the envoy reached him and conveyed the Tennô's orders for him to come to the court, *Myôren* seemed very arrogant and asked: "Why should I go there?" The envoy said: "The Tennô suffers from a serious disease that no one has been able to heal up to now. You must go to him and heal him through your prayers." In response, *Myôren* answered: "Then I will heal the Tennô, but without going there." The envoy replied: "When the Tennô is healed, how can we recognize that the miraculous powers come from you, holy man?" Then *Myôren* said: "When I have ended the prayers for healing, I will send the Tennô the guardian spirit of the sword. When he sleeps or daydreams, the Tennô will see him with a garment of woven swords and recognize him." In closing, he also said: "In no case will I go to the capital city," so that there was nothing else for the envoy to do but to return alone and give the Tennô his report.

Three days later, the Tennô suddenly feel asleep around noon and saw the guardian spirit of the sword, as was described to him. When he woke up, he felt refreshed and without pain. His disease was healed. The Tennô was so happy that he wanted to give *Myôren* the title of *Sôjô*[152] and much land. But *Myôren* refused both since the accumulation of possessions can bring bad karma with it.

Part 3—The Story of the Nun

During this time, the monk's older sister lived in Shinano. Since her brother had not returned to his hometown after the ordination as a priest, she went to the capital city to the *Tôdaiji* temple to look for him. But no one there remembered him since 20 years had already passed since his initiation into the priesthood. In despair, she spent the entire night in meditative practices before the Great Buddha and requested that he at least let her brother appear to her in a dream. As she fell asleep after many hours of prayer, she heard the Great Buddha speak in a dream: "The location of the monk you are looking for lies in the west. In the southwest direction there is a mountain with violet clouds. Search there for him." She woke up as it was just becoming light. There she saw in the far distance the weak outline of a mountain upon which violet clouds towered. She joyfully set out on the path.

When she went there, she actually found the temple hall. As she approached the place, she perceived a person there. He asked who she was, and she responded by asking whether the monk *Myôren* lived there.

---

[152] *Sôjô*: the highest rank of a monk; a type of Buddhist abbot.

Then he saw that it was his sister, the nun from Shinano. "Why are you visiting me so unexpectedly?" And she told him how this had come to be. In addition, she gave him a garment that he gratefully accepted because up to now he had only worn clothing made of paper. The sister also did not return to her hometown and lived there with *Myôren*. Together they performed many spiritual practices until the end of their days.

Myôren wore the garment until it disintegrated into shreds. Later, these little shreds, as well as the smallest pieces of wood from the rice granary, were used for talismans. Everyone who worshipped *Bishamonten* there became a happier and richer person. Consequently, people still go to this power place of healing today.

How Dr. Usui Was Able to Create the HS Symbol

As promised, here is an explanation of how the HS Symbol was created. While many of the details of the HS Symbol are based on Esoteric Buddhism in terms of its content, the way of creating such a symbol is anything but Buddhist. Although the making of talismans—as is also used for the HS Symbol—is included in the Shingon School of Esoteric Buddhism that Kûkai introduced to Japan, its roots come not only from the secret teachings but especially from magical Taoism and its talismans. The latter applies in particular in this case. Their origins are based on the energy work with light beings, whereby the magicians entered into a type of contract with the light beings to whom they promised, for example, that they would always work for the highest good of the whole and perform rituals for the light beings.[153] In return for this, the light beings provided the magician with healing energies or did other useful things. In addition, talismans were made from strips of paper, metal, or bamboo to symbolize this contract. Interwoven Chinese characters were written on it. In the Fourth Century, the Taoist Ge Hong provided more precise information about making talismans and their effect in his compendium on Taoist practices (Chin.: *Sanhuang nei wen*). The content, structure, and

---

[153] However, this procedure comes from the much older Wu Shamanism that later, especially in relation to its practical magic work, was integrated into Taoism.

number of the signs varies, depending upon what effect it is intended to have. For example, typical effects are making energetic contact with the light beings of the subtle world. The talismans were always created in a ritual manner. So there was a technical procedure, as well as the breathing of the power into it in a precisely defined ritual form. Wearing such talismans can have a great variety of effects such as the healing of diseases or protection from strange, harmful influences. However, they are also extremely useful on so-called shamanic journeys when it comes to gathering energetically high-quality medicinal herbs—such as those on sacred mountains. Talismans made of 18 signs provide protection against the wind and waves on the high seas or in raging rivers. The signs are written in red Chinese ink on silk and then worked into the garment. Master Wang Xizhi, who is famous in the area of calligraphy, is said to have once written the character for rain (雨, uppermost part of the character for Reiki 靈氣) with so much energy that it soon began to rain. The early Chinese character was originally, as shown by the oracle bones, used by the Wu Shamans for ritual purposes. They already contain certain magical power on their own. As described extensively in the chapter on how the script developed, they were not invented.

The combinations as in the Reiki character, the DKM Symbol, or the HS Symbol, are examples of how the original signs were arranged in the form of a talisman. Each of the Reiki symbols is such a talisman. However, without instruction and initiation, they are just simply characters. So, even today, the true power of the symbols remains concealed to most people because they only use the signs as script.

In addition to these belatedly visible talismans, there is also an entire series of other types that are not as easy to recognize for what they actually are. These may be made with water, Chinese ink, writing brushes, or stone. Since they have no visible traces of being characters, a layperson also cannot simply identify them as talismans. So a talisman can have a great many complex functions. People who are trained in the appropriate techniques and initiated into the necessary spiritual powers can use them. For others, such a talisman is only the material object. For example, the Rainbow Reiki Radionic crystal *Laya te yan* is one of these complex talismans with which powerful healings and fantastic rituals of energy work can be performed.

There are other talismans that are not bound to matter. This means that we cannot even see them during or after their use. But their effect can certainly be determined. The HS Symbol, as well as the other Reiki symbols, belongs in this category.

What all Taoist talismans have in common is that they are first drawn correctly and visualized at the same time; secondly, they must be activated through the proper mantra. A talisman in the form of a symbol is ritually created anew each time through this process. And how effective the synergy effect of the symbol is on the user is decided precisely by this process. More specifically, the user actually has the possibility to grow on various levels through conscious ritual work. One example of this is that especially through the ritual, slow, conscious, and attentive drawing of the symbols, the subtle perceptive ability develops immensely. In addition, it is a fallacy to believe that we can literally toss the symbols around like stamps if we have not already been on the consciousness-promoting path for years. In Japan, there is an interesting proverb about this: *Isogaba maware!* (急がば回れ). Literal translation: "When you are in a hurry, you take a detour." This obviously means "take your time," but especially the nuance that resonates in the Japanese is very appropriate here since many people want to achieve physical abilities as quickly as possible. However, short cuts here often lead into a dark dead end.

For both the subtle symbols and the water symbols, it is necessary to orient them in such a way as to produce a connection between the power source (such as the HS Symbol or a Reiki channel) and the recipient in a way that is as safe as possible and long term, if necessary. The connection and orientation of the sender to the recipient is produced by the CR Symbol.

A number of development steps are necessary for making a talisman, as well as for the HS Symbol. First, the goals that are to be achieved with the talisman must be determined. So this involves creating a symbol that serves as the source of the Reiki energy, that can be used for distant healing and making contact with other beings, and is available for all initiates and at all times. These three points may be the reason why Dr. Usui selected the energetic talisman method in particular. In the year after his vision on Mount Kurama, there was a terrible earthquake in and around Tokyo in 1923. This might have shown Dr. Usui the transitory nature of all things. Everything that has a material nature can be lost forever through various influences. This obviously also includes talismans of paper or other materials. Another reason is the availability of the materials. No matter how good the idea of a talisman is, it cannot be used if the necessary materials for making the talisman are not available. As long as human beings have existed, energetic talismans have been used by them at all times and everywhere, as well as being passed on to others through initiation.

In the next step, the question arises as to how it is possible to integrate the function into the talisman or the symbol. To do this, Dr. Usui did the above-described decoding of the HS Symbol backwards. During his extensive research, he had considered what he needed and included the above-described methods in the structure of the symbol. In addition, he intensively thought about the technical means for which this symbol can then be used. This obviously also applies to the other symbols. Although they originally came from various spiritual traditions, it is still possible to use them in a uniform manner.

Once the form of the symbol has been created, it must be incorporated in the right way into Reiki and the initiations, before it can be used by the Reiki practitioner.[154]

Goji No Myô–The Light of the Five Signs

I have already described how Dr. Usui created the HS Symbol himself and how this was possible. In its essence, the HS Symbol is based on a combination of the secret teachings of Esoteric Buddhism, Shugendô, and Taoism. Strictly speaking, it has many more levels than those of distant healing and the five elements. The HS Symbol is used for distant healing and as a source of Reiki. The Master Symbol is the DKM. Together (HS and DKM) they result in the Master Mantra. In the Reiki initiations for all degrees, the HS Symbol is used together with the DKM as the Master Mantra—directly in the Western tradition and in part as an inner practice (*Nei Gong*) in the authentic Japanese Reiki. Without this mantra, no traditional Reiki initiation would be possible. However, a contradiction to this is that Dr. Usui was able to initiate into Reiki even

---

[154] Please also compare this with the chapter on Symbols and Mantras as Tools of Spiritual Energy Work.

before conceived the HS for his students. The reason for this is relatively simple. Dr. Usui's goal was to find a method of healing that would result in much success with little effort. In order to achieve this ability, Dr. Usui had to take a long path himself. So that his students would not have to continuously re-invent the wheel, he created— on the basis of his years spent researching the secret teachings of various spiritual traditions—a method for achieving quickly visible results and for giving initiations. The tools for the specific treatments are the Reiki symbols, and those for the initiations are the Reiki symbols with the Master Mantra.

If someone is ill, it is as important to immediately be able to help him or her heal as it is to study the secret teachings for years. So Dr. Usui created the HS Symbol and made the deep knowledge of the secret teachings available on more of a technical level in order to quickly and simply be able to achieve success. However, the numerous additional applications remained concealed from most students—unless they were prepared to continue to develop themselves.

In the course of my own research, I came across a ritual complex of the secret teachings, which is called the *Goji no myô* (literally: the Light of the Five Signs). *Myô* is the same character as the third in the DKM Symbol. In addition to the meaning of "light" (from the sun and moon), *myô* can also signify wisdom[155]. The "five signs" refer to the individual characters concealed in the HS Symbol. There are nine levels of meaning and application beyond the five characters. For each individual character, there is a combination of five *Siddham* symbols that are directly related to the HS Symbol and *Dainichi Nyorai*. Dr. Usui created the HS Symbol as a simplified depiction of all nine levels and their *Siddham* in just one single symbol. Although the applications known in Reiki with the HS Symbol such as distant contact and the source of the Reiki power for space clearing and Reiki initiations are present in this ritual complex, we can be certain that the other levels are additional meanings and applications of the HS Symbol.

Each level involves *Dainichi Nyorai* as the source of power. Just as Reiki comes from *Dainichi Nyorai*, it is worth mentioning in this context that the spiritual traditions of East Asia related to Buddhism date back to *Dainichi Nyorai*. At the same time, it is noteworthy that before a hu-

[155]   *see next page*

man being can pass on the energy, he or she must always receive it from *Dainichi Nyorai* through a light being who is an emanation of him. In Reiki, these are *Dainichi Nyorai* and *Kannon*. In Shugendô, as well as in Esoteric Buddhism, these are *Dainichi Nyorai* and *Kongôsatta* or *Dainichi Nyorai* and *Dai Marishi Ten*.

Dainichi Nyorai in the sense of the Goddess, God, and Creative Force is also the central figure and source of many forms of magical energy work of East Asia. The HS Symbol is the source for the power of the wisdom light and the DKM is the symbol for its emanation. If this must be brought to a certain point and/or included or integrated from there, an additional CR Symbol is necessary.

In addition, the **nine levels of the HS Symbol** correspond with the nine fields of the Diamond World Mandala (Jap.: *Kongôkai*) and the nine mudrâs and mantras of the *Kuji Kiri*.

The **first level** deals with the HS Symbol in the sense of the mantra *a ba ra ka kya* of *Dainichi Nyorai* in the Mandala of the Womb World (Jap.: *Taizôkai*). In the various schools of Esoteric Buddhism, this level of the HS Symbol is used by the Master to initiate the students into spiritual powers (Jap.: *Reikanjô*).

[155] This meaning of the characters for sun and moon suggests the predominating conception in Asia that wisdom can only be attained by means of a sensible combination of masculine and feminine thinking. The sun symbolizes the masculine, more rational and logical thinking, with its yang qualities while the moon with its feminine yin quality represents the intuitive emotional and, in the narrower sense of the word, the spiritual way of thinking. It is also interesting that the apparently complete light can be attained only in the spiritual sense of enlightenment (Jap. *satori*) when the yin and the yang quality in a human being is integrated and fully developed. This means the fulfillment of spiritual ideals in our daily life that is characterized by material constraints. This philosophical approach is crassly contradictory to the patriarchal religion in its total orientation toward spiritualization, as it is manifested in the predominant expressions of Christianity, Hinduism, and Buddhism. There is apparently an older, more holistic approach in Hinduism and Buddhism that originated in the pre-patriarchal era. This approach recognizes and uses the spiritual forces of the feminine and masculine principle, understanding the individual representatives of these qualities, the Great God and the Great Goddess, as having an equal right. After all, the above-mentioned symbols of the Reiki System come from Esoteric Buddhism, Hinduism, Shugendô, and Taoism. This original approach is Tantric Shamanism.

The Sûtra of the Great Light (Jap.: *Dainichi kyô*) describes the way in which *Dainichi Nyorai* is omnipresent as the source of the Reiki power (HS) through his vast, radiant light (DKM). In the symbol *a, Dainichi Nyorai* is the life arising from the earth, which means the Great Goddess. The earth is like a richly endowed treasure house, filled with immeasurably abundant life and blessed with everything necessary for existing on it. In the symbol *ba, Dainichi Nyorai* bears the element of water, which causes everything to flow and permeates it. In the symbol *ra, Dainichi Nyorai* is the form for the element of fire, which has the effect of a cleansing flash of lightning. It can also manifest as the fire of wrath or will. In the symbol *ka, Dainichi Nyorai* is the form of the element of wind; he is the element of air in the symbol *kya*. The monk *Kûkai* extensively described the meaning of the five *Siddham* in his work *Sokushin jôbutsu gi* (On Attaining Enlightenment in This Life). It says here that everything develops from the symbol *a* as from the soil of the Great Goddess. It corresponds with the basis of all phenomena in the universe that is not subject to life and death. As in the Western alphabet, the *Siddham* symbol *a* stands at the beginning in the *Siddham* alphabet. The quality of the *a* comes from the spiritual heart, which is love in its highest developed form. Only love can connect the opposites of the feminine and the masculine, the spiritual and the material, into a meaningful functional unity. The *Siddham* symbol *ba* (Skr.: *va*) expresses the unspeakable (the mystical secret, for example, as revealed in the Egyptian spiritual tradition through the seven veils of the Goddess Isis). *Ba* is contained in the Sanskrit words of *vâc*[156] and *vâda*, containing every form of verbal expression. The *Siddham* symbol *ra* (Skr.: *ra*) is the first syllable in the Sanskrit word *rajas*, which means the "dust" that is burned away by the fire of *ra*. This means the impurities of the 108 attachments that arise through the desires such as greed. The *Siddham* symbol *ka* (Skr.: *ha*) is the initial sound of the Sanskrit word *hetu* (cause). The expanse of the cosmos is alluded to through the Siddham symbol *kya* (Skr.: *kha*). It stands for "hole" or "void" in Sanskrit. This means the space[157] that connects all beings with each other. Enlightenment is described in the *Sûtra of the Light* (Jap.: *Dainichi kyô*) with "I am awakened." This is the return to the natural original state and corresponds

[156]/[157] *see next page*

with the *Siddham* symbol *hûm*, which is comparable to the HS Symbol since it is composed of several signs. In addition, *hûm* is the syllable of the Bodhisattva Diamond Mind *Kongôsatta*, who has passed the teachings of *Dainichi Nyorai* on to human beings. It contains the perception that all phenomena are connected with each other in the expanse of the universe, even if they appear to be far removed from each other. All phenomenon comes from the one source of the Creative Force. The awareness of this is the cause for the practitioner, and the knowledge is the result for the enlightened one.

The natural original state is called the primordial consciousness in the *Sûtra of the Light*. This is a type of primordial soul, as well as the activity of the soul in immeasurable abundance, which means the oneness of all beings. Dr. Usui referred to this correlation with the sentence that he frequently said when healing: "Human being, Crown of Creation, return to your natural original state." Simply said, all beings could have a big party together if they would recognize this.[158]

---

[156] The Goddess in her quality as the Creator of the entire manifested universe is called *Vâc* in Indian Hinduism. She represents a manifestation of *Sarasvatî*, the Goddess of Wisdom and the Fine Arts. Even to this day, she must be called upon by every Hindu adept in order to attain enlightenment through the rising of the Kundalinî. Her secret mantra is used by a guru to trigger the rising of the Kundalinî in his student by means of *Shaktipad*, a spiritual energy transmission. In her manifestation as *Vâc*, the Great Goddess used the power of the world to create the material universe with all of its levels, including the spiritual. From the unbridled, chaotic waters of life she created the ordered structures of the world in which we live today. Consequently, the Great Goddess is also the source for the power of every single mantra. The chakras in the human energy system that bring the power of the word into this world are the 2nd and the 5th. This means the creative birthing force of sexuality from which the sensual ecstasy found in the loving union between the masculine and feminine brings new life into this world and the power of artistic self-expression that gives form and independence to this life. In the well-known *Gâyatrî* mantra, which was popularized by the internationally renowned saint *Satya Sai Baba*, this creative force of the Great Goddess is acknowledged.

[157] In this sense, "space" can be understood as the possibility of filling the time-space continuum with life processes and relationships.

[158] Please also compare this with the extensive explanations in the chapter on Spiritual Cosmology.

The **second level** involves the HS Symbol in the sense of the mantra *a ban ran kan ken*, which reflects the ecstasy of *Dainichi Nyorai*, of the Great God and the Great Goddess. Among other things, this mantra is used in a ritual to end the suffering of the purgatory realms. The *Siddham* symbol *a* is the most primordial principle of *Dainichi Nyorai* in the Mandala of the Womb World (Jap.: *Taizôkai*) and represents the Great Goddess and Mother Earth, as in the first level. From it, the great compassion is born, which is directed into the right channels by the other four *Siddham* symbols in order to have an effect at the proper time and in the right place. The symbols *ban ran kan ken* express the wisdom of *Dainichi Nyorai* in the Mandala of the Diamond World (Jap.: *Kongôkai*) and stand for the Great God who becomes active through the impulse of the Great Goddess. The Great Goddess—the symbol *a*—is the element of earth. *Ban ran kan ken* represent the elements of water, fire, air, and emptiness. All five together result in the five-level pagoda of the elements (*gorintô*). The above-mentioned activity of *Dainichi Nyorai* is shown with the symbol *hûm*, which is represented by the Diamond Mind *Kongôsatta*. *Kongôsatta* is the mediator of the teachings, which he has heard from the Great Goddess—here as *Dainichi Nyorai* in the *Siddham* symbol *a*. In most rituals of *Shingon*, he plays a significant role. *Ban* stands for speaking. *Ran* represents the dust that is burned away by the fire, which means the 108 attachments that cause the suffering of the beings. *Kan* means the cause, and *ken* stands for emptiness. The latter is the uppermost point in *hûm*, which describes the expansive and empty heavenly space and thereby symbolizes the gateway of meditation. This is where the wisdom can be brought to completion, through which the Mother of all Buddhas, the Great Goddess *Marishi Ten*, is reached. The cause *kan* allows the *Siddham* symbol for truth-cause to develop within the treasure of the heavenly space, which brings great protection with it. This is also related to the interaction of both symbols *kan* and *ken* together since they both resemble a general who crushes the power of the enemy. This ensures that no further obstacles remain. The power created in this way is as strong as a diamond. As a result, also inherent in the symbol *hûm* is the great power of joy that can be granted to each being in meditation, as it has been granted to the Buddhas of the past, present, and future as they all contemplate *hûm*.

The **third level** focuses on the HS Symbol in the sense of the mantra *an ban ran kan ken*. This may initially sound similar to the mantra of the second level. However, the written *Siddham* symbols have a different form, which means that their effect has also changed. This is about the Reiki initiations. The old texts describe how the Five Signs (HS) stand on a lotus blossom. This means the head of the person who is to be initiated. The big radiant light (DKM) shines in all directions and the world of the *Dharma* of *Dainichi Nyorai* illuminates the entire world. In order to focus the Reiki force onto the person to be initiated, this is followed by a CR Symbol and the Reiki Master channel assumes the role of a mediator between *Dainichi Nyorai* and the person to be initiated by means of an energy transmission. Through the Master Mantra HS-DKM, the power of *Dainichi Nyorai* with the energy qualities from the five elements of earth, water, fire, wind, and air is lastingly transmitted in the form of a general influence. This is an initial step in order to awaken through an inner process to the perception of being *Dainichi Nyorai*.

The **fourth level** is about the mantra *a bi ra un ken* of *Dainichi Nyorai* of the Womb World as a provider of contentment through the light of wisdom. This sounds very promising, and this is also what it is. Through the secret wisdom light of *Dainichi Nyorai*, it is possible to let almost every wish come true, as long as it is expressed by the heart for the highest good of all involved. This is the so-called high spiritual magic in the narrower sense of the word. It also includes Reiki initiations and healings with Reiki. The realization of the wish is born from the symbol *a*, which represents *Dainichi Nyorai*. The other four symbols of *bi, ra, un, ken* stand for the four aspects that protect from outside influences. This also includes the purification of the mind since as long as certain developmental steps are not taken in the personality, the fulfillment of a wish is hardly conceivable. Combining the symbols results in the symbol *hûm* of the purifying power of *Dainichi Nyorai* in the name of the Diamond Spirit *Kongôsatta*. Through the purification of the mind with the sacred nectar *Amrita*, all realms of existence are simultaneously charged with love and light, which has a protective effect.

The **fifth level** entails the most important mantra for the Diamond World Mandala (Jap.: *kongôkai*): *baku ri da do ban*. This mantra is among the few that have a coherent meaning, which is: *Dainichi Nyorai* of the

373

Diamond World. In subsequent times, the symbol *om* was also added at the beginning. While the symbol *a* of *Dainichi Nyorai* represents the earth and the Goddess, the symbol *ban* denotes water as a dynamic element that carries the divine emotional impulse and God. Water is the bearer of the channeled energy that is created from the earth and originates within it.

The **sixth level** involves *Dainichi Nyorai* with the Mantra of the Womb World (*taizôkai*): *baku ri da do a*. In subsequent times, the symbol *om* was also placed at the beginning here.

The **seventh level** focuses on all five transcendental Buddhas of the Diamond World, all of whom appear in one single mantra with their *Siddham* symbols. The mantra is *vam hum trah hrih a*. The use of this mantra involves the awakening of the five wisdoms, in which the individual wisdoms are realized in the opposite order of the mantra content. The symbol *a* represents transforming the consciousness of the five senses into wisdom, which makes it possible to act for the highest good of all involved in every case. The symbol *hrih* is the transformation of the six states of consciousness into the wisdom of seeing the separate individuals as one great whole. The symbol *trah* is the transformation of the seventh state of consciousness into the wisdom that all things, even if they appear to be so very different, form a oneness and should therefore be treated in the same manner. The symbol *hum* represents the transformation of the eight states of consciousness into the mirror-like wisdom of all things. The symbol *vam* stands for the ninth level of consciousness that unites all of the previous levels with each other in its totality.

The **eighth level** involves a mantra of the Womb World, in which the five variations of the *Siddham* symbol *a* are recited. As emanations of *Dainichi Nyorai*, these represent the five transcendental Buddhas. Four of the five *Siddham a* arise from the one for *Dainichi Nyorai*. This clearly illustrates the creative principle of *Dainichi Nyorai* since all of the Buddhas are created from him in the sense of the Goddess (Womb World). An additional meaning of the five symbols for *a* are the four steps to enlightenment: the development of the Buddha consciousness through the desire for enlightenment; walking the path; Enlightenment itself; and entering into Nirvana.

Finally, the **ninth level** is about the mantra *a ra pa ca na* (*a ra sa ha na*) of the *Monju Bosatsu*. This mantra subsequently also had the *Sid-*

dham symbol *om* added to it. *Monju Bosatsu* is both the mother and the father of the Bodhisattvas, as well as their spiritual friend and companion. Anyone who takes the path of the Bodhisattva, which means working for the highest good of all involved and wanting to help many beings achieve happiness, can learn a great deal from *Monju Bosatsu* and be initiated into many areas. *Monju Bosatsu* has a close relationship to *Dainichi Nyorai* because he also brings the wisdom of *Dainichi Nyorai* to the beings by means of the *Heart Sûtra*. At the same time, he also teaches that space connects the beings.

Practices with the HS Symbol

Preparation Practice for Consciousness Transmission

Connect with the Goddess **Dai Marishi Ten** *through the distant contact. Greet her with the words: "Dear Goddess* **Dai Marishi Ten,** *I come to you as a sick person and request healing. I come to you as an ignorant person and request teaching. I come to you as someone who does not know the way and ask for protection and guidance. I come to you as someone who is helpless and ask you for power in order to better serve. As compensation, I send you Reiki. Please use it as you wish for the benefit of all." Then draw several CR symbols and activate each of them with the mantra for intensifying the Reiki flow of power.*

*

Visualize yourself as *Dai Marishi Ten* in a red color and brilliant as a ruby with three faces, three eyes, and six arms. In your hands you hold a *Vajra* and an *Ashoka* branch, a bow and arrow, as well as a needle and a noose. Now imagine that your red body is hollow on the inside. Visualize a column of energy inside of you[159] that is open toward the top so that you can look up into the heavens.

*

---

[159] Skr.: *Sushumnâ nâdi* = rising energy channel that runs through the center of the spinal column.

*Also connect with **Kongôsatta** through the distant contact. Greet him with the words: "Dear **Kongôsatta**, I come to you as a sick person and request healing. I come to you as an ignorant person and request teaching. I come to you as someone who does not know the way and ask for protection and guidance. I come to you as someone who is helpless and ask you for power in order to better serve. As compensation, I send you Reiki. Please use it as you wish for the benefit of all." Then draw several CR symbols and activate each of them with the mantra for intensifying the Reiki flow of power.*

*

Visualize *Kongôsatta* floating above you. His body is also hollow. In his right hand he holds a five-pronged diamond scepter in front of his chest and a diamond bell in front of his belly in the left hand. Visualize a central energy column of wisdom rising up through his body[160]. The energy column within you now connects with that of the Diamond Mind, as if they were joined together.

The *Siddham* symbol *hûm* now appears in the heart of *Kongôsatta*, as fine as a hair and in a blue color, and another one takes shape in your own heart. Activate both symbols by repeating the mantra *hûm* three times. The *hûm* in your heart is the essence of your own spiritual consciousness. Now visualize how the lower part of the *hûm* in *Kongosatta* expands downward through the energy column until it reaches the *hûm* in your heart. Imagine how the *hûm* in your heart is slowly pulled upward by the *hûm* of the *Kongôsatta*. Inhale and exhale 21 times and loudly call out the sound of *heeg* every time you breathe out. With each breath, the *hûm* rises upward bit by bit until it has finally reached your crown chakra.

Now the *hûm* begins to flow downward again. Inhale and exhale 21 times and loudly call out the sound of *kâ* every time you breathe out. With each breath, the *hûm* sinks downward bit by bit until it has finally reached your heart.

---

[160] In the Cabbalistic Tree of Life—also see "Spiritual Cosmology"—there are three pillars. The middle one with the Sephiroth *Daath* (Secret Knowledge) is the pillar of wisdom because it simultaneously carries dedication to the whole and to the individual path, masculine and feminine forces, spiritual ideals and material constraints equally in its structure and combines them into a constructive functional unit in the sense of the divine order.

Feel what is happening inside of you for another moment. Finally, the form of *Kongôsatta* dissolves into light and falls into the *hûm*. This wanders through the dissolving column of light into the *hûm* in your heart, so that the two merge. Your form as *Dai Marishi Ten* now also dissolves into the light and falls into the *hûm*. The individual lines of the *hûm* finally disappear from the circular point on the crown. Keep your attention there for a while.

*

*Take leave by first giving thanks to **Dai Marishi Ten** and then to **Kongôsatta** and wish them all the best. Blow strongly through your hands and rub them together.*

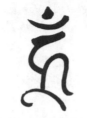

ILL. 143 – SIDDHAM HÛM

Advanced Preparation Practice for Consciousness Transmission

Only do this practice once you have spent adequate time doing the previous one.

The procedure is almost the same. During the 21 breaths, allow the *hûm* to rise up from your heart into the heart of *Kongôsatta*.

The Pagoda Meditation

*Connect with the Great Sun Buddha **Dainichi Nyorai** through the distant contact. Greet him with the words: "Dear **Dainichi Nyorai**, I come to you as a sick person and request healing. I come to you as an ignorant person and request teaching. I come to you as someone who does not know the way and ask for protection and guidance. I come to you as someone who is helpless and ask you for power in order to better serve. As compensation, I send you*

377

Reiki. Please use it as you wish for the benefit of all." Then draw several CR symbols and activate each of them with the mantra for intensifying the Reiki flow of power.

*

Now write the HS Symbol on a large piece of paper (as described in the chapter on calligraphy). Lay or place the HS Symbol in front of you and look at it for a while. Then imagine that the HS Symbol is turning into a pagoda. The curved diagonal lines form the multi-storied roof of the pagoda. A central pillar runs through the middle of the pagoda. It rises out of the pagoda a bit and connects heaven and earth. This is *Dainichi Nyorai*.

*

Then take your leave by giving thanks to him and wishing him all the best. Blow strongly through your hands and rub them together.

CHAPTER 16

The DKM Symbol

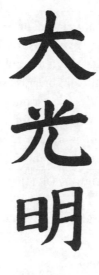

ILL. 144 – THE DKM SYMBOL

The DKM Symbol consists of the three *Kanji dai* 大, *kô* 光, and *myô* 明. In contrast to the HS Symbol, they are written separately. Together the three *Kanji* mean "Great Light" or "Great Enlightenment." The DKM Symbol has a close correlation with the Great Sun Buddha by the name of *Dainichi Nyorai* 大日如来. Like the HS Symbol, the pronunciation of the three *Kanji* of the DKM Symbol is Buddhist in nature. Just as the DKM Symbol is written and spoken in Reiki, it is also described in the sutras of Buddhism. This is the spiritual essence of *Danichi Nyorai* that embodies both the feminine and the masculine, as explained in the texts and mandalas of Esoteric Buddhism—especially in Shingon Buddhism.

The Origin of the Kanji in the DKM Symbol and Their Mystical Background

The Chinese Sign Dai 大

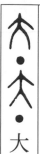 The *Kanji dai* 大 means "large" or "extraordinary." This sign is easy to remember not just because of the few strokes but also on the basis of the fact that this is a simplified picture symbolizing a person in his full height and breadth, standing with his arms and legs extended to the sides. This is one of the signs that apparently has "already always" existed. In comparison to this, the *Kanji* for "small" *shô* 小 also shows a human being, but this is someone who lets his arms hang down and stands with closed legs.

ILL. 145 – ORIGIN OF THE KANJI DAI

Readings of Dai 大

Sino-Japanese: *dai, tai*

Japanese: *oo, ookii, ooini, hanahada*

Japanese names: *o, oi, ooi, ooki, ki, takashi, takeshi, tomo, naga, hajime, haru, hiro, hiroshi, futo, futoshi, masa, masaru, moto, yutaka*

The Chinese Sign Kô 光

Kô 光 is also a Chinese character and means "light" or "lightning." This sign can also be easily remembered by imagining that the horizontal line is the horizon where the sun rises or sets. Although the sun itself cannot be seen, its light that shines upward in three rays and illuminates the sea through the two strokes beneath the horizon is visible.

However, the development of *kô* 光 is based upon a squatting figure that carries a bowl of fire on its head. This *Kanji* is also a fundamental sign that cannot be divided any further. Meanings: spiritual light, bowl of fire on the head = Crown Chakra, bowl = Great Goddess, three flames = three aspects of the divine, *kô*. The divine trinity above and the transition into the material level becomes yin and yang, *kô* = pentagram = spiritual humanness.[161]

ILL. 146 – ORIGIN OF THE KANJI KÔ

Sino-Japanese: *kô*

Japanese: *hikaru, hikari, kagayaku, kagayakasu*

Japanese names: *aki, akira, ari, kane, kanu, sakae, teru, hikari, hikaru, hiko, hiro, hiroshi, mitsu, mitsuru*

---

[161] For more information on the meaning of the three aspects of the divine and the pentagram, please compare the explanations in the chapter on Spiritual Cosmology.

381

The Chinese Sign Myô 明

Just like the other two, *Myô* is also a Chinese character. It means "bright." But in contrast to the previous ones, it is composed of the two signs for "sun" and "moon." The sun is located on the left side and the moon on the right. Based on the sign itself, there is a yin-yang polarity here. The moon represents yin and the sun stands for Yang. The sun is the same sign as the second sign of *Dainichi Nyorai* 大日如来 (Great Sun Buddha). The sun is smaller than the moon here since it is not as large in the sky when seen from the earth. The moon on the right is clearly recognizable as a half-moon because of its curved line on the left side. As we can see in the illustration, the sun was originally smaller since it is being pushed away by the moon. Both the sun and the moon shine. Together, they illuminate the earth, which results in the meaning of "bright." These two symbols indicate the Sacred Marriage (*Hieros Gamos*) of the Great Goddess and the Great God and the resulting liberation of the life impulse on the material plane. More precise explanations on this can be found in the chapter on "Spiritual Cosmology."

ILL. 147 – ORIGIN OF THE KANJI MYÔ

Sino-Japanese: *myô, min, mei*

Japanese: *akari, akarui, akarumu, akaramu, akiraka, akeru, aku, akuru, akasu, ake*

Japanese names: *aka, akari, akaru, aki, akira, akirakei, ake, kiyoshi, kuni, teru, tooru, toshi, nori, haru, hiro, mitsu, yoshi*

The Sign Combination Kômyô within the DKM Symbol

The signs *kô* and *myô* can appear as a combination and mean bright light or just simply light. However, the Buddhist Dictionary also says that *kômyô* is the light that emanates from the body of the Buddha. In many sutras, it is often explained that *Dainichi Nyorai* dwells at the center of the universe and light radiates from his pores into the entire universe. If this light is magnified manifold, it becomes discernable that this light is actually an infinite amount of little Buddhas who also emanate light or Buddha. After all, the Word "Buddha"" is also a Sanskrit term that means "the Enlightened One." If *dai* is additionally placed in front of *kômyô*, all three signs also mean "great, brightly shining light." This is related to the above-described background for the great light of all Buddhas. Since all Buddhas emanate from the cosmological Buddha *Dainichi Nyorai*, the DKM Symbol is the epitome of *Dainichi Nyorai* himself. When *Dainichi Nyorai* is mentioned in the following, this always also refers to the quality of the DKM Symbol.

When I was still at the level of Reiki 1, my first Reiki Master asked me for the Japanese character for "bright or great light." Although I already knew a bit of Japanese at the time, I did not initially understand what she was getting at and so I simply went to some dictionaries for advice. These revealed an entire series of terms for "light," all of which had various nuances such as daylight or electrical light. Since I thought that she was probably not looking for a light as in an electrical current, I simply presented her with the word *kômyô* 光明. Although she thought this *Kanji* was very beautiful, she thought that she could not use it since it was already taken. But she did not want to answer the question of why and for what. Otherwise, she would have revealed a big secret during a time when the symbols were still treated as a mystery. I had a premonition about this and she became quite embarrassed when I told her about it. This premonition was confirmed when I saw the Master Symbol for the first time a short while later.

In addition to the basic meaning of "light," *kômyô* can also signify "hope" or "ray of hope." In the Japanese dictionary of meanings, *kômyô* is described as illuminating even the darkest places. When someone has hope, he sees the chance of coming from the darkness into the light or shedding light upon the dark spot in his personality. When all of the dark spots within us are filled by light, this means the "great enlightenment" of *Daikômyô*.

Within this context, let us take a closer look at *myô*. As mentioned above, it consists of the sun and the moon. In Buddhism, the combination of the two represents the Buddha. However, this does not mean the historical Buddha *Shâkyamuni*. Before the Buddha of our era, there was already an entire series of other Buddhas who, as described in the *Brahmâjala Sûtra* and *Avatamsaka Sûtra*, arose out of the Great Sun Buddha *Dainichi Nyorai* since they are solely emanations of *Dainichi Nyorai*.

Among the emanations of *Dainichi Nyorai* are not only Buddhas and light beings but also humans. But most of them just do not know this.[162] Reiki is a method with which we can approach this state of consciousness. The Reiki initiations can help in this process at the beginning, but the practical applications of Reiki such as the laying on of hands and other practices are even better. The spiritual life energy of *Reiki* comes from *Dainichi Nyorai* through the Crown Chakra of the initiate, flows from there throughout the entire body to the heart and from there on to the hands and feet, the eyes, tongue, and other energy-sending chakras. This is where *Reiki* leaves the body and the aura once again in order to do something good for another being. In short, *Dainichi Nyorai* can develop this healing power through the initiated, who is an energy channel for Reiki. This form of energy transmission is called *kaji* (加持) in Japanese and is described in more detail below.

---

[162] The Indian Holy Avatar Satya Sai Baba frequently emphasizes in his speeches that the only difference between him and his students is that he is conscious of his divinity and they are not (yet).

The Spiritual Meaning of the Sun and Moon in the DKM

It is known from Esoteric Buddhism and Taoism that the power of the sun 日 and moon 月 is contained within the character of *myô*. In Taoism, the sun represents the masculine principle *yang*, and the moon stands for the feminine principle *yin*. Both are united here in one character.

When the *Sutras* of Buddhism were translated from Sanskrit into Chinese, the Chinese signs had already long been in existence and Taoism was also spread throughout all of China. So at least the influence of the Chinese usage may have been avoided. But I also think that the translators knew exactly what they were doing since there is something very similar in Esoteric Buddhism independent of *yin* and *yang*. And this is namely *Dainichi Nyorai* himself. *Dainichi Nyorai* is neither just masculine nor just feminine. He embodies, as described in the *myô* of the DKM Symbol, both the *yin* and the *yang*. This is seen in Esoteric Buddhism in the Mandala of the Two Worlds. In both mandalas, *Dainichi Nyorai* sits at the center and is surrounded by many light beings of Buddhism. The one is the Mandala of the Womb World (Jap.: *taizôkai)* and the other is that of the Diamond World (Jap.: *kongôkai*). The womb represents the feminine *Yin*—the Goddess, and the diamond stands for the masculine *Yang*—the God. In India, there were correspondingly two schools of Esoteric Buddhism. Each of the two is based on one of the two mandalas. The *Shingon* School says: "The two mandalas may be two, but they are

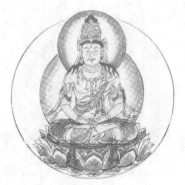

ILL. 148 – DAINICHI NYORAI OF THE WOMB WORLD

385

just one." *Kûkai's* teacher *Hui-kuo* recognized this since he was allowed to learn both forms of Esoteric Buddhism directly from the high Indian Masters. Many years ago, a monk of the *Shingon* School explained this phenomenon as follows: "...the right hand contains the Diamond World Mandala and the left hand holds the Womb World Mandala. Both are inseparable in the universe and are therefore depicted united in the Mudrâ of Wisdom, *Chiken in*, by *Dainichi Nyorai*. This mudrâ is always formed in front of the heart..." In both of the mandalas, *Dainichi Nyorai* sits at the center. In the Womb World Mandala, *Dainichi Nyorai* exhibits the Mudrâ of Teaching. In the Diamond World Mandala, *Dainichi Nyorai* shows the Mudrâ of Wisdom *Chiken in*.

The teaching is gained from the power of the highest single spiritual entity, the Great Goddess. She manifests the infinite abstract potential of the divine void in the infinity of the individual beings that are involved with each other in an unlimited material space and a time without beginning or end. Consequently, the Great Goddess brings the highest spiritual masculine being into the time-space continuum. Together with her, he constantly continues the creative act in the Sacred Marriage.

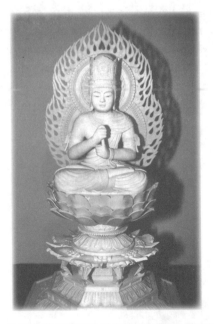

ILL. 149 – DAINICHI NYORAI OF THE DIAMOND WORLD

Examples of this creative act can be found in the *Yabyum* sculptures of India and Tibet, as well as in the symbol of the six-pointed star consisting of two triangles. This six-pointed star is also called Solomon's Seal in the Cabbala. Anyone who has read the Song of Solomon in the Bible will understand the Tantric background of this text. As a result, the Goddess Dai *Marishi Ten* is the spiritual mother of *Dainichi Nyorai,* who circles him with protection. Through his wisdom, *Dainichi Nyorai* then directs the teaching into the right channel. A very good comparison can also be made here with the HS Symbol and the CR Symbol in distant healing. As described above, the HS Symbol *Dainichi Nyorai* is the source of the Reiki energy. By using the CR Symbol, Reiki is then directed toward the appropriate person.

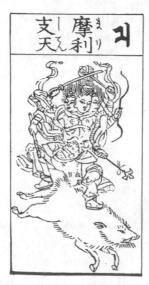

ILL. 150 – DAI MARISHI TEN

In Buddhism and Taoism there are apparently also parallels between the basic models of understanding for explaining the universe. Yet, the two philosophies of Taoism and Buddhism developed at very different times and completely independent of each other. Similar observations can also be made in other areas of the earth in the spiritual traditions than can be found there. Why is this?

Each philosophy that explains human existence, life, the universe, ultimately refers to the same things. As a result, the correct relevant thinking will always lead to the same insights time and again. This has also been sufficiently proved by the science of comparative mythology.

In East Asia, the moon was called the "light of the noble ones" in the literature of a very early period. Chinese scholars see the character and pure heart of the noble ones in the purity of the moonlight. According to the position of the moon, it is given various meanings. The moonrise develops the longing, and the setting moon indicates a sleepless night. However, the reflection of the moon is also a valued theme and, like the "wind in the pines," is compared with the personality of virtuous people.

In East Asia, looking at the moon at night is also a favorite activity for sensual-romantic hours, as well as for deeper insights in meditation. This is like the striving for enlightenment and expresses the wish to be free of the desires for earthly fame and personal advantages. When Dr. Usui meditated on Mount Kurama, he did this both day and night. So he had the sun during the day and the moon at night. However, the meditation that he performed was related to the planet Venus.[163] Through the light of the sun, Venus becomes just as visible as the moon for us people on the earth. Yet, it has a red-orange color that represents energy and passion. In addition, Venus appears directly next to the moon in the night sky. This is why both of these heavenly bodies are seen within a spiritual context in many cultures of the world. Dr. Usui allowed himself to be inspired by all three—the sun, moon, and Venus.—and had his experience with the great radiant light of *Daikômyô* after 21 days as a result.

The moon and its light also play an important role in both Buddhism and Taoism, even though this may not be in the same sense. In Taoism, it corresponds with the ideal of overcoming the fears about the transitory nature of life and with feeling our own soul within the world soul, the *Tao* 道. In Buddhism, the matter is somewhat more complex. If we look at the moon, we only see the moon. But it is reflected infinitely in the water, just as the light of Dainichi Nyorai radiates throughout the entire cosmos and illuminates every being and every place. The reflection of the moon in the water is a mirror image. In Zen Buddhism, the full moon is

---

[163] Cf. the chapter on Mount Kurama and the Morning-Star Meditation.

considered to be a symbol for perfect enlightenment, for the appearance of the Buddha. A human being who attains enlightenment will also appear to bc like the brilliant full moon, which means very pleasant light into which others can look. If he would shine as brightly as the sun, this would be too harsh. The light of the sun is also revealed through the moon, which in turn can appear at every place in the world through its multiple reflections. This is presumably the reason why many Buddhas are depicted in front of or on a moon disk.

The clear full moon is like the inherent Buddha nature of each being and is therefore a metaphor for enlightenment as the goal in Zen and Esoteric Buddhism. And this is precisely the meaning of the HS Symbol (see the chapter on the HS Symbol). This is why the DKM Symbol is always used together with the HS. The DKM Symbol also corresponds with the enlightened state, and the HS is the bridge for attaining this state. This is also one of the reasons why the Master initiation cannot be equated with enlightenment itself. The same also applies here, as always: The path is the goal. The human being returns to his natural state on this path and becomes like the luminous moon. His heart becomes as free as the clouds that travel across the heavens.

The surface of the water reflects the moon. This phenomenon can be compared with the spiritual heart (Jap.: *kokoro*). If the mirror is soiled, the reflection will not be clear. When the surface of the water is in motion or restless, the reflection is distorted. These inconsistencies symbolize the veil in front of our eyes, through which we subjectively perceive the world. However, the subjective perception does not correspond with the objective truth. So in order for us to see the world as it is, the water must be calmed and the mirror freed of dust. Mental healing and meditations with the SHK Symbol are good practices for perceiving the world as it actually is.

The Paradise Buddha *Amida,* who is the SHK Symbol together with the 1000-armed *Senju Kannon,* is called the "Full Moon Shining in All Directions" in his *Sûtra on the Pure Land.* This is an additional explanation for the *myô* in the DKM Symbol since *Dainichi Nyorai* stands for the sun and *Amida* represents the moon together with *Senju Kannon.* The spiritual heart is compared with the water itself in the same sûtra: "If the water is clear and calm, then the moon appears in it with its full form. If the water is cloudy and restless, the moon does not allow its radiance to appear in the water. The water-moon *Kannon* is also mentioned within this context.

The moon represents feminine power and the great knowledge of the Earth Goddess about life and the practical applications of spiritual principles, which reach us from the cosmos in the form of divine powers. Since these powers are too strong, too direct in order to help the beings of the material world, they are transformed through the kind power of the female moon in such as way that the needs and possibilities of her charges are taken into consideration. The female moon is an emanation of the Great Goddess, just as the Earth Goddess constitutes a part of the Great Goddess. Both of them work together harmoniously for the good of the whole.

So knowledge and wisdom are united with each other in the moon and the sun. It is only possible in this combination to fill the darkness with the great light. This thought is also expressed in one of the twelve famous Sun Angel mantras: *Om sûryaya Namahâ*. Spiritual seekers the world over have used this for thousands of years in order to drive away darkness and ignorance.

The Sun and Moon and the Siddham Vam and A

The moon is feminine, *yin,* and sun is masculine, *yang*. Related to the Mandala of the Two Worlds, the moon in the DKM shows the Mandala of the Womb World and the sun reveals the Diamond World. *Dainichi Nyorai* plays the most important role in both mandalas, also standing at the center as a result. Each of the Buddhist light beings have one or more *Siddham* associated with them. This classification was not made on an arbitrary basis. Instead, each *Siddham* corresponds to the quality of a light being. This can be compared with the colors in the chakras. Each color also has a special meaning here.

It is said that the Mandalas of the Two Worlds are separate and yet one. Exactly the same thing can be said for the DKM and *Dainichi Nyorai* as the Cosmic Buddha. Even if people speak of one symbol or one *Dainichi Nyorai*, there are always two. This is also one reason why Reiki is a non-polar energy form. However, this does not means that Reiki is an intelligent energy because other conditions would be required for this.

The Mantras of the Sun Angels

Om Adityâya Namahâ – A quality of the Hindu God Vishnu. The light of wisdom.

Om Arkâya Namahâ – The light that ends suffering.

Om Bhânave Namahâ – The source of the radiance that reveals the spiritual in material form, beauty in its highest perfection, for example.

Om Bhaskarâya Namahâ – The light of intellectual brilliance.

Om Hiranyagarbhâya Namahâ – The golden one: The healing gold that can bring forth what is most noble in every being.

Om Khagâya Namahâ – The light that penetrates everything, that cannot conceal itself from anything, that cannot be blocked.

Om Marîchâya Namahâ – This mantra contains the power of the Great Goddess *Mârîcî*, the fine, very special light of the dawn and dusk: the sunrise, the sunset. These are especially magical, romantic, and spiritual times of the day.

Om Mitrâya Namahâ – The light of the friendship that overcomes all differences and all obstacles.

Om Pûshne Namahâ – The light that radiates from the mystical fire, that produces the power of striving for oneness in the hidden places.

Om Ravaye Namahâ – The light of the winning being; the sweet, upright, clear, loving, kind, and wise character.

Om Savitre Namahâ – The light that emanates from enlightenment.

Om Sûryâya Namahâ – This mantra contains the power of the Great God, *Sûrya*, which is another name for *Dainichi Nyorai*. He drives away the darkness and ignorance. This clears the path for the perception and understanding of the divine truth, genuine knowledge, and the great radiant light.

In the Diamond World, *Dainichi Nyorai* has the *Siddham vam* (sun – *yang* – masculine) and in the Womb World he has the *Siddham a* (moon – *yin* – feminine). One of the most important practices in *Shingon* is meditating on the *Siddham a*. All knowledge is contained within this one symbol. We could say that it is discovered through this meditation, which means with the help of *Dainichi Nyorai*'s power. In order to direct this experience

391

into the right channel, the syllable *vam* is then added to it. In particular, this involves rituals with 37 light beings from 5 unities in the Mandala of the Diamond World. Among other things, this is one of the most secret practices in Esoteric Buddhism because of its complexity and its fantastic effects, but a more extensive description of it would go beyond the scope of this book. In short, among other things the *Siddham vam* is related to practices for attaining the truth behind the words, supporting the earth through communication through the element of water, death rituals with pagodas of the five elements, rituals for dissolving the causes of suffering such as possessions by entities and negative karmic influences (close connection with the 1000-armed *Kannon*), mandala meditations with light beings, power intensification, protective rituals, initiations, purification, the Heart Chakra, etc.

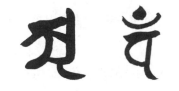

ILL. 151 – SIDDHAM A AND VAM

Kaji—The Secret of Energy Transmission in Reiki

Kûkai appears to have been the first Japanese to extensively comment on the energy transmission through light beings (*kaji* 加持). In his text on "Attaining Enlightenment in This Body" (*Sokushin jôbutsu gi* 即身成仏義), he describes *kaji* in terms of the sun of the Buddha *Daikômyô* 大光明, who stands for great compassion, being reflected in the hearts of all beings as in water. The practitioner experiences the sun of the Buddha in his heart when he meditates in a collected state on the meaning of this principle with the help of the Three Secrets (*sanmitsu* 三密). When the practitioner unites with *Dainichi Nyorai*, he receives extraordinary abilities (Skr.: *siddhi*), such as healing diseases (*kaji kitô*).

Healing itself is frequently called *kaji*. However, in the narrower sense *kaji* is the creation of flowing power.

Many years before his meditation on Mount Kurama, Dr. Usui was searching for a method to make the spiritual power, *kaji* of the life energy *Reiki* available in a lasting way. Without initiation into Reiki, this can only be achieved through difficult, longstanding ascetic practices. For example, mudrâs must be formed and mantras recited in order to prevent diseases and symbols must be visualized mentally in order to gather the power within ourselves in order to transmit it to other beings.

This energy is made useable in a lasting way through the Reiki initiation. In addition, the person is included in the *kaji*, which replaces the necessity of years of individual work and this person then becomes a lasting channel for the power of *Dainichi Nyorai*.

When we lay on hands after the initiation, Reiki flows. But this alone is not yet *kaji*. Although the flow of power from Reiki gradually becomes stronger, it is immediately there when we pray for healing on all levels for the being. When I (Mark) began with Reiki, I always had major fears during treatments for other people that it would not work and I would make a fool of myself. This is why I always prayed that Reiki would help this person, which then also happened without exception. At that time, I did not yet know that I unconsciously initiated the spiritual flow of power—*kaji*—with my prayer. *Kaji* is the blessing that *Kûkai* called the great compassion. This makes something possible that normally would not even function with Reiki. It works when we do it with the right attitude.

393

Despite this, spontaneous faith healings tend to be rare. Even if we want to heal, we cannot achieve every result. Not even Reiki can do everything right away. Some people require slow healing and support on the path in order to make their development possible. They receive help in understanding what they really need.

Incidentally, *kaji* can only occur when the actions are based upon decisions of free will. For example, it is possible to channel without *kaji* occurring, especially when this is done out of fear or greed. As long as human beings are ruled by fear and allow it to tell them what to do or as long as they give their power to the fear, there is no free will and *kaji* cannot take place.

The more we open up to the divine, the broader and more varied the support from the light beings will be. No development takes place on its own. If the surrounding field is very superficial and negative, a type of blessing is required. People caught in such a net require support. But this does not mean that the others are enemies. They are just on a different path. But if it is necessary, it can also help to understand why their path does not lead to happiness and oneness. At the same time, fighting and trying to convert others often leads to more tensions. If we receive support through *kaji*, we attract the appropriate people and the others move away from us. *Kaji* enables communication that brings understanding with it. We learn to wait, to put something aside, to change the way in which we speak to others, or no longer feel fear when someone has a different opinion.

The more we give Reiki, the stronger the spiritual energy flow of *kaji* will become over the course of time, in as far as we behave in a spiritual sense by integrating the three principles of personal responsibility, consciousness, and love—and include a divine being like *Dainichi Nyorai*. Then this light being will radiate support in the form of wisdom and power, which then enables the appropriate person to do things that are more meaningful.

By dwelling in the spiritual power of *kaji,* like during meditation, there may also be other occurrences in addition to the intensification of Reiki. This can lead to mystical experiences or sudden intuitions or insights inspired by light beings, fitting flashbacks to previous lives, and the like. Much of what I write or know about the symbols is based on such insights. I usually then discover only later while thumbing through books and searching for evidence in libraries that this knowledge was described in ancient religious writings from East Asia. My Master's thesis at the University of Heidelberg on "The *Siddham* Script in Japanese Art" is also an example of this. I usually knew the result long before I had found the text source as proof.

In the secret teachings—*mikkyô*—this phenomenon is explained in that just the presence of *Dainichi Nyorai* will also bring the teaching with it. So whoever opens up wholeheartedly to Reiki and therefore also to *Dainichi Nyorai* can be taught through the energy transmission—*kaji*—directly by *Dainichi Nyorai* in that sudden perceptions arise. To a certain degree, this state can also be deliberately produced if the respective person can let go at the same time. Only when Dr. Usui gave up the hope of solving the mystery on the 21st day of his meditation on Mount Kurama was he inwardly prepared to receive his vision. In Japanese, this is called *mushin* 無心, which is one of the expressions that can hardly be given a literal translation into English. It involves beginning something with the intention of success. Otherwise, we would not even do it. But then it says to not want to cling to the success. We have certainly all experienced at some point that we quite precisely know something but cannot remember it if we try to remind ourselves of it. The more we try, the more hopeless the situation becomes. Only when we let go, does it come to us. The channel for the information becomes free when we let go. *Mu* means as much as "nothing" or "emptiness." Within the context of the second character—*kokoro*—it describes the state of spiritual awareness that we can achieve if we strive for the appropriate success with the right intention and method; if this practice is blessed by the Creative Force; and the practitioner is prepared at the right moment, in the awareness of the divine presence, to completely give up the intention and fully trust in the higher guidance. So the word *mu* is also know as an exclamation of the Zen monks with which they endeavor to invite the teaching.

It is different from the memory because the messages from *Dainichi Nyorai* usually bring us something new. In the moment that we are practically connected with *Dainichi Nyorai* through the energy transmission, the information also comes through if we appropriately direct our attention to a goal. This state of fusion as a channel is then also called an "energy channel" (*kajishin* 加持身; literally: body of the spiritual energy transmission).

To give Reiki means receiving the spiritual life energy from *Dainichi Nyorai*, to channel it through our own body, and then transmit it to other beings through laying on of hand. *Kaji* is the power transference of the light being *Dainichi Nyorai* to other beings or objects. The only thing that is consciously done here is the technique, such as the laying-on of hands. The receiving and transmitting of Reiki cannot be consciously controlled. Since Reiki does not originate in the person giving Reiki but is first received from *Dainichi Nyorai*, those who are initiated into Reiki are also called Reiki channels. Even if the laying-on of the hands is a conscious action with which we can obviously increase the flow and promote the healing of a being if we do this in a skillful way, which means having a good training, it is also not possible to decide how much Reiki should be transmitted. Reiki is absorbed by the recipient. This process also takes place unconsciously and cannot be deliberately influenced, except for when the treatment and therefore the energy flow is broken off.

When Reiki Masters give initiations, an energy transmission takes place as well. In order to make Reiki or the symbols available to others in a lasting way, considerably more personal influencing is required than just laying on hands. However, the Reiki Master is also just a Reiki channel and additionally performs the initiation ritual. The actual energy transmission takes place through *Dainichi Nyorai*. In the process, the DKM Symbol—or an appropriate inner energy-work technique (*Nei Gong*) in the authentic Japanese tradition—plays an important role here because it represents the power of *Dainichi Nyorai* in its essence.

The third form of energy transmission consists of a person, such as Dr. Usui, receiving the Reiki initiation directly from *Dainichi Nyorai* without a human Reiki Master. To achieve this requires quite a bit of practice, much previous knowledge, and divine grace.[164]

---

[164] The appendix of the book *Reiki—Way of the Heart,* Lotus Press includes an astrological analysis of Dr. Usui's time of birth. When the transits are calculated for Usui on this basis during the time of his three-week meditation on Mount Kurama, it becomes obvious that there was an amassment of extraordinarily spiritual astrological influences makes the divine grace underlying this period clear.

There are many emanations of *Dainichi Nyorai*. These are other light beings such as Buddhas, Bodhisattvas, devas, or wisdom kings who are the same in their essence as *Dainichi Nyorai* but have special qualities. By means of special Rainbow Reiki techniques, it is possible to do energy work with these light beings.[165] Whenever an energy transmission with *Dainichi Nyorai* or one of his emanations takes place, we speak of the "protective power" that comes back from the Buddha spirit (*kaji riki* 加持力).

In addition, there are some other forms of energy transmission. The first is the power and energy of our own merits (*ga kudoku riki* 我功徳力). This energy is created by a being through the practice of *Dainichi Nyorai Kidô* and the Rainbow Reiki light-body work. Secondly, there is the power and energy in the world of Buddha's teaching (*hokkai riki* 法界力). This is the all-penetrating nature of things that is symbolized by the six elements and makes the Self and the Buddha essentially one and the same. The union of these "three forces" (*sanriki* 三力) is seen in Esoteric Buddhism as the energy of enlightenment. As *Kûkai* has described it, enlightenment—as a path that is accompanied by personality development—can be achieved in this lifetime through the combination of power transmission, individual effort, and the knowledge of things.

Related to Reiki, this means that the Reiki Master and Reiki practitioner must be initiated into Reiki for *kaji* to take place. In order to perform Reiki, our own effort is required when we lay on hands. And, in the final analysis, when we give Reiki we must also have the knowledge to use it in a skillful way. We must also know how to lead our clients to more love, personal responsibility, and awareness so that Reiki can work in an optimal way.

The DKM Symbol and Transference of Energy Through a Spiritual Being

The relationship between human beings and *Dainichi Nyorai* is embodied by the Bodhisattva *Kongôsatta*. *Kongôsatta* is considered to be a very special embodiment of *Dainichi Nyorai*. He symbolizes the enlightenment inherent to all beings, which is indestructible like a diamond. *Kongôsatta*

---

[165] Cf. *Rainbow Reiki* by Walter Lübeck, Lotus Press. Translated by Christine M. Grimm.

embodies both the enlightened beings and the beings on the path to en-lightenment. When we give Reiki and allow *kaji* to take place, we become *Kongôsatta* at this moment. In other words, *Kongôsatta* is the practitioner and at the same time the true Self that should realize what is to be practiced and which already appears in the translation of the HS Symbol. However, in the Reiki initiations the Reiki Master assumes the role of *Dainichi Nyorai* with the DKM Symbol. This means that *Dainichi Nyorai* works directly through him or her and the students of *Kongôsatta*. For Dr. Usui, the initiation into Reiki took place even more directly during his enlight-enment on Mount Kurama. Dr. Usui experienced not only *Kongôsatta* and *Dainichi Nyorai* but also *Senju Kannon*—the 1000-armed Goddess. As it is passed on to the students by the Reiki Master, Dr. Usui is said to have seen a light on the last day of his 21-day meditation.[166] This light approached him and then filled him completely. During this experience of enlightenment, he was given an understanding of the symbols in the form of clearly outlined spiritual truths and he was initiated into Reiki.

The ancient legend of the Iron Tower describes a similar transmission of the secret teachings to *Nâgârjuna*, the first human *Shingon* patriarch:

"After the death of the historical Buddha *Shâkyamuni,* there was an iron pagoda in India that no one could open for many centuries. As Buddhism appeared to be dwindling in Central Asia, the great Master *Nâgârjuna* came to this pagoda. For seven days, he walked around it, recited mantras, and scattered white poppy seeds. Then the door opened. A bright light shone from the pagoda, the air was filled with incense, flowers blossomed everywhere, and there was the sound of music praising the Buddha. As he entered, *Dainichi Nyorai* appeared to him in the form of *Kongôsatta*. During this experience, *Nâgârjuna* was initiated into the energy of Esoteric Buddhism and became familiar with the secret teach-ings, which are the basis for the *Kongô chô kyô*."

Although Dr. Usui did not set down a *sûtra* like the *Kongô chô kyô* for posterity, he did leave the Reiki symbols that conceal the wisdom and power of this and other sutras until the secrets could be revealed one day that Dr. Usui could not pass on during the four short years in which he taught Reiki.[167]

---

[166] Cf. the chapter on Mount Kurama for a more detailed description of the Morning-Star Meditation that Dr. Usui did at that time.

Kûkai explained that the iron pagoda was not created by human beings but by *Dainichi Nyorai*. In *Gyokuin-shô* (*Overview of the Precious Mudrâs*), the monk *Gôhô* (1306-1362) writes that the spirit (power) of *Dainichi Nyorai* comes from the iron pagoda. Within this context, the DKM Symbol represents the power of *Dainichi Nyorai* and the HS Symbol stands for the pagoda. We can also say that the pagoda corresponds with *Kongôsatta* and this, in turn, with the HS Symbol. This is why these two symbols play an especially important role in an initiation.

The pagoda symbolizes the entire cosmos of Esoteric Buddhism and the secret teachings. The pagoda (the HS Symbol) represents the totality of all things, beings, and actions in the past, present, and future. The five-storied pagoda, composed of the five *Kanji* of the HS Symbol, the five elements, and the five *Siddham a, ba, ra, ka, kya*, symbolizes the cosmological form of *Dainichi Nyorai*.

Each of the individual symbols has complex meanings and functions:

The **Siddham symbol** *a* is the source of spiritual power, the heart in human beings that connects the material with the spiritual. It is simultaneously the spiritual heart of the universe that links the realm of oneness with the realm of separateness. Esoteric Buddhism also speaks of dualism and non-dualism within this context. On the one hand, the mandalas of the two worlds are two mandalas, which are the Mandala of the Womb World (the Goddess) and the Mandala of the Diamond World (the God). But, on the other hand, they are an inseparable oneness, as the Chinese monk *Hui-ko*—the teacher of *Kûkai*—recognized and then reunited the two schools of Esoteric Buddhism. The symbol *a* represents the Divine Mother: not yet born, eternally alive. It is the sword that cuts through life and death. Every soul is the same—there are no hierarchies—just like when a raindrop falls into the sea. Nothing and no one is actually alive or dead. Life and death are an illusion since the creative force simply is. It cannot be born nor die. There is no specific place where something or someone exists. No beginning and no end. This is the state of true

---

[167] This was probably not necessary in the time after the Great Earthquake of September 25, 1923. Instead, Dr. Usui was busy with helping the many victims.

perfection. It is like the moon that reflects the sunlight. Spiritual element: earth.

The **Siddham symbol** *ba* stands for something that cannot be explained. Joy, happiness, desire, pleasure, sensuality, and the true secret of life. Spiritual element: water.

The **Siddham symbol** *ra* represents true innocence, wisdom, and enlightenment. Spiritual element: fire.

The **Siddham symbol** *ka* is not dependent upon conception and produces truth. Spiritual element: wind.

The **Siddham symbol** *kya* signifies absolute emptiness; absolute freedom; no boundaries. Spiritual element: space.

Meditation with the Mantra A Ba Ra Ka Kya

*Connect with **Dainichi Nyorai** through the distant contact. Greet him with the words: "I come to you as a sick person and request healing. I come to you as an ignorant person and request teaching. I come to you as someone who does not know the way and ask for protection and guidance. I come to you as someone who is helpless and ask you for power in order to better serve. As compensation, I send you Reiki. Please use it as you wish for the benefit of all."*

*

Then draw several CR symbols and activate each of them with the mantra for intensifying the Reiki flow of power.

Hold your hands in the Mudrâ of the Pagoda in front of your heart. Recite the mantra *a ba ra ka kya* 108 times or a multiple thereof. Silently enjoy the feeling for a while.

*

*Take leave of **Dainichi Nyorai** with the words: "I thank you for the contact and this beautiful meditation. I wish you the blessing of the Creative Force on your path." Blow strongly through your hands and rub them together. If necessary, ground yourself by giving your feet Reiki.*

Kaji and the Three Secrets of Body, Speech and Mind

Through the concentrated actions of body, speech, and mind, the practitioner activates the energy transmission of *kaji*. Since *Dainichi Nyorai* works through *Kongôsatta* in the practitioner, there is not just a one-sided but also a mutual transference of energy. In the secret teachings, this is also called the "Entering of the Self into the Great God/Great Goddess and the Great God/Great Goddess entering into the Self" (*nyûga ga nyû* 入我我入). There is an entire series of practices for this purpose, some of which are described below. Another practice for connecting with the life net of the Great Goddess can be found in the chapter on Spiritual Cosmology. But first, here are some advance explanations.

Since this union between the Great God/Great Goddess and the self symbolizes enlightenment, this practice is also called the Power Transference of the Three Secrets (*sanmitsu kaji* 三密加持). *Kûkai* wrote the following about it in his *Sokushin jôbutsu gi*:

"If the practitioner follows the instructions, forms mudrâs with the hands, recites mantras with the mouth, and dwells in *Samâdhi*[168] with the mind, then the Three Secrets will cause the energy transmission (*kaji*), and he will soon attain enlightenment."

Mudrâs are the secrets of the body, mantras are the secrets of the speech, and *Samâdhi* is the secrets of the mind. In the practice, symbols are used that are based on movements, forms, colors, fragrances, and sounds. Despite this, the Three Secrets symbolize an objective reality that cannot be limited to the body, speech, and mind of a human being. In the practices of the secret teachings, the Three Secrets are inseparably one. In *Dainichi kyô*, this is described as the body being equal to the speech and the speech equal to the mind, just as all parts of the great sea are equally salty."

Mudrâs, mantras, and visualizations are concretely integrated into practices such as meditations and rituals according to fixed rules in order to attain a specific goal. In addition, there are also the so-called "formless" practices. These include all possible actions that reflect enlightenment. These can also be integrated into rituals and meditations. But this is done in a more intuitive manner. The highest teaching of the secret teachings

---

[168] *Samâdhi* is a special state of consciousness in which thinking stops and which extends beyond the states of waking or dreaming. This results in a merging between the practitioner and a light being such as *Dainichi Nyorai* or another object of the meditation. Also compare the explanation of enlightenment and spiritual awakening in the corresponding chapter.

becomes reality when every word is a mantra, every movement a mudrâ, and every thought a meditation. This is why things with and without form are inseparably one.

Basic Meditation from the Sûtra of the Great Light (Dainichi Kyô)

ILL. 152 – SIDDHAM SYMBOL A ON A MOON DISK

Go to a calm place that is neither too light nor too dark. Sit in a full or half-lotus posture or in Japanese *Seiza* position on your knees. Your eyes are neither open nor closed.

Place your hands together in front of your heart in the way that you know from the initiations or the *Gasshô* meditation. Calm your mind by concentrating for a while on breathing into the Hara and the Reiki power in your hands.

Visualize in front of you a fully opened lotus blossom with eight petals. There is a round mirror on the bottom of the flower. The *Siddham* symbol *a*—the energetic essence of the DKM—stands on it. It makes the lotus blossom vibrate with astonishment. Out of the symbol *a,* a great radiant light now shines in all directions and to all beings like that of 1,000 flashes of lightning. From the depths of the round mirror, embodiments of the symbol *a* now go in all directions. Like the moon in clear water, the symbol *a* appears in front of all living beings.

Now the forms dissolve in the great radiant light. Continue to feel this for a moment and give thanks.

Meditations of the Three Secrets with the DKM Symbol

The following section introduces various meditation practices that have been taught by well-known monks through the centuries. They all refer to the monk Kûkai's ritual handbook on meditation with symbols. According to *Kûkai*, his texts were profoundly studied and his teaching was passed on orally. During the course of the centuries, some monks then wrote down the practical applications in explanatory commentaries. The Meditation of the Three Secrets is well known as one of the most outstanding practices for laypeople, advanced students, and professionals.

Performing these meditations promotes a strong ability to visualize and concentrate, which is why it is considered a good precondition for the above-described meditation by Dr. Usui on Mount Kurama.

The three following meditations are described here in the way in which they were written in the sutras and taught by the monks. Of course, they can also be performed using the distant contact to *Dainichi Nyorai*.

Meditation with the Symbol A Using the Writing Brush,
According to the Monk Kakuban (1095-1143)

Go to a calm place that is neither too light nor too dark. Sit in a full or half-lotus posture or in Japanese *Seiza* position on your knees. Your eyes are neither open nor closed. Place your hands together in front of your heart in the way that you know from the initiations or the *Gasshô* meditation. Calm your mind by concentrating for a while on breathing into the Hara and the Reiki power in your hands.

Using a writing brush, draw an eight-petaled lotus blossom of medium size on a large piece of paper. Above it, draw a moon disk in the form of a circle. Now write the symbol *a* on the moon disk (in the circle). Look at this picture as long as you like. Continue to feel this for a moment and give thanks.

Meditation with the Symbol A,
According to the Monk Myôe (1173-1232)

Go to a calm place that is neither too light nor too dark. Sit in a full or half-lotus posture or in Japanese *Seiza* position on your knees. Your eyes are neither open nor closed. Place your hands together in front of your heart in the way that you know from the initiations or the *Gasshô* meditation. Calm your mind by concentrating for a while on breathing into the Hara and the Reiki power in your hands.

Visualize in your heart a fully opened lotus blossom with eight petals. A moon disk stands on top of it. Within the moon disk that stands on top of the lotus blossom, the symbol *a* is now created stroke for stroke in a golden color. The symbol *a* radiates white, clear light to all living beings, eliminating ignorance and delusion in all beings.

Now the moon disk transforms into a crystal ball. It contains the golden symbol *a*. The crystal ball is the wisdom, and the symbol *a* is the truth. Hold this state as long as you can.

Now the forms dissolve in light. Continue to feel this for a moment and give your thanks.

ILL. 153 – STROKE SEQUENCE FOR THE SIDDHAM SYMBOL A

Dainichi Nyorai Meditation of the Three Secrets with the Symbols Om A Hûm

Connect with **Dainichi Nyorai** *through the distant contact. Greet him with the words: "I come to you as a sick person and request healing. I come to you as an ignorant person and request teaching. I come to you as someone who does not know the way and ask for protection and guidance. I come to you as someone who is helpless and ask you for power in order to better serve. As compensation, I send you Reiki. Please use it as you wish for the benefit of all." Then draw several CR symbols and activate each of them with the mantra for intensifying the Reiki flow of power.*

*

Hold your hands in the Mudrâ of the Pagoda in front of your heart. Visualize how *Dainichi Nyorai* meditates in front of you. He wears a crown on his head. His legs are crossed in the full-lotus position. His hands assume the Mudrâ of the Pagoda in front of his heart. His body is radiant gold.

From his forehead (6th Chakra), a white light now shines into your forehead and fills your entire head. As the white light spreads within your head, the *Siddham* symbol *om* arises on a moon disk within your head. Now sing the mantra *om* nine times. The light, the symbol, and the sound dissolve blockages and knots in the head area. Harmful habits—the cause of much suffering and disease—now leave you. This will make your body a powerful tool of love and protection for you and others. Your actions will promote love, personal responsibility, and consciousness.

From *Dainichi Nyorai's* throat (5th Chakra), a red light now radiates into your throat and fills your neck completely. While the red light spreads into the area of your neck, the *Siddham* symbol *a* arises on a moon disk there. Now sing the mantra *a* nine times. The light, the symbol, and the sound dissolve blocks in speaking. Words that bring suffering now leave. Harmful habits—the cause of much suffering and disease—now leave you. Your speech will become a means of compassion and wisdom, promoting love, personal responsibility, and consciousness.

From *Dainichi Nyorai's* heart (4th Chakra), a blue light now radiates into your heart and fills your chest completely. While the blue light spreads in your upper body, the *Siddham* symbol *hûm* arises on a moon disk. Now sing the mantra *hûm* nine times. The light, the symbol, and the sound dissolve knots, blockages, and obstacles in the mind. Rigid concepts that lead to dead ends now leave you. Your mind now represents boundless joy and realizes self-responsibility, love, and consciousness.

Now you see how the three rays of white – red – blue light all flow into you at the same time from *Dainichi Nyorai*. As you do this, recite the mantra *a ba ra ka kya* 108 times or a multiple thereof. Silently continue to feel this for a while.

Finally, *Dainichi Nyorai* dissolves into the light that radiates into you. Your own form eventually disappears as well. Time and consciousness are now one unity. Stay in this state as long as you can.

*

Take leave of **Dainichi Nyorai** *with the words: "I thank you for the contact and this beautiful meditation. I wish you the blessing of the Creative Force on your path." Blow strongly through your hands and rub them together. If necessary, ground yourself by giving your feet Reiki.*

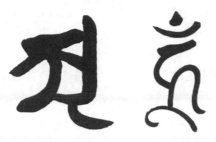

ILL. 154 – SIDDHAM A AND HÛM

The Reiki Initiations and the Master Symbol

There are initiations on many different spiritual paths. These are mostly rituals in which the adepts are introduced to the spiritual path. In Buddhism, there are the initiations of the so-called "Crossing Over" (Jap.: *tokudo*). This corresponds with the preparations and the ordination as a monk. However, such rituals tend to be more of a matter of form in many cases. This means that certain ritual actions such as the tonsure stand in the foreground.

In addition, there are additional forms of initiation rituals in the schools of Esoteric Buddhism and these correspond with the Reiki initiations in their effects. Among other things, this is because the Reiki initiations are very closely related to Esoteric Buddhism and have also been derived or assumed in part from it. Such initiations are called *kanjô* in Japanese. These always involve an uninterrupted continuation of a lineage that can be traced back to *Dainichi Nyorai*. Consequently, *Dainichi Nyorai* and *Kongôsatta* are initially followed by the Eight Shingon Patriarchs in the Shingon School until Japan. At the same time, the monk *Kûkai* is the eighth patriarch, followed by many others during the course of the centuries. Lineages like these also exist in Reiki. For the Reiki that first came to the West, these are *Dainichi Nyorai – Kannon – Usui – Hayashi – Takata*. But since Dr. Usui initiated about 20 Reiki Masters, there are now accordingly more lineages since Dr. Usui than people have assumed up to now, even if not all of them have become known or some have also ended. Dr. Hayashi also trained about 20 Reiki Masters. Among them were Mrs. Takata, and another well-known Reiki Master who he trained was Mrs. Yamaguchi (her son, Tadao continues the lineage). In both the Shingon School and Reiki, this lineage plays an important role within the initiations. The individual masters of the lineage or the patriarchs—and just the ones who are no longer alive—are integrated into the ritual, beginning with *Dainichi Nyorai* and *Kannon* in Reiki or *Kongôsatta* in Shingon. This is especially important for the success of the initiation. What is "transmitted" in the initiations is nothing that can be acquired by reading books. It is a special energy form that can only be transmitted to a person from a spiritual being like *Dainichi Nyorai* through a master of the lineage. This means that what is called the secret teaching (*mikkyô*) is not only a teaching put into words, which is why the term "teaching" often causes confusion within this context. It is also worth mentioning at this point that there are generally two forms of the secret teachings. The first is what is transmitted through initiations. But that is just the beginning. Afterward, what is much more significant is the path that we take or what we make out of the initiation. Consequently, that the important thing is not the techniques, the secret teachings, but that what is secret conveys itself through regular involvement with it and through application of the methods acquired in the training. Because of the connection to the lineage that goes back to *Dainichi Nyorai*, only the true essence of the secret teachings can be received through it. In order to achieve this, it is useful to have a spiritual teacher for a longer period of time who can help us progress in an individual way on this path and who is ready and capable of pointing out when we have possibly gone astray. When students are also ready to integrate these things, they will soon be able to take the path alone because they have become true masters in the meantime.

A lineage dies out when it is not followed in a way that is authentic and has integrity or when the rituals and/or symbols are not correctly transmitted to others—when the ability to function is no longer adequately present. Unfortunately, this is very difficult for most people to understand and grasp. In order to check this, there are various methods in relation to the Traditional Usui System of the Healing. The simplest consists of examining the lineage of their own master to see whether it can truly be traced back without interruption from person to person to

Dr. Usui. But then it only becomes a problem when disastrous mistakes in the initiation rituals or symbols have occurred within the lineage.

The fact that the symbols and rituals had been kept secret for decades, connected with the completely unfounded prohibition of making written or other recordings of the training contents has unfortunately promoted this problem. Second, it has happened that some Reiki Masters have, without knowing it, become Masters outside of the lineage but had been correctly initiated into the First and Second Degrees of Usui Reiki somewhere else so that although they can now practice Usui Reiki but their students who have been trained with the faulty or completely different initiations cannot. So I recommend that anyone who is serious about Reiki should thoroughly examine whether the package contains what the label claims it does.

The writings of Esoteric Buddhism describe how the *Kanjô* initiations can be traced back to the ancient Indian crowning ritual. But it is also quite probable that the history of this Indian ritual also has a long prior history, which is perhaps a good topic for another book. What did such rituals look like? Visible to the human eye, it primarily appeared that the head of the new king was ritually sprinkled with the water of the four seas, which was intended to symbolize his rule over the entire kingdom. Correspondingly, the head of the person to be initiated into Esoteric Buddhism was sprinkled with the water from five containers. So first four, then five? This process was explained in *Dainichi kyô*. *Dainichi Nyorai*, the King of All Buddhas and therefore also the Cosmic Buddha who rules over the entire cosmos, is the only Buddha to wear a crown[169] and jewelry. In the mandalas of Esoteric Buddhism, which depict the cosmos in an abstract and simplified form, *Dainichi Nyorai* sits at the center and is initially surrounded by four additional Buddhas. These four correspond with the four seas and the four directions. With *Dainichi Nyorai* as the king, this results in the number five. The four Buddhas and the Buddhas that follow in the mandala, the Bodhisattvas, etc., are his emanations. In the Shingon and Reiki initiations, this part is replaced by the symbols. For making the contact with *Dainichi Nyorai* and transferring energy with him, this part is the same in all initiations for a lasting transmission. Depending on the

---

[169] In Tibetan Buddhism, *Dainichi Nyorai* is replaced by the Root Lama, who also wears a (black) crown.

function and purpose of the initiation, the following steps may vary. In *Dainichi kyô*, the various types and levels of the initiations are described. Listing them all here would go beyond the scope of this book (although I do discuss them in my own seminars). One form of the initiation is the first contact with an area of the secret teachings. This may be a meditation or even the experience of receiving Reiki from someone. But this does not correspond with any type of Reiki initiation in the actual sense since Reiki is still not available in a permanent manner afterward.

Only through the initiation into the First Degree does the actual contact with the secret teachings (*mikkyô*) take place. In the process, the lasting connection to the source of the Reiki energy—*Dainichi Nyorai*—is created, through which the student is included into the spiritual power (*kaji*). Such initiations are also called *Reikanjô* in Shingon and *Reiki kanjô* in Shintô. Sometimes the initiations are also called *Reiki ki* in Shintô. This may be somewhat confusing because Reiki is written with the character 麗氣 here, which literally is translated as "pretty energy." The first sign is also different from the one for Dr. Usui's healing method of Reiki (靈氣). So *Reiki ki* is simply another word for *kanjô* (initiation).

The sequence for the main portions are the same in Shingon and Shintô. Only the setting, as well as the preparatory practices, are different. Both of them are initiations into the Reiki power. In Shintô, this type of initiation has been assumed from Shingon. However, there is a difference in the types of explanations given for precisely what happens there. In Shingon, a person becomes a channel for Reiki through the connection with *Dainichi Nyorai*. In Shintô, the god *Tenshô Daijin*, who slumbers within every living being, is awakened by being implanted in the person. In turn, this god can be compared to our own primordial Buddha nature that is innate within every being and can be awakened. *Tenshô Daijin* is the Shintoist *Dainichi Nyorai*, and simultaneously also an emanation of him. In turn, this god corresponds with the *T'ai-I* of the Wu shamans of ancient China. It is quite possible that through the great variety of developments during the course of the centuries the qualitative power of the energy has changed in the initiations. Depending upon which partial aspects and light beings the emphasis is placed upon, the type of energy can be different. But the personal connection, as well as the adept's ability to resonate, can cause the energy form to appear differently. As a result, the experiences in the initiations and treatments, as well as the meditations, can be completely different in nature.

In Shingon, there is an entire series of different initiations into greatly varying aspects. The emphasis here is initially upon the meditation with light beings for the development of the mind, which represents the precondition for health on all levels. This approach is also similar in Shintô, which focuses on the purification with the light being *Kami* in shamanic rituals. The direct healing of physical diseases is usually just reserved for the adepts of the higher levels. In keeping with this, Dr. Usui emphasized in his three principles of healing that the mind should first be treated and then the body. In Reiki, treatments within the scope of Reiki energy transmissions already begin at the First Degree. So we can also treat ourselves and others while we develop our minds.

In order to use Reiki in a specific and intensified form, the initiation into the Second Degree is very useful because it teaches the symbols CR, HS, and SHK, in addition to many fundamental applications. Since the symbols can be traced back to the individual light beings, who are emanations of *Dainichi Nyorai*, the connection between Reiki and the quality of the light beings makes special applications possible. The initiation into the Second Degree is called *Jumyô kanjô* (Receiving of Light-Filled Symbols Through Initiation).

The initiation into the Degree of Master and the DKM Symbol ultimately make it possible to also pass on Reiki to other people by means of the above-described initiations. This so-called Master Initiation has the Japanese name of *Denpô kanjô* (伝法灌頂) and means something like "Transmission of the Teaching Through Initiation." However, not everyone can immediately attain this degree in Esoteric Buddhism and also not with Dr. Usui. In order to become a Master, a certain degree of personality development and personal devotion is required. Unfortunately, this point is no longer valued by many Reiki Masters today so that an entire series of extremely brief trainings make it possible to become a Reiki Master in a day or on a weekend. The result is a very low standard and hardly any know-how. Although these initiations include the people in the spiritual power, each person must take the path on their own.

In Esoteric Buddhism and in the Usui System of Natural Healing, the requirements can also be recognized in the so-called Principles of Dr. Usui,

among other things. It is interesting to mention in this respect that the five
principles already appeared in the *Sûtra of the Great Sun Buddha Dainichi
kyô,* which are extremely similar to those of Dr. Usui.

Life Principles in Dainichi kyô	Principles According to Dr. Usui
Stay away from everything that is impure.	Just for today do not get angry.
Create trust in the understanding of the law of cause and effect through insight.	Just for today work hard on yourself (while taking into consideration the law of cause and effect, which means karma).
Be careful but without worries	Just for today do not worry.
Develop a deep belief that overcomes all boundaries.	Just for today be thankful.
Always work for the good of others.	Just for today be nice to your fellow human beings.

For the Master Initiation of Reiki Masters there are two basic forms, but
these are frequently lumped together since Reiki Masters can initiate both
students and Masters. When someone has just become a Reiki Master,
he has—if he was lucky—had a good training. Initiating students into
Reiki One and Two is not a problem then. However, the ability to guide
a student who wants to become a Master can only be achieved through
the experience of teaching and initiating beginners in the First and Second
Degree. I therefore believe it is meaningful to divide the Master training
into the appropriate levels. This is the standard in Rainbow Reiki, for
example. Incidentally, the same also applies to the initiations in Shingon
Buddhism. The Master, who is called *Ajari* there, has this title only as a
basis for further studies. There are also even higher *Ajari* Degrees. Only
those who appropriately distinguish themselves can finally carry on the
lineage and train both students and Masters. This point is also where
there is a difference in Japan between the Master and Grand Master. The
Master can teach students and the Grand Master can additionally train

teachers and provide them with advanced training. This Grand Master title is in no way limited to just one person. Fortunately, we rarely hear such stories and in the rule it usually turns out that just some form of ego-aggrandizement and the greed for power are involved when someone wants to solely bear this title.

Many of the individual initiations may be similar in the Reiki initiations and Shingon, yet they are still quite different. There are a great many different types. In Shingon, Reiki initiations are called *Reikanjô* (靈灌頂). A monk and friend on Mount Kôya told me that the monk *Kûkai* once brought this form of initiation to Japan. But it is far from being the only initiation that there is in Shingon. In addition to the healing aspect and the path of enlightenment, there is also an entire series of other initiations with numerous functions and effects. However, the initiation doesn't make things necessarily better since it always depends upon which path we take and how much we are prepared to develop ourselves, with all of the consequences that entails.

There are fixed rules for the various initiations. Actions, postures, standing positions, symbols, mantras, and mudrâs are always used, all of which have their meaning and specific effect. A great common factor is the so-called symbol and mantra of the Five Syllables of the Light (Jap.: *Goji no myô* 五字ノ明). In Shingon, this is the secret name for the HS Symbol.[170] However, it is used in alternating combinations of the five *Siddham* in Shingon, which are related to the five elements and the five transcendental Buddhas. But a sixth element is also mentioned, with which the monk *Kûkai* explained consciousness. This, in turn, is the esoteric meaning of the HS Symbol itself. This is the basis of the secret teachings. Moreover, there is a description of how the five syllables rest on a lotus blossom (the head of the person to be initiated) and from there the great radiant light *Daikômyô*, which illuminates the entire cosmos, is transmitted to the students with the help of the master, who assumes the role of the channel *Dainichi Nyorai*. In this manner, the spiritual life energy Reiki and the secret teachings are transmitted to the students on a spiritual level and make it possible for them to open up to the source of enlightenment.

---

[170] Cf. the explanations in the chapter on the HS Symbol.

Another form of the initiation is the transference from heart to heart. It is sometimes also called the initiation from forehead to forehead in Japanese, which classifies it under the term of *Himitsu kanjô* (secret initiations). The special characteristic of this initiation is that it is not a fixed ritual and also does not use any external aids. This is a direct, partially intuitive transference of the teaching, as well as a very personal process between the teacher and the student. I (Mark) believe that I once had an experience like this as I spoke with my Master about whether I had been a certain person in an earlier life, as people have often told me. Among other things, the initiation took place within the question: "What would change for you in this life if this were so?" Here in this book, this question may sound like a normal sentence, but at this moment so much happened that it is very difficult to put into words. However, in all of my chakras—particularly in my heart chakra—I felt an unbelievable sense of happiness and a simultaneous increase in power. I had the impression that I was merging with my Master and expanding in space at the same time. In my mind, I immediately found the answer but it took a while for me to express it in words. The *Kôan's* solution was that nothing at all would change since the only thing that is important is what I make of my possibilities in this life, no matter who I was and who I am ... At the same time I recognized something else in my Master, something that still was hard to grasp... Perhaps I also personally encountered a manifestation of *Dainichi Nyorai*. I believe that I grasped a deeper level of personal responsibility, love, and awareness in this initiation. Even now as I write these lines, tears of joy and liberation come to my eyes.

The secret teachings say that initiations touch very deep layers of a being. The change that occurs through the initiation happens on another level than the conscious work on ourselves. The latter is a developmental process from bottom up. However, an initiation is an experience from top to bottom that penetrates to the innermost self in a way that can only be fully and completely grasped through our own experience.

CHAPTER 17

The CR Symbol

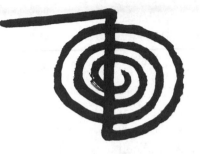

ILL. 155 – CR SYMBOL

Explanation of the Characters of the CR Symbol

The CR Symbol has the Japanese pronunciation in *Choku rei*. In contrast to the other three symbols, the CR Symbol does *not* simultaneously involve characters[171]. It is also possible to associate the CR Symbol with an entire series of characters. This is meaningful in so far as the pronunciation is so Japanese or Sino-Japanese that there must be Chinese characters for it. However, this in no way implies that the CR Symbol can be replaced by Chinese characters. In order to grasp the meaning, the question arises here as to which characters are the appropriate ones. Fortunately, there are just a few possibilities here and only two of them are applicable within this context.

The following three characters are possible for *choku*:
直・勅・捘

The following characters are possible for *rei*:
霊・靈・例・礼・令・零・玲・鈴・怜・麗・黎・伶・隷・苓・
禮・齢・嶺・冷・蛎・砺・戻・励・澪・礪・蠣

---

[171] The CR Symbol illustrated above corresponds with the way that Hawayo Takata wrote it.

It would be extremely futile to translate all of the possible combinations of *choku* and *rei*. Besides, most of these combinations do not exist, which also considerably simplifies the selection.

The following sign combinations are available for *Choku rei*:

勅令   Imperial decree/command

直靈   Intuitive consciousness, the consciousness/the mind is immediately there

直隷   Submitting to the government

勅励   Urging someone to do something

Only the first two sign combinations have something in common with the CR Symbol. In the West, the first combination of "Imperial Command" (勅令) has already been spread by word of mouth in many places. The pronunciation of *Choku rei* is very rare in Japan. On the one hand, this is because there are few combinations; on the other hand, this is because the combinations listed here are rarely used in everyday spoken language. Only the first combination appears in most of the Japanese dictionaries because this is a term that has a historic context for Japanese. Asking a Japanese person about the meaning of *Choku rei* usually results only in the response of an "imperial command."

Strictly speaking, this is not just a command but also a decision made by the emperor, which in any case became a command that must be executed. Accordingly, this term already appeared four times in the first Japanese Constitution of 1889 and was described there as an extremely urgent command by the emperor. Until 1945, the Japanese Emperor (*Tennô*) was not only worshipped like a god but it was actually assumed that he was a god of the original Japanese religion of Shintô because he, as has been handed down historically, descended from the Sun Goddess *Amaterasu*. However, on the occasion of the Japanese capitulation of the Second World War, the Tennô was forced to announce on the radio that he was only a human being. Consequently, the words *Choku rei* do not even appear once in the current constitution from the year 1946. Related to the CR Symbol, this means that this does not refer as much to the command of an emperor but instead to the command of the highest goddess of the Japanese Shintô religion. This is the Sun Goddess *Amaterasu*, who is comparable with the Great Sun Buddha *Dainichi Nyorai* of Esoteric Buddhism. *Dainichi Nyorai* is the spiritual being represented by the DKM Symbol. The Japanese already recognized early on that the various names of the light beings are the archetypes of the Japanese gods (*Kami*). It is believed that one light being incarnates itself as another or that they are emanations and forms of manifestations of each other. The same applies to *Amaterasu* and *Dainichi Nyorai*. This is why the various spiritual traditions were connected with each other in Japan instead of destroying the other religions and their followers with the sword, torture, and burning at the stake.

When the name of the Great Goddess *Amaterasu* (天照大神) is written in Chinese characters, it becomes apparent that these are the same characters as those for the highest god in Taoism. According to the pronunciation, her name is purely Japanese (Shintô) and the script is based on the Chinese (Taoism) script. Consequently, this involves a three-fold archetype of Shintô, Taoism, and Buddhism. And the origins of the CR Symbol can also be found in precisely these three spiritual traditions. In Japan, there is also an additional spiritual tradition that contains the magical aspects of the above-mentioned three traditions—*Shugendô*[172].

The second sign combination of the CR Symbol (Jap.: *Choku rei* 直靈) cannot be found in any common dictionary. Nevertheless, this word exists. 直靈 is a specialized term of Japanese magic (*Shugendô*). Its meaning cannot be translated in one word and requires a more detailed explanation. It refers to the Creative Force, which appears at any moment. In other words, it is the power that ensures that something manifests itself. Through applications of the CR Symbol, the Creative Force is invited to become active in the here and now. The sign analysis of 直靈 should clarify this within this context:

---

[172] Cf. the chapter on *Shugendô*.

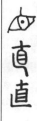

Choku (直) has the following meanings: "momentarily, to heal, immediately, upright, straight ahead." It also appears in the Japanese word for intuition (*chokkan* 直観・直感, literally: "that which is immediately seen/that which is immediately felt"). As can be seen in the illustration at left, the original sign is an eye. The vertical little stroke above the eye indicates that only what is actually there is seen when the mind does not wander.

ILL. 156 – KANJI ORIGIN FOR CHOKU

Rei (靈) is the first character of Reiki 靈氣 and represents the work of the shamans and magicians here. The basic meaning is "the pure mind of the Creative Force".

ILL. 157 – KANJI ORIGIN FOR REI

Rei, the Chinese *Ling*, is understood in Chinese Qi Gong as "the secret, spiritual meaning" that works secretly behind the directly perceivable life processes and energies and the force that promotes life itself. It is the highest that organizes life according to the laws of the Divine Order. In ancient times, it was the main task of the shamans to bring power into this world on a regular basis and for special occasions. This was intended to synchronize human beings and nature, as well as the spiritual and material worlds with each other to create a meaningful harmony. As a spiritual energy organ, the heart is seen in the Chinese spiritual teaching as the dwelling of the human mind. Here, heart means the psychic and mental center of a human being. The mind (Chinese: *shen*), the spiritual, conscious intrinsic nature, shows itself through the spirituality (Chin. *ling*) that a being expresses in thinking, emotions, decision-making, and taking action. *Shen* and *ling* relate to each other like yang and yin. In this respect, *ling* is essentially one feminine quality of the divine. Incidentally, all of this with its great, radiant light that illuminates spiritual consciousness is called *Lingjue* in Chinese. If the form follows the mind, the form will not be harmed. If the mind follows the intrinsic nature, the mind will not be harmed. We can become aware of our intrinsic nature and then

417

develop the potential of our intrinsic nature for spiritual perfection. By doing this, we attain our essential life energy that is the source of all of the body's spiritual life force and resides in the kidneys. The energy is the so-called original substance of the empty void of eternal duration. If it is present and strong, it can rebuild the intrinsic nature, the mind, and the other, secondary forms of the life energy.

In everyday Chinese, the attribute of *ling* describes someone who copes well with life, has a sharp, clear mind, and can quickly build and keep good emotional relationships with others. *Ling* is also seen as the divine portion of the *shen*, which does not die with a being but is retained by the world as a potential for doing good. The Wu shamans of ancient China were famous for being able to draw wisdom, love, and meaning from this source. The more *ling* a person collects, the greater the spiritual power and abilities of perception will be developed by his *shen*. Because of his extraordinarily strong *Ling*, a spiritually realized human being becomes a *Shen Ming* (the second word—*Ming*—consists of the symbols for sun and moon) after his death. This is a charitable spiritual being who helps the needy to leave the astral world or is reincarnated just to provide help to others. In Buddhism, such a being is called a Bodhisattva. If the *Ling* is very strongly developed in a person, he will live longer than usual, is more capable, and can even travel outside of his physical body with his spirit body and do good. He may appear to people in dreams as a teacher and healer, as well as performing magical feats through his pure presence to support the Divine Order. During his lifetime, such as person is called a *Xian* (god, immortal, fairy being) but *Shen Ming* is used upon his death. *Shen* resides in the uppermost of the three *Tantiens*, in the 6th Chakra. If the *Ling* in the *Shen* is not strong enough, the *Shen* scatters throughout the body and the mental and spiritual functions suffer. By learning and practicing wisdom in thinking, coping with emotions and actions, as well as appropriate energy work, the *Ling* can be strengthened and the *Shen* then collected again. A developed, spiritual *Shen* expresses itself through wise use of the willpower that is oriented upon the divine order. The proper use of the Qi—the life energy—for outer and inner activities of all types that correspond with our own spiritual path, nourishes the *Ling*.

The following acupuncture points of *Du Mai* have a close resonance with the *Ling*: *Du* 10 (*Lingtai*) – foundation of the soul; *Du* 11 (Shendao)

– path of the mind; *Du* 12 (*Shenzhu*) – support of the character; *Du* 4 (*Mingmen*) – gateway of life; *Du* 2 (*Yaoshu*) – directs the Qi to the hip; *Du* 23 (*Shangxin*) – following our own star; point outside of the meridian system 12 (*Wuming*).

The Origin of the CR Symbol

Since we know now that the CR Symbol is a term from *Shintô* (Path of the Gods) and *Shugendô* (Path of Magic), it is helpful to take a closer look at the rituals of both spiritual paths. These both have a very long history.[173] Since the CR Symbol stands in direct correlation with the *Tennô* as a Shintoist light being (Jap.: *Kami*), it is quite probable that the term *Choku rei* already appears in much earlier texts. The earliest work that I could find is the *Engi Shiki* (延喜式), a text compiled by scholars in the 10th Century describing many of the Shintoist rituals at the old Court of the Tennô. This states that *Choku rei* was originally a *Kotodama* (言靈). The term *Kotodama* is used for words or sentences whose recitation releases spiritual powers with practical effects. In this regard, the term *Kotodama* corresponds with the description of the word mantra that is familiar to us from the Indian spiritual tradition.

Even today, there is still a Shintoist festival in Japan by the name of *Choku sai* (勅祭). This involves the imparting of welcoming words through an imperial messenger (*choku shi* 勅使) in the form of *Kotodama* to a shrine and its spirits (*Kami* 神).

During his search for a method with which the life energy can be made available in a lasting way, Dr. Usui had studied Shintô and Shugendô in addition to Esoteric Buddhism and Taoism. In the chapter on ritual prayers for light beings (*norito*), the *Engi Shiki* describes the applications of the CR Symbol in a very detailed way. *Norito* are the ritual prayers that are based on the language of Japanese mythology. It is said that the words in the *Norito* are also inspired (*kotodama*). *Norito* can be used for various purposes such as expressing thanks, blessing, protection, individual needs, or festivals. The earliest preserved collection of *Norito* has been

---

[173] Also see chapter on Shintô in Japan.

handed down in the *Engi Shiki* from the year 927. The spelling of *Norito* has been determined according to specific rules in which the root of the word is written with large signs and the ending of word, as well as verbs, are written with smaller signs. Throughout the centuries, many *Shintô* priests have created new *Norito* for various purposes time and again.

However, it is now common to use the collections that already exist.

The language of the ritual prayers was apparently already considered to be archaic in the Seventh Century. The methods that are used there consist of equating the pronunciation of a word made of several Chinese characters with a symbol. This also applies quite precisely to the CR Symbol. Incidentally, the same is also valid for the HS and DKM Symbols. The pronunciation of *Hon sha ze shô nen* represents the five Chinese characters 本者是正念. In their interwoven combination, they result in the HS Symbol. The pronunciation of *Daikômyô* stands for the three Chinese characters 大光明, which result in the DKM Symbol when read in the order of top to bottom. This method also reveals the reason why in Reiki the SHK Symbol—which, after all, is an Indian *Siddham*—has the Sino-Japanese pronunciation of *Sei heki* with the Chinese sign 正癖 (healing habits) instead of the Indian pronunciation of *hrih*.

The text in the *Engi Shiki* becomes even more interesting because it is described there that the imperial instructions, meaning the CR Symbol, follow the application of each individual symbol to breathe its effect into it. This shows the correlation between the above-explained character combinations for the CR Symbol. The spelling of 勅令 relates to the imperial (or rather divine) commission of the Sun Goddess *Amaterasu*, who is identical with the Great Sun Buddha *Dainichi Nyorai*. *Dainichi Nyorai* embodies God, Goddess, and Creative Force in one. This means, that the CR Symbol becomes active as the Creative Force in the sense of the second spelling of 直靈 *Dainichi Nyorai*.

This corresponds precisely with many Reiki techniques, such as distant healing, space cleansing, mental healing, and the Rainbow Reiki Shower. If, for example, I would like to perform a mental healing, I would first draw the SHK Symbol on the crown of the person to be treated. Then I would activate this by saying the mantra three times. Next, I would draw a CR Symbol in the same place and also activate it by saying the mantra three times. Only then would I say the name three times and, if necessary, the affirmation. Of course, there are additional methods of this application that also work; however, the ones described here appear to have proved especially effective throughout history.

In ancient Shintô (*koshintô*), it was assumed that the human being who lives in the great universe is not just a part of this great universe but himself a little universe in which the big universe is depicted. The great universe is the world of the Japanese gods and they have also breathed life into it (*rei kon*). Some of the gods came down to the earth many millions of years ago and breathed life into it. Human beings, who continue to be connected with the gods, then developed from this. Within them works the life-giving power (*Choku rei*), that is sent directly from the gods through the crown into the center of human beings. Without them, a human being cannot live. In the four directions—just like a mandala—there are four souls that enable human beings to live in the material world and yet still remain connected with above at the same time. The Soul of the Wondrous (*kushimi tama* 奇魂) lives in the area of the pituitary gland. It is responsible for the inner and outer abilities of perception and action. At about the height of the heart lives the Soul of Happiness (*sakimi tama* 幸魂). It is responsible for wisdom and the ability to use wisdom constructively. Around the area of the 1st Chakra is where the Soul of harmony (*wakimi tama* 和魂) lives. It takes care of the energy equilibrium and that all parts of the person work together in harmony. At the back, somewhere between the shoulder blades, lives the Soul of Coarseness (*arami tama* 荒魂). It strives for fulfillment of the wishes and needs in the material world. The four souls are nourished by the Inner God (CR Symbol), who in turn receives his life force from the gods in the universe. This also explains the function of the CR Symbol, which permits the subtle energies to be anchored in the material world.

The first three souls are in resonance with the three *Dan-tians*, of which the best-known is the Hara.

The Esoteric Meaning of the CR Symbol's Form

The chapter on calligraphy introduces some practices for writing the symbols. The CR Symbol is usually drawn like a flat disk, consisting of a horizontal, vertical, and spiral-shaped line. When numerous CR Symbols are drawn in a row with the writing brush on a white piece of paper, a type of 3-D effect gradually occurs. Then it looks as if the vertical line is coming out of the picture. In other words, the spiral is like a disk upon which the vertical stroke stands. In Esoteric Buddhism, there is an entire series of rituals and meditations in which a similar phenomenon appears. In this process, a flat-laying moon disk is usually visualized—within light being or within ourselves—upon which a *Siddham* syllable such as the SHK Symbol (*Siddham*: *hrih*) stands. Each *Siddham* carries the energy of at least one light being. For the SHK Symbol, these are the 1000-armed *Kannon* and the Paradise Buddha *Amida*. In exactly the same way, a HS Symbol (*Siddham*: *hûm*) may be there. The light beings of the HS symbol are the Bodhisattva Diamond Mind *Kongôsatta* and the Imperturbable Wisdom King *Fudô Myôô*.

At the foot of the *Siddham*, a spiral begins from the syllable of a long mantra or *Dhâranî*. Seen in this light, the CR Symbol conceals visualization instructions in a somewhat complicated meditation cycle. The energy of the creative force comes through the horizontal stroke in the CR Symbol. This touches the uppermost part of the Siddham, which, as described by the monk *Kûkai*, depicts a connection to the heavenly realm. This is why the *Siddham hûm*, which portrays the Esoteric-Buddhist equivalent of the HS Symbol, has its upper area associated with the element of emptiness within the Buddhist context. The elements of air, fire, water, and earth follow beneath it. The correlation with the HS Symbol becomes more clear when we remember that the form of the Buddhism elements described here corresponds with a pagoda (Jap.: *gorintô*).

With the help of the *Siddham* (the vertical stroke), the Creative Force of *Dainichi Nyorai* has the possibility of materializing step by step. The function of the mantra in the spiral therefore describes the direction in which the energetic impulses of the Creative Force are effective. In other words, the effect of the meditation or the ritual changes depending upon which mantra and *Siddham* are used.

At the same time, the applications of many Reiki techniques become clearer through this interpretation of the CR Symbol. It should first be mentioned that the Reiki channel in a human being has a similar function as that of the CR Symbol and HS Symbol itself. The Reiki power comes from *Dainichi Nyorai* through the Crown Chakra into people who have been correctly initiated. From there, it assumes the function of the *Siddham* syllable *hûm* (the HS Symbol) because it becomes the bridge between *Dainichi Nyorai* and the material plane in which we would like Reiki to have an effect. *Dainichi Nyorai* can initially become generally active through the purposeful laying on of hands. If additional symbols are used individually or in a series, they extend the possibilities. Then Reiki can be applied very specifically. In addition to power intensification, the latter also corresponds to the second main effect of the CR Symbol; this occurs through the orientation of precisely where Reiki should now flow.

ILL. 158 – THE SIDDHAM OF THE FIVE-ELEMENTS PAGODA

The situation is similar with distant healing. Here as well, the Reiki channel is the bridge between heaven and earth. In addition, *Kongôsatta* becomes active as the light being of the HS Symbol. In order to create a connection to the client, another additional bridge is produced through the HS – CR – client.

In the mental healing, the 1000-armed *Kannon* becomes active in the form of the SHK Symbol. The connection occurs through the SHK – CR – client.

Kotodama–Inspired Words

Even before Buddhism reached Japan in the 6ᵗʰ Century and, accordingly, the tradition of the Indian *mantras* developed, *Shintô* had already long used the *Kotodama* —the so-called "inspired words." A spiritual power resides within them. The CR Symbol is such a *Kotodama*. It already appeared in *Nihon shoki* 日本書紀, the second-oldest Japanese historical work from the years 720.

When comparing the symbols, it becomes apparent that the second character of *Kotodama* (言靈) is a *rei* 靈 like the character for Reiki 靈氣; however, the pronunciation is different here. This is a phenomenon that quite frequently occurs in Japan since there can be various readings for one and the same character. A differentiation is also made between a Chinese reading (*on yomi* 音読) and a Japanese reading (*kun yomi* 訓読). Chinese characters (*kanji* 漢字) are usually also used for ancient Japanese terms because Japan had no script of its own at the time when it was introduced to Buddhism and the sutras in the Chinese language. However, this does not mean that every word with a Chinese reading can be traced back to Buddhism since Taoist and Confucian texts were also imported over the course of the centuries in addition to the Buddhist *sutras*. In addition, there are also exceptions and combinations in which the Chinese and Japanese pronunciation is mixed within a word that has several characters.

The *Kotodama* appeared in the earliest Japanese sources as a magical language in which spiritual powers and light beings reside. The special thing about it is that it is not a language created for this purpose alone but pure Japanese. If Japanese is spoken in a normal manner, nothing at all happens at first. Expressed in special forms such as ritual prayers (*norito*) or magical songs (*majinai uta*), the Japanese language is still used to this day for shamanic purposes.

Majinai uta are magical songs, frequently in the form of the Japanese *Waka* poem. This can be recognized in the fixed number of syllables (31 syllables) per verse and in the form per line of 5-7-5-7-7.

Since ancient times, *Waka* have been related to *Shintô* because poetry is derived from the religion.[174] We owe much of what we know

---

[174] Sokura, T. *Nihon shiika no kigen ronsô, shukyô kigen setsu.* In: *Kôya nihon bungaku nosôten.* Volume 1. Tokyo, 1969. P. 64f.

about light beings from Japan's early age to an ancient poetry collection—*Manyôshû*.[175] Since the introduction of Buddhism, and especially of Esoteric Buddhism, to Japan, it did not take long until people recognized that the Buddhist and Shintoist light beings are archetypes that have manifested in different forms in various countries and are given other names elsewhere. This means that they are identical and can be equally integrated into the energy work. The same also applies to the Shintoist *Waka* and Buddhist mantras.

This type of word magic is integrated into rituals of active magic such as *daiji, kaji, kaji-kitô, hihô* etc. or written on amulets. They are accompanied by mudrâs and frequently stand before or after the mantra to be recited (Jap.: *shingon*). Parts of the mantra are sometimes also woven into the text of the poem, such as the widespread mantra *Om abira unken sowaka* of *Dainichi Nyorai*. On the whole, these magical songs are limited to the following four types: recited, written on paper, ingested as medicine, worn as an amulet on the body or as inner or outer magical songs.

In Japan, these useful things were and are gladly integrated into the native culture. For example, Shintô priests and scholars took over powerful spiritual instruments from the Chinese advanced civilization, which already pointed the way in many respects for the development of the Japanese culture and civilization. So it is understandable that in the *Kotodama* the readings of Chinese characters and Indian *Siddham* were also included.

With the introduction of Esoteric Buddhism to Japan, some monks such as *Kûkai, Saichô,* and *Gyôki* discovered that the light beings of Shintô (Jap.: *Kami*) were interchangeable with those of Buddhism. For example, the Sun Goddess *Amaterasu* is a manifestation of the Great Sun Buddha *Dainichi Nyorai*. It appears as though various religions have arisen at different times throughout the world. However, when the cultural and power-political influences are removed, the individual religions are actually not that different from each other. Since in Japan—in contrast to most Western countries—the old cultural assets, religions, and traditions were retained when new ones were introduced, it did not take long until the

---

[175] The *Manyôshû, Collection of Ten-Thousand Petals* is a 20-volume poetry collection with 4516 *Waka* poems that were written down from the Fifth Century to 759 A.D.

common grounds could be determined. At that time, the greatest difference was seen solely in the names. The function or task was frequently quite similar. In ancient Rome as well, it was the custom when conquering new areas to give the deities of the people living there names that were equivalents of the Roman deities.

There is much evidence that there was once a unified religion throughout the world in the distant past, which the science of compared mythology proves. This religion was matriarchal and oriented itself upon the natural order of things, in which human beings had their place, their responsibility, and their rights. It was the Golden Age, which can be found throughout the world in the legends—the time of the Great Goddess. Shamanism and the Tantric teachings, as well as the Huna tradition that can be found in the Pacific, are relics of this period that hand down parts of the ancient wisdom.

The question of why Dr. Usui placed such great value upon the *Waka* Poems of the Meiji Tennô[176] was on my mind for a long time. Dr. Usui used these poems in the training of his students. In Japan, there is also a Reiki school that the Reiki Master and book author Frank Arjava Petter learned about, in which the initiations are performed through these poems. The explanation lies in their power as magical songs—*Majinai uta*—and the inspired words that they contain—*Kotodama*.

The *Kotodama* (inspired words) have an effect similar to that of the Reiki symbols. By means of initiations and through their correct applications, the symbols and *Kotodama* are awakened so that their effects can be manifested here in the material world. The learning of the symbols is already difficult enough for people in the West. Otherwise, so many deviations would not have taken place in the course of the last decades. If Mrs. Takata had also taught her Western students the *Kotodama*, it would probably have been a perfect catastrophe, especially since she was not capable of reading or understanding the Japanese texts herself. This shows just how little of Dr. Usui's Reiki System has actually reached the West.

The initiation rituals are structured in such a way that Reiki can also be transmitted lastingly without the *Kotodama*. This means that either

---

[176] The translation of the Meiji Emperor's poetry can be found in *The Spirit of Reiki*, Lotus Press.

there were and are several forms of the initiation for various purposes within Reiki or that the initiation rituals were changed either by Dr. Usui or by Dr. Hayashi without a loss of quality. The situation of the *Kotodama* is similar to that of the symbols. Just as each symbol has its own effects and applications, the various *Kotodama* also have their own way of working. Through the applications of the *Kotodama*, the spectrum of the possibilities with Reiki can be considerably supplemented.

The Effects of the Kotodama

In order for a Japanese song such as the above-mentioned Japanese poem form of *Waka* with its 31 syllables to become a magic song (*majinai uta*), certain preconditions must be fulfilled. As a result, not all *Waka* can be used as magical songs. To this day, many are written in literary form or simply as a pastime in card games, in competitions, or for writing love letters. Even more popular than the *Waka* are the so-called shortened forms like the *Haiku*, which are well-known in the West.

Waka poems, which depict a form of the *Kotodama*, have been associated with *Shintô* since ancient times as a religious means of expression. Through the absorption of the Japanese spirits (Jap.: *Kami*) into Esoteric Buddhism and the Buddhist light beings into *Shintô*, the Japanese *Waka* poems were also equated with the Indian *Dhârânî* (long mantras). In addition to the *Waka*, there is an entire series of additional poems that can all be summarized under the term of song (Jap.: *uta*). In the foreword of the much-quoted poetry collection *Kokinshû*[177], the following has been written on this topic: "The song contains the heart (*kokoro*) of the people and many thousands of words as petals. The light beings feel touched by what moves heaven and earth without violence, what leads men and women together in love, what sweetens life, and what can comfort the heart of the tough warrior. This is the Japanese song. It was created with the beginning of heaven and earth. In as far as it has been handed down into our world, it began in the heavens with the Princess of Light (*Shi-*

---

[177] The *Kokinshû* 古今集 is one of the poetry collections commissioned by the *Daigo Tennô* of the Engi Period from the year 905, with a preface by *Ki no Tsurayuki* (868-945). It was the first anthology commissioned by the Tennô (*Choku rei*) *Daigo Tennô* (885-930).

tateru hime)[178] and on the earth with the God of Storm (*Susa no o no mikoto*)[179]. In the Age of the light beings, the number of the syllables was still unlimited. But in the Age of the Human Beings, 31-syllable poems have been written since *Susa no o no mikoto*..."

It took until the 12th Century for the poems in Esoteric Buddhism to be seen as identical with the mantras. For many centuries, Japanese poetry was considered to be one of the ten evils (*juaku*) because some followers of Buddhism came up with the idea of justifying Buddhism by trying to ban other things. For this purpose, they used means that would have been at home in the religious history of Europe. This included the threat that those who became involved with untrue things would go to hell. This lead to a death ritual for *Murasaki Shikibu*, the woman author of the *Story of Prince Genji*[180]. Fortunately, this prudish attitude could not be maintained for long in Japan, which spared the Land of the Rising Sun many interpersonal problems and diseases of body and mind.

In *Shasekishû*[181], a Buddhist text from the 13th Century, the correlation between *Waka* and *mantras* is explained in several places. The Zen monk *Mujû*[182] of the *Rinzai* School has written the following here: "The light beings of Japan are avatars of Buddhas and Bodhisattvas. Already the God of Storm composed the 31-syllable poem *Izumo yaegaki*, which is comparable to the words of Buddha. The *Dhâranîs* of India consist solely

---

[178]   *Shitateru hime* is the Princess Who Lets the Light Shine Upon the Earth.
[179]   *Susanoo no mikoto* is the younger brother of the Sun Goddess *Amaterasu*. He is the God of the Storm, the Underworld, Farming, and Diseases. The element of water is attributed to him. His greatest achievement was the victory over the sea monster *Yamata no Orochi* with 8 tails and 8 heads. In the freeing of a girl from the monster, the sacred sword *Kusanagi* also appeared, which then became one of the three imperial insignias of the *Tennô*.
[180]   The *Genji monogatari* is the *Story of Prince Genji* by *Murasaki Shikibu* of the 11th Century in prose. The 1000 pages describe the many love stories of a prince by the name of *Genji* who constantly falls in love with new women.
[181]   The *Shasekishû* is a collection of 134 stories that the monk *Mujû* (1227-1312) wrote down between 1279 and 1283. They largely describe the customary life of the *Kamakura* Period (1185-1333). In addition, this is an important document for the popular Buddhism of this time.
[182]   *Mujû* (1226-1312) is often called the Monk of the *Rinzai* School of Zen Buddhism. But considering his tendencies when writing, it is conspicuous that he was additionally occupied with Esoteric Buddhism and *Shintô*.

of the words of that country's language, which Buddha used in order to explain the *mantras*." For this reason, the monk *Ichigyô Zenji*[183] said in his commentary to the sûtra *Dainichi kyô*[184]: "The languages of the various places are all *mantras*. If Buddha had appeared in Japan, there is no doubt that he would have used the language of our land as a *mantra*. The syllables that record everything did not originally know any characters."

In their quality, *Kotodama* (here *Waka*) have an all-embracing effectiveness that manifests itself in various ways. In addition to the inner effects such as the calming of the mind, the activation of the powers of self-healing, or spiritual development, some poems have very concrete effects attributed to them such as the healing of snakebites.

Probably the most important precondition for an effective magic song is that a type of life must be breathed into it or that it must be inspired. This becomes understandable when the content of such magical songs is compared. The following examples are just a small selection:

[183] *Ichigyô Zenji* (683-727) was a monk of the Tang Period (618-908) and the sixth Patriarch of the *Shingon* School. He studied Esoteric Buddhism under *Zenmui* and *Kongôchi* and wrote some commentaries on the most important *sutras*.

[184] *Dainichi kyô* is the fundamental sûtra in the Esoteric Buddhism of the Shingon School. *Dainichi kyô* is actually an abbreviation for *Dai birushana jôbutsu shinpen kaji kyô*. The original text in Sanskrit no longer exists today. However, there is a translation into Chinese by *Zenmui* and his student *Ichigyô*, as well as a translation into Tibetan. Covering seven volumes, this sûtra discusses the Womb World (Skr.: *Gharba dhâtu*; Jap.: *Taizôkai*). In addition, it systematically describes how we can achieve enlightenment in this life through personality development with the help of practices with *Dainichi Nyorai*. As a young man, *Kûkai* discovered the *Dainichi kyô* inside the east pagoda of the *Kumedera*. Unfortunately, he was not capable of understanding the text or the *Siddham* that it contained, which sparked the desire within him to go to China in order to study Esoteric Buddhism there. *Saichô*, who left for China together with *Kûkai* and brought the *Tendai* teaching of Esoteric Buddhism to Japan, concentrated especially on the *Dainichi kyô*. The translation by *Ichigyô* was explained by the *Shingon* School in the 20-volume 大日経疏 and by the *Tendai* School in the 14-volume 大日経義釈...

Protection against Colds

Waga na aru kado ni wa tatsu na kaze no Kami na naki kado ni wa to ni
mo kaku ni mo
"Gods of the Cold, go away from my door here, where my name stands.
Go there where no one lives, where no name protects the house!"

Stopping Bleeding

Tenjiku no ô ga hara no chidome gusa nanto zo hayaku naorase tamu.
Abura unken sowaka
"With the grass that stops bleeding, which grows in the heavenly plain *Ô*,
it will somehow heal quickly with the oil of *Dainichi Nyorai!*"

This magic poem is an example of the fusion between Japanese magic and
Esoteric Buddhism. The last three words *abura unken sowaka* are derived
from the Mantra of the Great Sun Buddha *Dainichi Nyorai* (DKM). His
mantra is usually *abira unken sowaka*. Through the conversion into *abura*
instead of *abira,* the mantra receives the meaning of "oil of *Dainichi Nyorai*". This is intended to strengthen the magical effect of the poem.

Easy Birth

Dai hannya harami onna no kitô ni wa ichi ni wo sunde
san no himo toku
"If the *Heart Sûtra* is recited by the pregnant woman, one and two are
accomplished. This undoes the belt then at three."

Protection Against Falling from a Horse

Ikazu kozu tatazu hashirazu todomazu ikazu ya kozu ya
naka ni fusu ran
"Not walking, not coming, not standing, not running, not stopping. The
horse does not come or go, it lies quietly in the stable."

Increasing Wealth

Chihayaburu Kami no tsutae no kono tsuchi wo ware utsu tabi ni tomi to
narikeri
"The hammer that you tough gods have handed down brings me certain
wealth every time and with each blow."

430

Applications of the Kotodama with the CR Symbol

For the application of the *Kotodama* and the CR Symbol, the *Kotodama* is always followed by the CR—as in the application with other symbols. The *Kotodama* determines the quality of the effect. It expresses what should be accomplished. Then the CR Symbol follows. It determines the direction in which the effect should be manifested. At the same time, the power is increased as a result.

Mental Healing with Kotodama and the CR

Select an appropriate *Kotodama* from the above-mentioned magical songs or from another one with which you are familiar.

Begin the mental healing as accustomed with the SHK, CR, and the first name/last name. Place your initiated hand on the head, recite the *Kotodama* three times, and then use a CR Symbol. Repeat the *Kotodama-CR* application for several minutes.

A magic song that we use in Rainbow Reiki is *Hey loa, key loa*. The lyrics and notes are included on page 459. It is a request of the Creative Force in its boundless love and wisdom to help out with whatever the person making the request is doing at the moment. This is very easy to use as part of every Reiki treatment, so be sure to try it out.

CHAPTER 18

The Characters for Reiki

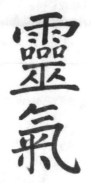

ILL. 159 – THE TRADITIONAL CHARACTERS FOR REIKI

Reiki is often translated as "universal life energy" in the esoteric scene. This translation appears to be referring less to the character itself as to the explanation of Reiki's healing energy. Instead, the precise analysis of the Reiki character leads to a translation like "spiritual life energy."

The word Reiki consists of the character *rei* 靈 and *ki* 氣. In addition to these characters, the new simplified characters *rei* 霊 and *ki* 気 are now being used. Furthermore, there is an entire series of additional ways of writing them and types of script (see the Excurse on Calligraphy). The advantage of the simplified signs for Reiki 霊気 is that they have fewer strokes, which makes them easier to write and remember. However, the disadvantage is that they lose their original meaning and the energy of the sign. While repeatedly writing the characters with the writing brush according to the traditional rules of Chinese and Japanese calligraphy,[185] I have had good experiences of the energy that emanates from the characters themselves. When writing the new characters 霊気, it feels as if I were writing any other sign. But when I write the old characters 靈氣, something really happens while writing. An objectively perceivable spiritual power is released.

[185] Cf. chapter on calligraphy.

The Explanation of the Character Rei

ILL. 160 – ORIGIN FOR THE KANJI REI

The uppermost part of the *rei* 靈 means rain (Jap.: *ame* 雨). This is easy to remember by noticing that there are four drops in the stylized cloud. This means that the water, which is ready to fall upon the earth, has been blessed by the heavens and has already manifested within the cloud. There are three squares beneath the rain. Each individual square describes the sign for mouth (Jap.: *kuchi* 口). Three mouths mean prayer because the three archetypal partial personalities of the Inner Child, Middle Self, and Higher Self express the same wish to the divine. Of course, the three partial personalities have different names in the Chinese teaching. Here they are known as the three *Hun* souls. Beneath the three praying mouths is a type of reclining H with two points in it. The reclining H represents work (Jap.: *kô* 工). In earlier times, there were farming devices that had a similar form. The lower horizontal stroke is the earth, the vertical stroke is an axis that is inserted into the ground, and the upper horizontal stroke is a leverage beam that is being moved by the working people. The two points to the right and left next to the axis are two people (Jap.: *hito* 人). Human beings and work in this combination result in the character for shaman (Jap.: *miko* 巫). When joined together, this means that the people who work on the earth need water so that the plants can thrive and grow. In Asia, where much rice is cultivated, especially large amounts of water are required. But since it does not always rain when the water is needed, the people must do more than just work hard. Latin expresses this quite beautifully in the words *Ora et labora*—pray and work." This is why the

433

shaman 巫 now appears on the scene and prays 口 口 口 so that the heavens will give the people rain 雨 in both the literal and the figurative sense in the form of favorable occurrences. This results in the character of *rei* 靈, which can be translated as the "soul" and "spiritual mind." Through the work of the shaman, who communicates between the heavens and earth, the things on the earth—such as the rice—can be , inspired. The Chinese character *Ling*, which is the equivalent of the Japanese *Rei*, is the earliest written depiction of a female shaman performing her work.[186]

How is this related to the second character *ki* 氣?

The Explanation of the Character Ki

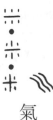

ILL. 161 – ORIGIN FOR THE KANJI KI

The character *ki* 氣 consists of the components of energy (the steam that rises from the cooked rice) (Jap.: *ki* 气) and the grain of rice (Jap.: *kome* 米). In this simplest form of the *ki* 气, we cannot yet speak of a concrete energy form. This is the case when this sign is combined with another sign that imparts a specific quality to the energy. As a result, the Japanese has the 气 as the radical, which establishes the pronunciation of *ki* and gives the character the meaning of an energy form. However, which energy form this exactly is has not yet been clarified. This can only be deduced from the combination.

An individual grain of rice is the seed of a plant, but not the plant itself. The grain of rice becomes a plant when the energy of Mother Earth

---

[186] Source: *Die Religionen Chinas* (The Religions of China), Werner Eichhorn, Kohlhammer Verlag; page 56 f.

and Father Sky are united. This occurs as soon as the rain brings the energy of the skies to the earth. Consequently, the grain of rice can only grow into a plant through this act of creation, bringing much life energy *ki* 氣 with it. This is also precisely the moment where a grain of rice 米 appears beneath the *ki* 气.

The Combination of the Characters Rei and Ki

The farmers toil in the field and do their earthly material work. In order for the seed to thrive—which is mostly rice in Japan—much water is necessary. Water is associated with the 2nd Chakra—the so-called Sacral Chakra. This is a sacred chakra because new life is created through it. The shamans pray for rain so that the fields receive the water they need. Through prayer and rain and the work of the farmer, the divine energies from above and below (heaven and earth) are combined. From the Tantric perspective, an act of creation takes place through which the spark of life is breathed into the grain of rice. In this way, new life arises. The rice plant grows from it, producing in turn many grains of rice.

As we often say: The life energy Reiki promotes living processes, and this is already reflected in the descriptive *Reiki* character. By giving Reiki, we transmit the life energy produced by this creative act to ourselves and others, contributing to more love, peace, and wisdom in this way.

Excursus: A Brief Introduction to Calligraphy

What Is Calligraphy?

Calligraphy is an artistic form of handwriting. In East Asia (China, Japan, and Korea), it has always been seen as the queen of all the arts. In these countries, it surpasses the term of "handwriting" used in the West to a considerable degree since calligraphy also includes writing with *ki* 氣, which can even be seen centuries later in a successful work. Learning this ability requires much practice. My calligraphy master always emphasized this point in particular. He also separated calligraphy (Jap.: *Shodô* 書道), which he interprets as writing with *ki*, from pure handwriting (Jap.: *Shûji*, literally: practicing signs), even though both should be practiced at the same time to a certain degree.

Handwriting is solely concerned with the correct order of the individual strokes and the form. If the emphasis is only upon the writing of correct spelling and form, and the aura or power of expression and energy do not play a role, pure handwriting is obviously adequate. This is also how it is taught at the schools in Japan. Unfortunately, there are very few masters in Japan who are in command of both arts. Most of the true masters of calligraphy in Japan are Buddhist monks. Their calligraphies can virtually animate a room and captivate the viewers. The main methods of writing with *ki* consist of copying the calligraphies of the old masters. There are obviously also many technical exercises such as proper breathing in order to achieve this ability. If the old masters, beginning with *Wang Xizhi* (303-361) are not studied through many repetitions of copying, a development in this direction is hardly possible. In short, East Asian calligraphy is concerned not only with the *right* technique but with much, much more.

Anyone in the West who learns 2nd Degree Reiki for the first time will initially practice writing the symbols correctly by focusing on the stroke sequence and form. This is very important for the application of all techniques with the symbols since they can only be reliably effective their full power and in the quality established by Dr. Usui when executed in their correct form and stroke sequence, as well as the number of strokes.

436

For the Reiki symbols, writing them with a quality of *ki* that is clearly far beyond the normal degree is also very significant. As a simplification, I (Mark) denote this as "writing with *ki*" in the following text. The more we succeed in writing the symbols with *ki*, the greater their effect will be in the applications on one hand; on the other hand, this also promotes our personal, subtle, and spiritual development. Moreover, such symbols also are considerably more beautiful in appearance. Further below in the practical section is a description of how we can write the symbols so that they are beautiful and also have *ki*. However, it is first helpful to have a deeper understanding of how this script originated.

The Reiki symbols and characters have been used in many different variations since the time of Dr. Usui, and in part also long before throughout centuries and even millennia. The knowledge about the origin and history of the symbols in this book is being completely made accessible to the public for the first time. Although many hundreds of thousands of people use the symbols and the characters, they may not know the precise meanings and background for most of them. This is also a feature of the Chinese and Japanese calligraphy. It may be beautiful, but not absolutely necessary, to also understand the content of calligraphic works of art. The form, expression, and necessary function of the individual works of art are much more important.

It is possible to consider the Reiki symbols and characters as works of art. Then the form and esthetic appeal stands in the foreground. If the Reiki characters, which we can hang on the wall like a piece of art, also have expressive power—if they are also written with *ki*—then this is even better. Then even someone who is not familiar with a sign, let alone able to read it, can enjoy it and feel the healing vibration.

Even in East Asia, where the people understand the content, this does not always play such an important role. For example, the Chinese Emperor Ming (58-75 A.D.) of the Eastern *Han* Period (25-220 A.D.) sent a messenger to the deathbed of an exemplary calligrapher to ask him to write ten more letters. The Emperor was less concerned about the content than the script itself. With the help of the script as the "seal imprint of the mind," the Emperor was able to mentally connect with the artist by looking at the signs.

Since the *Tang* Period (618-906 A.D.), people in China also speak of the Chinese ink or writing brush traces (Jap.: *bokuseki*) that reveal something about the personality of a calligrapher[187]. A similar approach is also used in the West, where the handwriting is analyzed to draw conclusions about the personality. However, the writing is usually not done with the intention of creating a work of art.

Furthermore, the symbols and sometimes even entire texts have specific functions for the various types of rituals that extend beyond the content. Healing is in the foreground in the word *Reiki*, whereby other goals can be achieved with it. In Taoism, for instance, sacred texts are received from the gods in a ritual, whereby the calligrapher is the medium for the texts to be written down.[188]

In addition to the completed works of art, writing the symbols, characters, and texts like the sutras can also fulfill numerous functions. For example, these include meditation, the awakening of the subtle abilities of perception, or even the accumulation of good karma because writing a sutra contributes to the dissemination of Buddhism or the teaching of the light, creating the precondition for a pleasant future. Expressed in simple terms, karma is just the law of cause and effect and copying a *sûtra* is like a potential seed for a good harvest since it teaches how the beings can be led to happiness.

However, the Chinese characters—which are the components of the Reiki symbols—existed long before Buddhism. And Buddhism does not come from China but India. Many of the roots of Buddhism, such as the ancient Indian *Siddham* script (which includes the SHK symbol), mantras, and dhâranîs had their origin in the Vedic texts[189], which also existed long before Buddhism. If we research beyond the boundaries of one country, it is conspicuous that the history always seems to somehow go further back until the origin is found. But in terms of the Chinese

---

[187] The phenomenon of the Chinese ink traces is described in a very beautiful and clear way in the book *Erleuchtung ist überall* (Enlightenment Is Everywhere) by Peter Zürn, Windpferd Verlag, Germany.

[188] Ledderose, Lothar (1984). *Some Taoist Elements in the Calligraphy of the Six Dynasties*. In: *T'oung Pao* 70: pages 246-278.

[189] See chapter on the *Siddham* script.

script, it appears as if a certain number of the signs have always existed since they appeared quite suddenly. This will be discussed in more detail in the next section.

Origin and Structure of the Chinese Characters

During a very early phase, it was customary to tie large and small knots into bands of plant fibers in order to note approaching events in the sense of a calendar. Since the Emperor *Fu-Hsi* (28th Century B.C.), the phenomena of the nature between heaven and earth were recorded with a system called *Bagua* (eight-field pattern). In this system, there are two signs ▬▬ and ▬ ▬, which stand for yang and yin. *Fu-Hsi* developed these into eight combinations, which represent heaven, earth, thunder, wind, water, fire, mountains, and rivers. Later, in the 12th Century B.C., this system was further developed by Wen Wang, the first king of the Western *Zhou* Period (1045-771 B.C.). It forms the basis for *The Book of Changes* (Chin.: *I Ching*). From the knot technique to the 64 combinations, a development can be followed from simple methods for noting events to a method of directly depicting human thoughts.

However, this type of sign bears little relation to the Chinese character itself. The history of the character can be traced far back, yet it appears that a certain number of signs have always existed, especially since these signs suddenly appeared without any evidence of a previous development. The oldest Chinese characters found up to now have been discovered on ceramic shards that are up to 6,000 years old. These were followed by bronze objects. Not until the so-called oracle bones of the late *Shang* Period (1600-1045 B.C.) could entire connected texts be recognized.

Oracle bones were mostly bone plates and tortoise shells that had signs scratched onto them for the purpose of an oracle. In

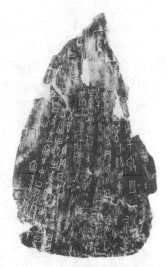

ILL. 162 – ORACLE BONE

439

this process, a precise question on a topic is raised, such as whether it is meaningful to cross the river in order to attack another state. By heating them in the fire, the bones developed tears and cracks. Depending upon where the bone cracked in relation to the sign, the people at that time could read what would be the sensible thing to do.

So the Chinese signs were originally used exclusively for religious purposes. Earlier sources of Chinese script have not been discovered up to now. It is conspicuous that the signs in the early time were mainly used within a ritual context. It is also obvious that they are the ideal carriers of spiritual energies for use in symbols such as the HS and DKM Symbol, as well as the Reiki character itself. According to my experience, the characters of Reiki have a strong power and affect me like symbols as long as they are left in their original form—meaning as they are seen on the tombstone of Dr. Usui, for example. Within this context, "original" does not mean an individual type of script but the form and number of the strokes within one sign that shows its characteristics. Strictly speaking, this means how an unbiased observer would recognize it. This refers to the self-similarity, which is typical in examples from modern math such as the fractals, Julia numbers, and Mandelbrot numbers. Humans are beings that reproduce in a self-similar manner. None of us looks exactly like another person, but we can determine without a doubt that an individual belongs to the species of human beings. As long as there is a self-similarity in the Reiki symbols, they basically function in the sense of energy work. Yet, the versions that have a stronger thematic similarity with the original form possess a much higher functionality than symbols that only have a very superficial resemblance to the "blueprint." As in all things, there is also a limit here: If we write a "C," we will not be able to convey an "A" to another person.

The original signs are symbols for rituals. Only later did they experience a further development into a script as carriers for information. Calligraphy then developed from the symbols and the script. Because of the complexity of the signs, they were frequently abbreviated during the course of the centuries. This may sound practical at first, but it did not lead to a real simplification because the new signs did not assert themselves everywhere. As a result, there was a doubling in the amount of signs. For example, the simplified "short signs" have been used in Mainland

China since Mao Tze Dong, but the old long signs are still employed in Hong Kong, Taiwan, and Japan. In addition, the signs were frequently simplified at a much earlier time so that there were also very lengthy long signs and somewhat shorter long signs that were used differently in the above-mentioned countries. The Reiki characters, the HS Symbol, and the DKM Symbol—as taught by Dr. Usui—consist of the old long signs as can be found in the Buddhist sutras. As a result, they have retained their full effect. All forms of simplification contribute to a change or dilution of the effect.

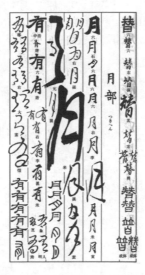

ILL. 163 – WRITING VARIATIONS FOR "MOON"

Another special feature of the Chinese script is that it cannot be replaced by letters. If this script was abolished, it would not be possible to communicate clearly through script in either Chinese or in Japanese. This is because there are many characters and combinations of characters that may be written the same way in letters but vary dependent upon the tone of their pronunciation. So this script is an indispensable system. Another factor is that the old characters are symbols whose form is indispensable in combination with their pronunciation for their effective application in rituals. In relation to the Reiki symbol, this means that every change leads to a loss of its effectiveness.

However, there are still some variations possible in the spelling. In the course of the centuries, various types of script have developed in China. Each type is subject to certain rules. Some of these can be easily changed but others cannot. Therefore, it is even possible to vary the symbols slightly as long as the rules for the individual types of script are followed. But the types have nothing to do with the writing variations of other types of script or simplifications of the script itself. Before the development of the various types of scripts is explained, here are the various ways to write the Reiki signs as an illustration. Although all of the variations are correct, they differ greatly in their power of transmission. It is interesting to meditate with the various signs as a practice and as an experiment. To do this, look at each individual spelling for a while and let it have its effect on you.

靈氣 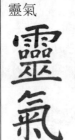	This is how the signs appear on Dr. Usui's tomb. The original meaning of the signs can be deduced and explained through them.
霊気 霊 気	This is how the script is usually written today in Japan. Here the characters are greatly simplified. The original meaning of the signs can no longer be recognized in them. However, they can still be used to find the old signs in a good sign dictionary.
レイキ レ イ キ	This is how Reiki is written today in Japan. The signs have lost all of their power or never even had it. Although these signs can be traced back to the Chinese signs, they are a Japanese invention and are called *Katakana*. These signs are popular in Japan for several reasons. First, they are usually used for foreign words. Since Reiki was also re-imported to Japan, Reiki has been labeled a Western healing art with Japanese roots. But another, much more important reason is that the original signs were also related to poltergeists and ghosts of the dead so that many Japanese are filled with fright and prejudices when just looking at these signs.
灵 气	This is how Reiki is written today in Mainland China. These signs have also lost all of their power.

In addition, there are further variations of the Reiki characters. Although all of these are correct despite the differences in their components, they express various nuances and have diverse energetic effects. For example, here are the various ways of writing the *Kanji Rei*.

ILL. 164 – WRITING VARIATIONS FOR REIKI

The Development of the Types of Script

	Sun	Moon	Fire	Water	Wood	Metal	Earth
Oracle Bones	⊖	☽	ᘒ	沈	米	ᐱ	ᘯ
Bronze Ritual Objects	⊙	ⅅ	ᘒ	ᘔ	米	金	ᘯ
Seal Script	ᘖ	ᘰ	火	沝	米	金	土
Chancery Script	日	月	火	水	木	金	土
Cursive Script	日	月	火	水	木	金	土
Regular Script	日	月	火	水	木	金	土

ILL. 165 – TABLE OF ALL TYPES OF SCRIPT

During the course of thousands of years, the signs have developed from a pictographic system to their current form. However, this development has not always taken place in a uniform manner and new characters were constantly added. In addition to the increase of characters, various types of script also developed. This can be compared with the fonts in the computer. According to requirements and taste, fonts are used today such as Times, Century or Arial. The signs are always the same while the form is slightly varied. The Chinese characters are very similar in this respect, whereby the individual types of script used up to this day are more than 1700 years old.

After the oracle bones, the next characters were found as inscriptions on bronze ritual objects from the late *Shang* Period (1600-1045 B.C.). **Bronze ritual objects** are pieces of bronze in the form of wine and food containers or musical instruments. Since they cannot be employed for daily use because of their unwieldy size and weight, we can assume that they were solely used for ritual purposes. On the outside, they are generally decorated with animal figures such as dragon motifs. Short inscriptions of a few signs sometimes appear on the inside of the containers. In the following *Zhou* Period (1045-221 B.C.), not only the decorations on the bronze objects changed but also the type of the inscriptions. They became longer with time.

445

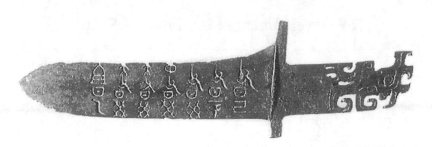

ILL. 166 – INSCRIPTION ON A BRONZE KNIFE

The type of script used here is called **Seal Script** (Chin.: *zhuanshu,* Jap.: *tensho* 篆書). For many generations, people also wrote on bamboo, wood, and silk until these materials were replaced by paper during the Western *Han* Period (206 B.C.-9 A.D.).

The Seal Script is still used today for seals. In the East Asian countries, it is an official and business custom to "sign" with a seal of one's own. Since the modern seals are computer generated in Japan, they correspond with something like a person's fingerprint and are very difficult to forge, even when several individuals have the same name.

The first emperor of China, *Qin Shi Huangdi*, had seven steles of stone with inscriptions erected in his kingdom. These were the works of art in China, into which historical events were chiseled. They are the models for millions of other steles. Although the originals now have been lost, there is a replica from the year 993 on the Yi mountain. People believe that the type of script there, which is called the **Little Seal Script** (Chin.: *xiaozhuan*) corresponds with the original. This type of script was created by *Li Si* (?-208 B.C.), the emperor's closest advisor. He is said to have standardized the script of various region with it. The signs all fit into a pattern of evenly distributed squares, the individual strokes are all equally thick, and the number, as well as order, of the strokes was precisely determined. This has a direct relationship to the Reiki characters and the DKM Symbol. Like all Japanese and Chinese texts, they are also written in this pattern. The order is also precisely determined and, according to the rules the calligraphy, should not be changed. This pattern can only be used to a limited extent for the HS Symbol since its five basic signs are interlocked with each other according to an ancient Taoist method of spiritual script.

In the Little Seal Script, all of the signs are composed of a phonetic part (related to pronunciation) and a semantic part (related to the meaning). The individual modules[190] (with a total of 540) are exchangeable among each other, which means that new signs are created time and again.

These 540 modules, as well as the amount of strokes, were gradually reduced to simplify matters. In the 2nd Century, the Little Seal Script was replaced by the **Chancery Script** (Chin.: *lishu*, Jap.: *reisho* 隷書). In the Chancery Script, the modules were reduced to about 200. Of these, many belong to the so-called 214 radicals.

ILL. 167 – THE 214 RADICALS

However, since some of the radicals just consist of individual strokes, not all of them can be called modules. Even today, many dictionaries are sorted according to these 214 radicals, which makes it possible to quickly and simply find any of many thousands of signs. This also applies, of course, to the Reiki characters and the DKM Symbol. This is somewhat more difficult for the HS Symbol because it is necessary to initially break down the symbol into the original signs.

In the 4th Century, three additional types of script developed in Chinese calligraphy under the famous calligrapher *Wang Xizhi* (303-361).

---

[190] The module system in the Chinese script and other areas of art are very beautifully and clearly explained in the book *Ten Thousand Things* by Professor Lothar Ledderose, published by the Princeton University Press.

But it is not certain whether all three types actually came from *Wang Xizhi* since no works by his own hand have been preserved. However, because he has been copied and revered as the most outstanding calligrapher of all times by so many famous masters, it is certain that the peak of the development for these types of script occurred with his works. All three types are still in use to this day, and no newer types of script have been developed. Of course, there are personal styles of writing that are based upon these three types. How do these types of script look, and which of them are significant for the Reiki symbols?

The **Semi-Cursive** (Chin.: *xingshu*, Jap.: *gyôsho* 行書; literally: running script) and the **Full Cursive** (Chin.: *caoshu*, Jap.: *sôsho* 草書; literally: grass script) developed from the above-mentioned Chancery Script for more unofficial purposes such as letters. What both types of script have in common is that some strokes are abbreviated, but without omitting them. This may sound somewhat paradoxical, but the abbreviation consists of the individual, original separate strokes now blending into each other and virtually merging. So these cursive scripts are a somewhat less formal type for letters and calligraphies, but it is not allowed in official documents, classic works, and sutras. The differences between these two types are that the Full-Cursive Script is even more difficult to read at first glance because the individual strokes blend into each other even more and some signs are even connected with each other in this way. It is sometimes hard to know where one sign ends and the next begins. This is a clear parallel to the HS Symbol because the five original signs are also interwoven with each other here. Yet, the HS Symbol is not taught in the cursive scripts since the form and stroke sequences are in the forefront when learning it.

In calligraphy, as well as for writing the Reiki symbols, there is no point in practicing in these scripts from the start because these types of abbreviations are also subject to strict rules. Some people may think that rules exist so they can be broken. However, it is hardly possible to progress without practicing the exact form and stroke sequence. There is also the danger of mistakes creeping in that make the symbols useless in their effect.

The third and last type of script from the 4th Century is the so-called **Regular Script** (Chin.: *kaishu*, Jap.: *kaisho* 楷書). This is exactly the type that is taught even today in the schools as the standard handwriting. In contrast to the cursive scripts, the Regular Script is clear and easy to read because the strokes are distinctly separated from each other. In comparison to the Chancery Script, there are more modulations here in the brushwork. The individual strokes can vary in their width, depending upon whether the writing brush is set on the paper in a light or firm way. Some strokes come to an end by getting thinner until just a hair can be seen. Other strokes have little hooks that hint at where the writing brush will go next. These details have probably developed more from the Semi-Cursive Script by leaving out the abbreviations but hinting at the transitions with the little hooks. Depending on factors such as the quality and execution, this is an indication of whether it was written with *ki*. However, this certainly does not mean that all of the signs with little hooks were written with *ki* since this can also be reduced to a technical level. The Regular Script is the standard type for practicing the Japanese and Chinese script, as well as the symbols. Before they have barely mastered the Regular Script, most people tend to use the **Semi-Cursive Script** in order to write faster by letting the individual strokes blend with each other. The printed types of Standard Scripts in books and newspapers are based on the Regular Script without abbreviations. The same obviously applies to this book.

Legends About Writing with *Ki*

There are many stories about the great calligrapher *Wang Xhizhi,* two of which will be briefly told in the following. They can give us a glimpse of what it means to write with *ki*.

Piercing a Board with Chinese Ink

One day, *Wang Xizhi* is said to have written on a wooden board with his writing brush. Because of the moisture, people are accustomed to having some of the Chinese ink seep through thin paper onto the backside. But this is hardly possible with a wooden board. A close examination showed that the Chinese ink used by *Wang Xizhi* went through the entire board. This is an example of writing with *ki*.[191]

We could obviously claim that this story is just a legend. But because I (Mark) experienced something similar in the summer of 2003 in Japan,

[191] Please note here that the seeping of the Chinese ink is not always a sign of writing with *ki*. Depending on how the back looks, the chaff can be separated from the wheat.

449

I have once again become aware that many legends have more truth to them than many people want to believe. I watched a calligrapher at a festival as he presented his art there. When I observe such people, I am initially always very skeptical since very few of those who hold a writing brush in their hands can also use it properly. But I liked this calligrapher, so I asked him to write the Reiki characters on a fan made of firm mulberry-tree bark paper. As a draft, I first—as is the custom in Japan—wrote the Reiki characters on a normal piece of paper. When he saw the characters 靈氣 and the way in which I had written them, he looked at me with skepticism but also delightful surprise. Then he said: "For you, I will write in a very special style. Watch closely!" In contrast to his previous approach, the calligrapher went into a state of meditative absorption. He raised the writing brush as if he had a sword in his hand. And with the same intention, he lowered the writing brush to the bark. At the same time, I felt a vehement but very pleasant vibration that came from the Heart Chakra. Despite the black Chinese ink, I had the impression as if golden light were illuminating the room with every stroke. When the calligrapher was done, I instinctively raised the fan and looked at the back. The Chinese ink had gone through it...—A true master of calligraphy had written with *ki*.

The Foreword of the Orchid Pavilion

There is a well-known story about *Wang Xizhi* regarding the emergence of the Regular Script within the context of writing with *ki*. In the year 353, *Wang Xizhi* celebrated a garden party in the so-called Orchid Pavilion. A little stream flowed through the garden, and the guests sat at its banks. To amuse them, filled sake cups floated on the water. When one of the cups floated toward a guest, he was permitted to not only empty it but also to write a poem. In the evening, all of the poems were collected and *Wang Xizhi* himself wrote a foreword of 324 characters for them. In terms of the type of script, this is a mixture between the Regular Script and the **Semi-Cursive Script**. The forms of the individual strokes vary in a great many nuances. The free and yet balanced composition of the signs, as well as the lively flow in the arrangement, show the art of writing with *ki*. When *Wang Xizhi* copied his own work a number of times on the following day, he did not succeed in this brilliant feat a second time. His foreword was created in an intensive mood of happiness where he was completely centered.

The Use of the Script Types

The Chancery Script (*lishu* 隸書) was first found on little bamboo panels that came from around the 3rd Century B.C. During the 1st Century B.C., it replaced the Seal Script as the script for general usage. The Semi-Cursive Script (*xingshu* 行書) and the Full-Cursive Script or Grass Script (*caoshu* 草書) were already found on the bamboo panels of that time. After the *Han* Period (206 B.C. to 220 A.D.), the Chancery Script was standardized into Normal Script (*kaishu* 楷書), after which the development of the script types came to a halt until the 20th Century.

Apart from this, the Seal and Chancery Script are only rarely found and only in certain functions of a monumental, emblematic, and decorative character. This includes stone inscriptions, trademarks, equipment inscriptions, and book titles such as the very beautiful one on the cover of *The Spirit of Reiki*. By way of contrast, the other three types have been used without interruption and in a general manner since their creation. The Normal Script serves as a printing and writing script while the two cursive scripts are used exclusively for handwritten texts such as letters.

During the time of the Six Dynasties (3rd-6th Century), a fundamental change occurred in the development of the script. While the script had previously been used in an anonymous way, it now became a cultured form of art in the class of the literati civil servants. The most famous master of this time, as well as in the entire history of calligraphy, is *Wang Xizhi* (303-361).

Since the conclusion of the development of the scripts, many different period-related, school-related, and individual styles have developed. Both the writer and the viewer were aware of the various stylistic layers within a work. Although a good script required its own individuality, it also had to make it evident that the writer mastered the history of the art of script in both a theoretical and a practical manner. As a result, we can speak of an increasingly scientific development in the calligraphy since the time of the Six Dynasties.

Consequently, there are primarily three phenomenons that have a special significance within this context: The collecting of calligraphy, the theoretical literature, and the esthetic appeal of the writer.

Throughout history and even today, the Chinese script has been used for ritual purposes in Buddhism and Taoism. This book is an example of all the beautiful things that can be done with this script.

Introduction of the Script to Japan

Since Japan had no script of its own despite its long history, the Chinese script was adopted at the latest in the Sixth Century with the introduction of Buddhism from Korea to Japan. Because of the active contact with the mainland, we can assume that Chinese texts had already been passed on since the Third Century to Japan. The script was especially important within the context of Buddhism since the sutras (sacred writings) translated into Chinese played an extraordinarily important role in the propagation of the Buddhist teaching. In addition to the Chinese characters (Jap.: *kanji*), two additional Japanese script systems were also developed in Japan, *Hiragana* and *Katakana*, which are both still in use today. Anyone who has ever seen a modern Japanese text will probably notice that it has very complex signs (*kanji*), rounded and curved signs (*hiragana*), and angular signs (*katakana*).

The structure and grammar of the Japanese language is so different from Chinese that the Chinese script in no way fits the Japanese language. Yet, the Japanese have still succeeded in integrating this script in particular into their language and have continuously used it to this day. This is one of many examples for the ability of the Japanese to assimilate foreign things and then adapt them to their own needs.

Apart from the grammar, the pronunciation of both languages is also completely different. Because of this, the Chinese characters within the Japanese language still have at least one purely Japanese (*kun yomi*) and one Chinese (*on yomi*) pronunciation. The Chinese pronunciation of the signs in Japan hardly has any remaining similarities with modern Chinese today. It is therefore more appropriate to speak of a Sino-Japanese pronunciation (*Sino* means China). For example, *Reiki* is pronounced in modern Chinese as *Lingchi* (*rei* = *ling* and *ki* = *chi*). Even today, Chinese texts in Buddhism have a Sino-Japanese pronunciation. The symbols HS and DKM, as well as the Reiki character, are examples of this. Strictly speaking, these are purely Chinese words.

In terms of the Chinese texts, a method was additionally developed for reading these Chinese texts in Japanese. This means that anyone who can speak Japanese can also read and understand classic Chinese without ever having learned it using this technique. This is really fun.

During his stay in China, the monk *Kûkai* (774-835) studied not only Esoteric Buddhism but also calligraphy. Years of practice enabled him to finally write in the style of *Wang Xizhi*. As a result, *Kûkai* also had a profound influence in this area of Japanese culture.

It only became possible to write texts in the Japanese language with the development of the Japanese Syllable Script (Jap.: *kana*). The Syllable Script was developed on the basis of the Full Cursive Script, where the number of strokes and form were abbreviated through the quick writing. It took almost 200 years after *Kûkai* for the Japanese calligraphers to develop a typical Japanese style.

ILL. 168 – LOVE POEM IN THE JAPANESE STYLE OF THE 12TH CENTURY

453

The current name of the Syllable Script—*hiragana*—only came much later in the *Edo* Period (1603-1868), after many developments had taken place through the centuries.

Because of the simplifications of the original sacred signs from China, the Syllable Script can hardly be used for ritual purposes such as the Reiki symbols. Not even the Japanese *Kotodama* (inspired words) are an exception here since these orally transmitted magical songs had already existed long before the introduction of the script. Of course, the *Kotodama* have been written down since the use of script. Similar to the Reiki symbols, their power arises only through their direct application in the practice.

Calligraphy in the Practice

The Four Treasures

In order to do calligraphic work with the Reiki symbols, there are some traditional tools that greatly facilitate this possibility. They are also called the Four Treasures and include the writing brush, Chinese ink, ink stone, and paper (or silk).

The original implements from China, Japan, and Korea have especially proved themselves in the practice. If these are not at hand or not available anywhere, you can also start out with a paint box with a normal paintbrush. However, you will very quickly discover some major limitations with this approach.

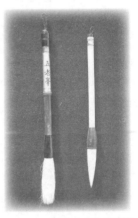

ILL. 169 – CALLIGRAPHY WRITING BRUSH

The **writing brush** should not be large—but also not too small. With a bit of practice, a medium-size writing brush can be used to draw quite large and even very small signs. In addition, the hairs should neither be too hard nor too soft. If they are too bristle-like, it will be difficult to smoothly guide the writing brush. If they are too soft, it will be difficult to maintain the form of the writing brush, which will immediately affect the signs.

When they are first pur-
chased, the brush hairs are
still firm and pointed. They
become supple by washing
and **gently** bending them.
After that, the hairs generally remain loose.

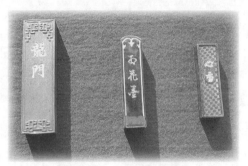

ILL. 170 – INK STICKS

In terms of the **Chinese ink,**
there are two basic possibili-
ties in calligraphy. The first consists of buying
ready-made Chinese ink. This is for people
who are in a big hurry and would prefer to
dispense with the ritual aspects of calligraphy.
This also includes developing the ability of
writing with *ki*. The second variation, which is
also traditional, consists of using an ink stick.
This is usually a rectangular stick of dried
Chinese ink, with which you can make the
Chinese ink yourself. Most ink sticks are black.
This is also the customary color in calligraphy.
For special purposes such as correcting or for
rituals, the color red is also used. Sacred texts
are sometimes gold or silver. Other colors do
not tend to be customary. When selecting an
ink stick, it is best to take one that not only
looks beautiful but also smells good.

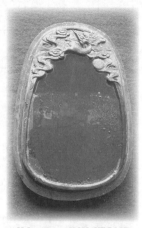

ILL. 171 – INK STONE

The **ink stone** is a stone with an indentation.
Water is added and the ink stick is made into
Chinese ink in it. Whether it is round, square,
or decorated does not play much of a role.
The important thing is that you like it. But
not every stone with an indentation is usable.
It should actually be one that has been made
especially for calligraphy.

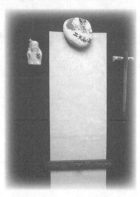

ILL. 172 – AIDS FOR
WRITING

455

Finally, **paper** is the material that is written on. Traditional rice paper is very well suited for calligraphy. Depending upon the quality of the paper, it will be either easy or difficult to write on it.

Other Writing Utensils

In addition to the Four Treasures, there are other useful writing utensils that can make life easier for a calligrapher or practitioner of the Reiki symbols. The utensils presented here are useful, but not essential. Many of them can be improvised.

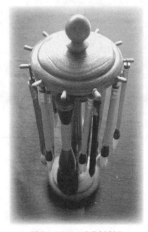

ILL. 173 – BRUSH HOLDER

The first one is a desk pad. Since the paper is very absorbent and some of the Chinese ink usually seeps through, a thin mat of felt is especially good for this purpose. This will save Chinese ink and avoid a mess on the table or carpet. In order to stop the paper from slipping, it is useful to place a weight on the upper edge. This can be a stone or a piece of metal. A brush-holder can be used for putting down the writing brush when taking a break. Placing the writing brush into a glass of water for this purpose will ruin it. A little container with a spout for adding water when making the Chinese ink is also very practical.

The writing brushes will be very happy when they are hûm with the tip downward on a brush stand after having been washed. This also allows the remaining Chinese ink to drip off and the vertical position helps maintains the original shape.

The Spiritual Meaning of Calligraphy

Calligraphy is comparable to Qi Gong in many respects. Already during the preparations, we strive for a meditative state of absorption in order to completely open up to the process of drawing. In the ideal situation, the body, mind, and soul equally participate in what happens. As in Qi Gong, we consciously work with the flowing power of the life energy. Consequently, good Chinese or Japanese calligraphy always has a Qi charge that is strong and unique in its quality, which makes it a spiritually effective symbol that supports the viewers in meaningfully integrating a specific, important quality into their personalities. Through the practice of calligraphy, an increasingly better ability to focus attention, to concentrate, and to direct the Qi develops over time. However, there is a major and very important difference to Qi Gong: The effects of the calligraphy can also be seen outside of the practitioner in a lasting form—namely, as an ink drawing on paper. So calligraphy is an art that produces considerable longer-lasting results. Through writing a certain term, such as "love," the practitioner can receive more and more insights into the wide spectrum inherent to the meaning of this word. Many great masters of calligraphy practice just one single character for years because they have understood that this is a key to their spiritual realization that will cause all of the other qualities within them to blossom.

The sensitive approach to the writing brush while drawing also enhances our perceptive faculty with increasing practice, even to the point of becoming a medium. An important rule of calligraphy is that each hair of the writing brush should touch the paper. By training the psychic perception, an increasingly complete transference of the *ki* is learned. Strictly speaking, the writing brush in Japanese and Chinese calligraphy is an extension of the practitioner's self. Through this expansion, which draws the multi-leveled symbols of the Chinese script, the being of an individual is basically shaped while executing a subtle, spiritual gymnastic exercise through the process of drawing because of the many different levels of meaning in the symbols and practices uniting with this special quality.

Preparatory Practices

In addition to the Four Treasures, the preparation and atmosphere also play a very important role; they are also decisive in terms of the result.

Practice 1: The Choice of Location

Look for a place in which you feel good, you can relax, and where you can be as undisturbed as possible. Attune yourself to it. It is a good idea to always practice in the same place in order to gradually draw upon its full power.

I personally prefer to write at dusk on the balcony with a view of the mountains. The fresh air, the sounds of the wind and the birds, as well as the lighting, are all my ideal prerequisites for a mystical-meditative mood that leads to successful calligraphies.

Practice 2: Preparation of the Place of Practice

After selecting a suitable place, prepare it in the following way: A thin felt pad is best to write upon. Then arrange on it the Four Treasures— which include the writing brush, Chinese ink, ink stone, and paper—together with the model that you are copying and a longish weight so that the paper does not slip while writing.

Practice 3: Energetic Preparation

It is quite possible, and also customary in Japan, to energetically upgrade the place of practice. For example, this can be done with appropriate flower arrangements, incense, calling upon a light being, or a special altar. Reiki offers a whole series of practical possibilities.

Reiki Shower

When you create a Reiki shower above your place of practice, you can provide yourself with Reiki the entire time. To do this, draw a large HS Symbol above the place where you would like to set up the Reiki shower. The symbol forms a pagoda, the source of energy. Starting here, draw a CR Symbol with the back of your hand facing the HS Symbol and the palm directed toward the place that you would like to have sprinkled by the Reiki shower. This will promote your concentration, patience, and spiritual development.

Crystals

It is very helpful and refreshing to set up one or several beautiful crystals in front of you. Activate them beforehand with Reiki or the *Goddess Crystal Radionic Tool*.[192] Here is a simple method for activation: Take the crystal between your hands in front of your heart. Now thank Mother Earth for creating this crystal in order to help human beings. Thank the crystal for coming out of the earth in order to help human beings. Sing the power song *Heyloa keyloa manaholo* nine times from your heart, then nine times with the crystal in your hands raised to the sky, and then nine more times to the earth. Once again, hold the crystal briefly in front of your heart and give thanks. Through the spiritual activation, the crystal now has a much stronger, more profound effect. Because of the sacred geometry of its special crystal structure, it is capable of supporting its surrounding environment—in as far as it is prepared to enter into resonance with it—in becoming oriented upon certain important areas of the divine order that the crystal embodies. In addition, energetically active crystals increase the vibration of their surroundings and facilitate, for example, contact with a light being or our own spiritual essence.

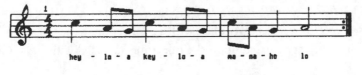

hey - la - a key - lo - a ma - na - ho lo

ILL. 174 – HEY LOA KEY LOA MANAHO LO

---

[192] This is a spiritual radionic device with which healing stones and minerals of any type can be energetically cleansed in a quick and very effective way, freed of programming and energetically activated—in other words, helped to be 100% effective. The latter is achieved by connecting the crystal with the earth's power lines, the Ley Lines. Crystals can also be regenerated with the GCRT and programmed with the information of a Bach Flower or a homeopathic remedy, for example.

Crystal quartz supports clarity when writing. Fluorite opens us for new impulses. Amethyst promotes a meditative mood. Rose quartz is good for the heart. There are obviously other crystals that can be used within this context, so be sure to experiment with them. It is very interesting to experience how the individual vibrations of the various healing stones can influence calligraphy. If space permits, you can also set up a crystal mandala on the table or close by in an intuitive way for this purpose.

Salt Lamps

Salt lamps provide not only a romantic touch but also energize the room by transmitting negative ions into the surrounding area through the warming of the salt crystal. This is comparable to those generated in a waterfall. Negative ions are very beneficial for good health. It is also very beneficial to place three crystal quartzes and three rose quartz stones around the salt lamp.

Reiki Chinese Ink

Very interesting results can be achieved if you charge and activate the water for the Chinese ink or the Chinese ink itself. The activation works in exactly the same way as described under the section on "Crystals."

Ink-Stone Activation

Since the ink stones are made of stone, they can also be activated. Follow the procedure described under "Crystals." The transmitter function with the *Goddess Crystal Radionic Tool* can be especially interesting here. This allows you to create a power place with a connection to the Great Goddess for the calligraphy based upon the ink stone activated with the GCRT.

Inviting Light Beings

You can also invite a light being with the distant contact methods of the 2nd Degree and request that it support you in your calligraphic intentions. When you do this, do not forget to express your gratitude afterward and offer Reiki as compensation.[193]

---

[193] This precise way of working with light beings is described extensively in Walter's *Rainbow Reiki* book.

Incense

Incense can also help to enrich the mood and the atmosphere for the calligraphy. In East Asia, incense is also used as a type of clock. For example, you can light an incense stick and write the symbols until it has burned down. Although this does not take particularly long, it is a good amount of time for everyday practice. Experience has shown again and again that regular and brief practicing leads to great success.

Practice 4: Preparation of the Mind

Gasshô Meditation

Before you get started, consider doing the Reiki *Gasshô* meditation. It is not so important to meditate for hours at a time. But to calm the mind and as an attunement for working with the writing brush, this meditation is very helpful.

To do this, place your hands together in front of your heart and bow briefly. Breathe into your *Hara* and concentrate on the tips of your middle fingers as they touch. When you have the feeling that the right moment has come to begin with the writing, pick up the writing brush and get started.

Incidentally, the *Gasshô* meditation is one of the key components for writing with *ki*. The more you succeed at remaining in your center while you write, the more beautiful and expressive your style of writing the symbols will be.

Ink-Rubbing as Meditation

If you do not work with ready-made Chinese ink or prefer the traditional method, you can also use the ink-rubbing as a preparatory meditation. To rub the ink, you need an ink stone, ink stick, and a little bit of water. Dribble some water into the flat area of the ink stone. Now hold the ink stick vertically and rub it where the water is with a minimum of pressure on the surface of the ink stone until the water turns into Chinese ink.

Depending on the quality of the ink stone and the ink stick, this process will vary in the amount of time it takes. In any case, ink-rubbing has the pleasant side effect of developing a fragrance pleasant to the nose that very gracefully uplifts the calligraphic mood.

Within this context, I would also like to explain a bit more about the direction of the rubbing. There are various directions that are more or less effective when rubbing the ink. A circular motion is usually used in China for the Chinese ink, while vertical strokes are more common in Japan. My first calligraphy master from Shanghai, a Zen monk with one Chinese parent and one Japanese parent, explained to me that the circular movements can be meaningful in many respects because the technique of writing the character is also based upon the circular movements. Without this approach, it is hardly possible to write with *ki*. By making circular movements while rubbing the ink, the hand becomes accustomed to them. Anyone who practices this a great deal will one day discover that it is less the hand than the entire body that gives the impulse for the circling vibration and that this impulse comes from the *Hara*.

I have spoken with many Japanese people about the vertical rubbing direction. They were all surprised that I do it with a circular motion. As a result, many of them thought that I am a so-called *Hen na gaijin*[194] who does not know how to do it the right way. However, no one has yet been able to give me a meaningful explanation for the vertical direction. In response to the question "why?" I always just receive the response that they all do it like this and that is just how they learned it. When I then explain why I rub the Chinese ink in a circle, I either meet with astonishment or I am "as expected" (*yappari*) a *hen na gaijin*.

Be that as it may, I recommend the circular motion in ink-rubbing for the symbol practice. This is actually an outstanding practice for the CR Symbol. Drawing circles with the writing brush is really not all that

---

[194] *Hen na gaijin* is a disparaging term for foreigners in Japan; unfortunately, it is still used quite frequently. The literal translation is something like "strange (perverse) person from the outside." It also contains the word *gaijin*, which is a discriminating variation of the word *gaikokujin* and simply means "foreigner." If you should hear this term, it is best to not take it personally since it is not meant in a personal or offensive way. Many Japanese appear not to realize that the use of such terms is not in keeping with the polite Japanese manner and can have a hurtful effect. This becomes especially conspicuous when Japanese outside of their own country are told that they could themselves also be *hen na gaijin* there. Once they become aware of this, it saddens them so that they only use this term with extreme caution from that time on. Moreover, this term is usually not meant to be as deprecating as it sounds. So take it easy.

easy. This is why I also consider the CR Symbol to be the most difficult. This not only involves drawing a circle but also a spiral from the outside to the inside at the same time.

Writing Techniques

There are simple rules for writing the character in the HS Symbol and DKM Symbol, as well as for the Reiki characters. When these rules are followed, there is actually very little that can go wrong. Nevertheless, similar rules apply to the other non-Chinese CR and SHK Symbols.

Although the practices listed in this chapter are coordinated with the symbol practice, they correspond with the rules of Chinese calligraphy according to the master *Wang Xi zhi* of the Fourth Century that are still applicable today in China, Japan, and Korea.

Sequence of Strokes

The HS Symbol

The version of the HS Symbol used by Hawayo Takata consists of 21 strokes. This version corresponds to such a large degree with the rules of traditional Chinese calligraphy that it is completely functional in the sense of energy work. However, Hawayo Takata's version is very Westernized—which is not surprising because she did not know the Japanese script. She grew up on Hawaii and learned English as her native language with its English script. Below, as well as in the chapters on the Symbols, there are many examples of calligraphically exact variations of the symbols that all function in the sense of energy work. The order of the strokes for the HS Symbol corresponds with the signs 本 者 是 正 念, whereby joining together the characters abbreviates some of the individual strokes. Because of the many strokes, the sign appears to be very complicated. Yet, with a little practice you will soon be able to remember it if you simply notice the order and writing rules that apply to all of the Chinese characters.

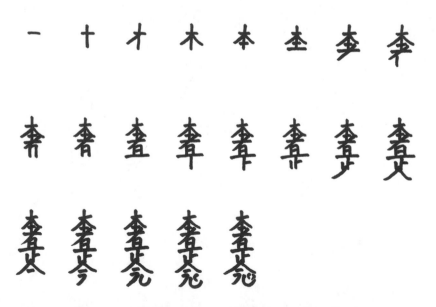

ILL. 175 – STROKE SEQUENCE FOR THE HS SYMBOL

464

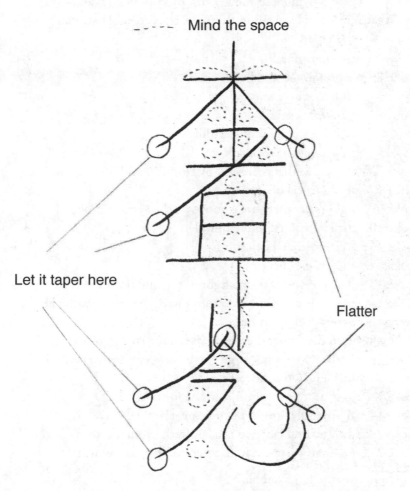

ILL. 176 – WRITING TIP 1 FOR THE HS SYMBOL

The HS Symbol in the version by Hawayo Takata
that is most widespread in the West consists of 21 strokes.

Strokes

Stroke 1: large horizontal

Stroke 2: vertical in the middle

Stroke 3: left large curve

Strok 4: right large curve

Strok 5: small horizontal in the middle

Stroke 6: large horizontal beneath it

Stroke 7: large curve that is crossed by strokes 4 and 5 at a right angle

Strok 8: small vertical beneath it

Stroke 9: begin the corner stroke above on the vertical stroke

Stroke 10: small horizontal in the middle

Stroke 11: large horizontal beneath it

Stroke 12: large vertical beneath it

Stroke 13: small horizontal to the right in the middle of the vertical

Stroke 14: small vertical to the left from the large vertical at the height of the small horizontal

Stroke 15: begin the left large curve between the two verticals

Stroke 16: also begin the right large curve between the two verticals

Stroke 17: small horizontal beneath it

Stroke 18: make a stroke beneath it in the form of a "J"

Stroke 19: an upwardly open semicircle next to the "J"

Stroke 20: small vertical curve to the left in the semicircle

Stroke 21: small vertical curve to the right of it in the semicircle

This completes the HS Symbol.

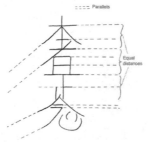

ILL. 177 – WRITING TIP 2 FOR THE HS SYMBOL

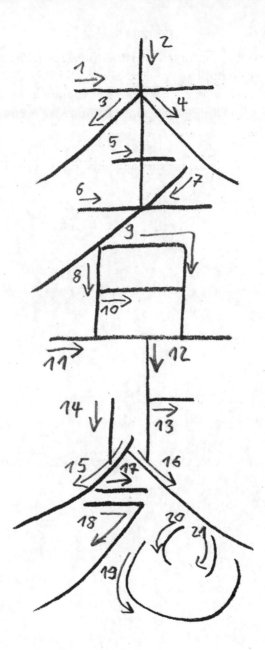

ILL. 178 – WRITING TIPS 3 FOR THE HS SYMBOL

The DKM Symbol

The DKM Symbol consists of three individual Chinese characters, each with a different number of strokes. Like the HS Symbol, it is written from above to below. In contrast to the HS Symbol, the three signs are separated by a small distance from each other, as is customary in the Chinese script.

Order of strokes for the individual signs in the DKM

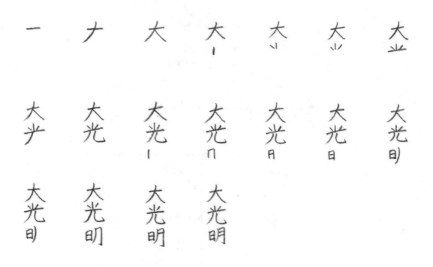

ILL. 179 – STROKE SEQUENCE FOR THE DKM SYMBOL

468

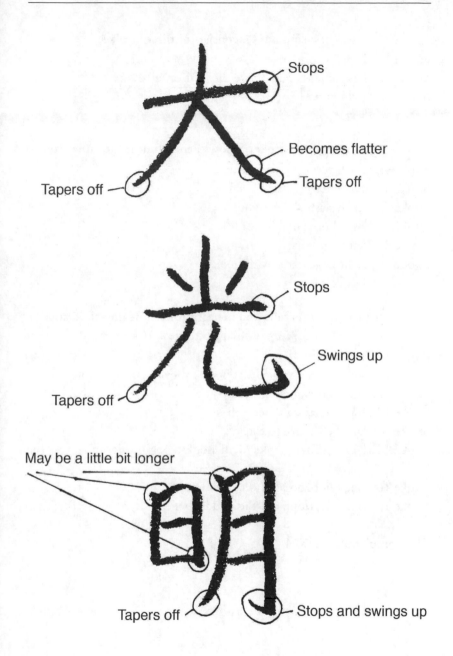

ILL. 180 – WRITING TIP 1 FOR THE DKM SYMBOL

The first sign *dai* 大 consists of three strokes.

Stroke 1:   large horizontal
Stroke 2:   left curve (begins above the horizontal)
Stroke 3:   right curve

The sign *kô* 光 of six strokes follows beneath it in the same size.

Stroke 4:   small vertical in the middle above
Stroke 5:   small diagonal above left
Stroke 6:   small slash above right
Stroke 7:   large horizontal beneath it
Stroke 8:   left large curve
Stroke 9:   right large curve with hooks

In conclusion, this is followed beneath it by the same-sized sign *myô* 明 of eight strokes.

Stroke 10: small vertical
Stroke 11: small corner stroke that begins above at the vertical
Stroke 12: small horizontal in the middle
Stroke 13: small horizontal beneath it
Stroke 14: large left curve to the left of it
Stroke 15: large corner stroke with hooks, beginning above on the
            curve
Stroke 16: small horizontal in the middle
Stroke 17: small horizontal in the middle beneath it

This completes the DKM.

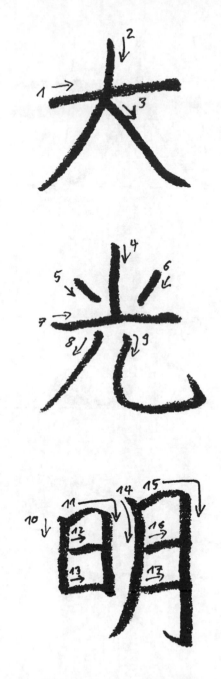

ILL. 181 – WRITING TIP 2 FOR THE DKM SYMBOL

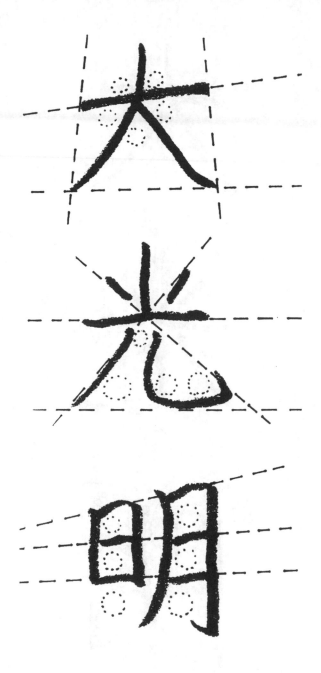

ILL. 182 – WRITING TIP 3 FOR THE DKM SYMBOL

The Characters for Reiki

The word Reiki consists of the two characters *rei* 靈 and *ki* 氣. The number of strokes for the individual signs varies here as well.

In calligraphy, the characters—just like the symbols—are written from top to bottom. But when you do not use the Reiki characters as a symbol in the sense of the *kotodama*, you can also write them from left to right or for headings in the old way of writing from right to left.

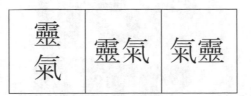

ILL. 183 – SIGN SEQUENCE OF THE REIKI CHARACTERS

ILL. 184 – STROKE SEQUENCE FOR THE REIKI CHARACTERS AS A SYMBOL

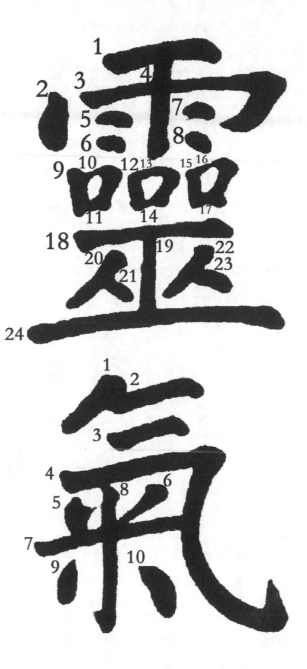

ILL. 185 – WRITING TIP 1 FOR THE REIKI SIGNS AS A SYMBOL

The sign *rei* 靈 consists of 24 strokes, in which there are also many repetitions.

Stroke 1: horizontal above
Stroke 2: small diagonal somewhat to the left beneath the horizontal
Stroke 3: begin long corner stroke at the slant
Stroke 4: begin vertical in the middle of stroke 1
Stroke: 5: small dot to the left next to the vertical
Stroke: 6: small dot beneath it to the left next to the vertical
Stroke: 7: small dot to the right next to the vertical
Stroke: 8: small dot beneath it to the right next to the vertical
Stroke 9: small vertical to the left
Stroke 10: begin small corner stroke above at the vertical
Stroke 11: small horizontal beneath it
Stroke 12: small vertical left to the right next to it
Stroke 13: begin small corner stroke above at the vertical
Stroke 14: small horizontal beneath it
Stroke 15: small vertical left to the right next to it
Stroke 16: begin small corner stroke above at the vertical
Stroke 17: small horizontal beneath it
Stroke 18: large horizontal beneath all three mouths
Stroke 19: vertical at the middle of the horizontal
Stroke 20: small curve to the left at some distance left of the vertical
Stroke 21: begin right of the curve in the middle and a small slash to the right below
Stroke 22: small curve to the left at a little distance right of the vertical
Stroke 23: begin right of the curve in the middle and make a small diagonal to the right below
Stroke 24: large horizontal beneath it

The sign for *ki* 氣 consists of ten strokes.

Stroke 1: small slash left above
Stoke 2: begin horizontal at about middle to the right at a slant
Stroke 3: small horizontal beneath it
Stroke 4: large corner stroke with curve and hooks beneath it
Stroke 5: a slanted dot to the left beneath the horizontal part of the large corner stroke

475

Stroke 6:   a slanted dot to the right of it

Stroke 7:   horizontal beneath it

Stroke 8:   vertical between the two dots through the horizontal

Stroke 9:   a slanted and longish dot to the left beneath the horizontal

Stroke 10: a slanted and longish dot to the right beneath the horizontal

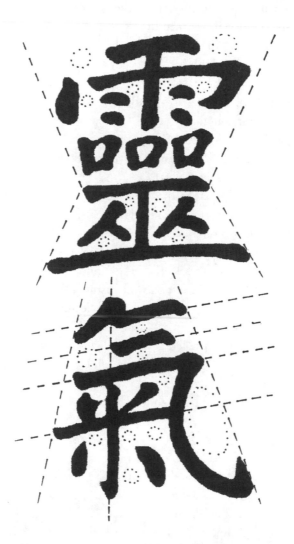

ILL. 186 – WRITING TIP 2 FOR THE REIKI CHARACTERS AS A SYMBOL

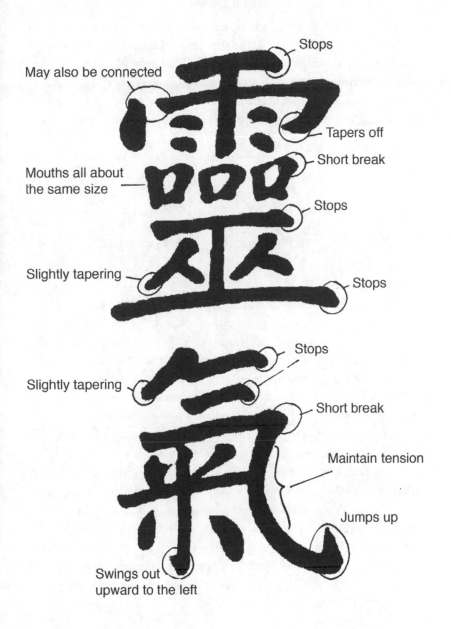

Stops

May also be connected

Tapers off

Short break

Mouths all about
the same size

Stops

Slightly tapering

Stops

Stops

Slightly tapering

Short break

Maintain tension

Jumps up

Swings out
upward to the left

ILL. 187 – WRITING TIP 3 FOR THE REIKI CHARACTERS AS A SYMBOL

The CR Symbol

Since the CR Symbol is not a Chinese character, the same rules do not apply as above. Despite this, the sequences of the strokes and direction must be precisely complied with, as for all Reiki symbols.

The CR Symbol is carried out in one line. In keeping with this, there is also no sequence of strokes. The one important factor here is to precisely adhere to the beginning and end point, as well as the direction.

ILL. 188 – STROKE SEQUENCE FOR THE CR SYMBOL

Proceed as follows:

Begin the horizontal stroke at the left top. It should be so long that it juts out far beyond the following spiral. Without a break, now guide the writing brush vertically downward. The vertical stroke should be long enough to that you can draw the spiral in such a way that allows for the entire composition. Continue to guide the writing brush further down counterclockwise in a right angle to the right and write the spiral in such a way that it crosses the vertical stroke beneath the horizontal three times to the left and three times to the right. The spiral should end to the right of the vertical stroke but the stroke should not be too close short.

Since the CR Symbol points to a spiral that continues into infinity, small variations in the length of the spiral are not a problem for its meaning. The vertical stroke should be approximately in the middle of the spiral. The horizontal stroke has a right angle at the top where it meets the vertical, and there is also a right angle at the bottom where the horizontal stroke turns into the spiral. In China and Japan, there are different variations of this sign that more or less have the whorls of a spiral and the horizontal strokes are much longer or shorter. From the appearance of the symbol, it should basically be possible to deduct the meaning of the spiritual yang energy coming from the right (seen from the perspective of the sign) that descends into matter, the yin, and passes through all seven

478

major chakras (essential, spiritual life themes) in order to disappear into a point (Hara, *Tan Tien*) after it has been transformed and enriched.

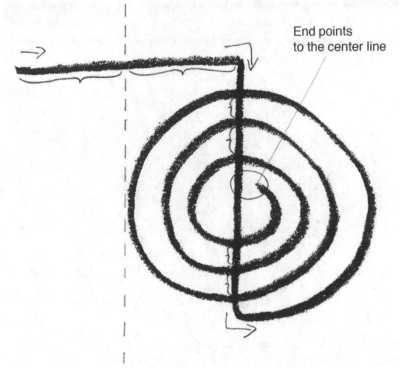

End points
to the center line

ILL. 189 – WRITING TIP FOR THE CR SYMBOL

The SHK Symbol

The SHK Symbol is also not a Chinese character but an Indian *Siddham* symbol. As a Reiki symbol, it is slightly abstracted so that a stroke sequence similar to those of the characters can be used. They are only similar because there are no semicircles that start to the right in the Chinese characters.

The *Siddham* were originally drawn with a narrow wooden brush. However, in East Asia it is quite customary to draw the *Siddham* with a writing brush for calligraphy. Because of the various shapes of the brush tips, the lines of the symbols are varied.

ILL. 190 - STROKE SEQUENCE FOR THE SHK SYMBOL

The SHK Symbol is drawn in four strokes:

Stroke 1: Pull the writing brush downward at a slant to the left and then horizontally to the right. The horizontal ends beneath the starting point of the slanted part. From there, the line continues at a slant downward to the left. Both slanted lines should be parallel to each other. Then move downward vertically and horizontally to the right. The vertical should not be too long. The corner points should correspond with the upper ones. End the first stroke now by moving the writing brush downward in a curve to the left that has about the doubled height of the vertical.

Stroke 2: Begin with the writing brush above stroke 1 to the far left above the left part and draw a large curve downward to the right that ends in a vertical right next to the end of stroke 1.

Stroke 3: Draw a semicircle on the right side of stroke 2 so that the center of the semicircle lies at the height of the first horizontal of stroke 1.

Stroke 4: Draw another semicircle beneath it on the right side of stroke 2 so that the center of this semicircle lies at the height of the second horizontal of stroke 1.

This completes the SHK Symbol.

Writing Direction

The tendency of the writing direction in the Chinese characters always moves from left to right and then from above to below, in as far as this is permitted by the sequence of the strokes. Horizontal strokes are always written from left to right. Vertical strokes are always written from top to bottom. The strokes that go around the corner start with the horizontal portion by moving from left to right and from top to bottom without removing the brush. The large curves ending at the left are always begun by writing from the top right down toward the left. The large curves ending at the right are always begun by writing from the top left down toward the right.

Individual strokes within a character are written after the main one. So first create the framework and then the inner portions. Also see: 雨 • 氣 • 日 • 月 • 明

ILL. 191 –
STROKE SEQUENCE FOR THE ORIGINAL INDIAN SIDDHAM FORM OF THE
SHK SYMBOL: HRIH

Basic Exercises for Correctly Writing Shûji 習字

Exercise 1: Writing a First Sign

Before you begin practicing the individual strokes, select any sign or symbol and copy it. Be sure to save this if it is your first work of art since this will allow you to later recognize how much you have improved through the following practices. You may also want to write all of the symbols once in order to compare them as evidence of your progress.

Exercise 2: Writing a Sign at Different Speeds

Once again, select any sign or symbol and copy it as quickly as you can. When you are done with it, write the same sign or symbol again but this time as slowly and concentrated as possible. As you do this, attempt to copy the model as precisely as possible. Then compare your two examples.

Is there a difference? The signs that are written slowly should look more beautiful and more similar to the original. In fact, it is very important in calligraphy to write in an extremely slow and conscious way. The same principle is also very important for a successful symbol practice and the development of your subtle perception. Also keep these two works of art.

Practicing the Individual Strokes as Components of the Symbols

As a basic practice, many people who begin with the study of calligraphy spend quite a few years writing the first character from the famous foreword of the *Orchid Pavilion* by *Wang Xizhi*. This is the sign for "eternal" and is called *ei* 永 (chin: *yong*). It actually contains all of the important strokes of calligraphy. However, you really have to look for these strokes.

Since all of the stroke forms are also contained in the Reiki symbols and the Reiki characters, the emphasis here should be on practicing the characters that are important for Reiki. The following illustration shows all of the strokes that appear in the Reiki symbols and Reiki characters and how to write them. The color black shows how the form of the strokes should look. The arrows are intended to help guide the brush in order to create the exact form of the stroke.

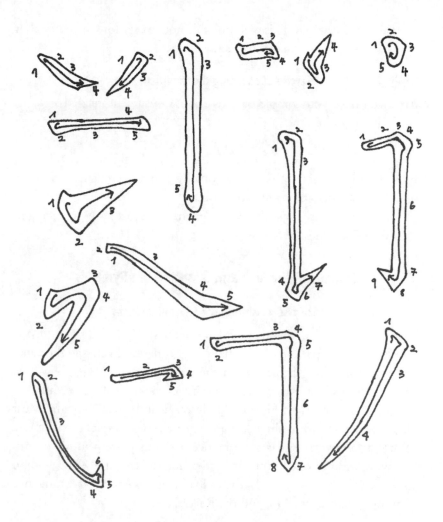

ILL. 192 – TYPES OF STROKES IN CALLIGRAPHY

Exercise 3A: Practicing the Individual Strokes

Now select the strokes for the signs or symbols that you have just written from the chart. Practice each individual stroke by filling an entire piece of paper with it. Please also note here that the art does not consist of filling the page as quickly as possible but of dedicating yourself to each individual stroke attentively and consciously. Try to draw each stroke as

483

it looks in the original. This will probably not be easy for you at first, but as you know, practice makes perfect.

Exercise 3B: Writing the Complete Sign

After you have you completed Exercise 3A, write the related signs or symbols one more time.

What has happened now?

If your ability has deteriorated, this is completely normal. This is a type of initial worsening as in homeopathy. Just keep practicing and the result will be outstanding at some point.

If you have improved, this is very good. Then just keep practicing in this way to become even better.

Practicing the Size and Shape of the Symbols

Exercise 4: Writing the Signs in Patterns

This exercise involves the size and shape of the symbols and signs. Divide your paper into a pattern of six equally large squares. If you fold the paper and then run along the edge with the writing brush, the paper will be smooth again when you unfold it because of the moist Chinese ink.[195]

An individual character should always fit into such a square. Most characters are somewhat higher than they are wide. Despite this, they are traditional drawn in squares as practice. Use this pattern until you can also write without one in this size and form. You can apply this method for the CR and SHK symbols, the individual signs of the DKM, the five beginning signs of the HS, and the Reiki signs.

Exercise 4A: The HS Symbol

Because of its 5 joined characters, the HS Symbol has a longish shape that does not fit into a square. You can make a pattern for it by dividing your paper lengthwise in the middle into two halves. Now write the symbol from top to bottom without individual parts sticking out too far to the left or right.

---

[195] My first calligraphy master *Hôon Kenmyô* thought up this technique in order to create a time-saving pattern.

Exercise 4B: The DKM Symbol

You can practice two DKM Symbols on a piece of paper with a pattern of six squares. Draw one of the signs of the symbol from top to bottom in the individual squares.

Writing with Ki

Up to now, the main topic has been the technique of writing called calligraphy. However, the technique obviously just forms the basis for writing with *ki* since the writing brush is not guided by the technique but by the mind.

Sometimes I am also not so certain what has actually put the symbols on the paper. Then I can no longer differentiate between whether I guided the writing brush or whether the writing brush guided me. At this point, I would like to share a brief experience from my first hour of calligraphy: After I had repeatedly made pathetic attempts to write as beautifully as my master, and he had explained to me that writing with *ki* is as important as the form, he encouraged me to use his writing brush.

What happened next was an absolutely brilliant experience. I could do whatever I wanted, but the writing brush guided me and my hand instead of my hand moving the brush. The results were very striking signs. Later, it was not possible for me to repeat such results with my own writing brush for a long time. How is this possible? Because my master had the ability to write with *ki*, the brush had become type of "energy channel" that had filled itself up or become permeated with *ki*.

This is obviously very similar to Reiki. All those who are initiated into Reiki and practice it are Reiki channels. As a channel, we can transmit Reiki to other living beings, objects, and ourselves. The only precondition is that this Reiki is absorbed. Under special conditions, such as the programming of healing stones or initiations, it is then possible to make the effect of Reiki available on a lasting basis.

Exactly the same principle applies for writing with *ki*—transmitting the *ki* with the Chinese ink through the writing brush onto the sheet of paper. Depending upon the quality of the *ki* (and this does not mean

485

good or bad), the expression, shape, and appearance of the calligraphy also changes.

This may lead us to think that this is probably very simple since we are Reiki channels and the Reiki from our hand permeates the writing brush with the Chinese ink onto the paper when we write. Although this is correct, unfortunately it is not quite so simple since this is not the exact equivalent of writing with *ki*. If this were the case, all Reiki channels would soon become masters of calligraphy without even practicing it.

Just as receiving a Reiki initiation does not make us enlightened but we have to take the path of personality development on our own, we must also walk the "path of calligraphy"— *Shodô*—for this same purpose by ourselves. In calligraphy, just as in Reiki, the techniques are obviously just the foundation. When we master this basis, we must still climb up the ladder to reach the roof at some point.

In traditional calligraphy, it is customary to spend years copying the works of the old master from earlier generations. Through the continually new contemplation on the form and style of the old masters, it becomes possible in the course of time to get closer and closer to them. There are also calligraphers today who can write in the style of a long-deceased master. This is a high art. As a result, there are a great many forgeries of old works of art and it is difficult to differentiate between the originals and the copies.

In the history of Chinese calligraphy, there are occasional references to the fact that some of the very famous calligraphers were criticized during the course of their careers because they lacked verve and creativity. In addition to the art of copying one's models as a path to mastery, it is also necessary to one day develop our own style in order to truly become a master. Although the mastered techniques continue to be used, creativity also comes into play as well. This approach can obviously also be applied in many other areas, such as Reiki. Using Reiki and the symbols according to the motto of "it should work out somehow" can easily lead to a dead end. But developing a personal style too early can also lead to making fundamental mistakes. The more and longer we practice the symbols according to the rules of the art, the more the global standard will rise and therefore the higher the chances of one day applying Reiki and its symbols in a creative way. Rainbow Reiki is an example of this. The more we test it, the more we discover that it works.

The following section reveals how you can achieve this by using methods based on the individual symbols by combining *Shodô* and *Reiki*. Please let me know if you have interesting discoveries that you would like to share. Enjoy!

Selecting a Symbol for Personality Development

First select a symbol for yourself. Do this however you like or even include your Inner Child in the process, which can be done using the pendulum or the symbol cards that you should prepare in advance.

Personality Development with the CR Symbol

I have frequently observed in seminars how students or even Reiki Masters write the CR Symbol. This is extremely exciting. But only in very rare cases do they succeed in having the vertical stroke of the CR Symbol in the middle of the spiral. It is just as rare for the circles of the spiral to be truly circular. The more you are centered, the better you will succeed at drawing round and even CR Symbols that do not look like they will tip over at any moment.

To the same extent, I have also observed that the personal development of an individual is accompanied by the improvement of the CR Symbols. As a result, the CR Symbol is a type of personality and/or mood barometer. Of course, similar observations can also be made for the other symbols.

In previous time, I was surprised that there were long phases in which I made no progress at all. But this changed abruptly when I recognized that the shape of the symbol reflected my inner state and tried to tell me what I could work on within myself. So writing the symbols and their interpretation is like a type of aura/chakra reading. In this sense, it is therefore also quite possible to connect *Reiki* and calligraphy with the life principles of Dr. Usui.

The CR Symbols that I write are also not always perfect. But by studying the form, I can examine whether I am centered or how I relate to yin and yang, for example. If the symbol leans too much to the left or right on a regular basis, this also has a meaning. So I use the practicing of the CR Symbol as a means to measure my personality development.

When the CR Symbol is used in a way that functionally strengthens our energy and points us in the right direction, it also has fulfilled its task completely since it shows us our path by means of its shape. And that is wonderful!

Exercise 1: CR Symbol and Chakra Energy Cards

In order to find out more about the spiritual meaning of the form you have drawn, you can also consult the *Chakra Energy Cards*. So, if you also would like to discover more details about the cause or the spiritual lesson for your personality development found in the form of your CR Symbol, draw a card with the question: "What is my spiritual lesson related to this form of the CR Symbol?" Give yourself a mental treatment with the affirmation on the card until you clearly notice changes while writing in the following days.

Exercise 2: Chinese Ink with Bach Flowers

Put some drops of the Bach Flower listed under your affirmation of Exercise 1 into the water before you rub the Chinese ink next time. By rubbing the Chinese ink, a part of the water always evaporates. This promotes the effect of the Bach Flower, triggering healing through the nose and the aura.

Exercise 3: Chinese Ink with a Healing Seal

Program the water for the Chinese ink with the healing seal on the card. The healing power of the seal will also have an effect through the nose and the aura.

Exercise 4: Yin and Yang in the CR Symbol

Check to see whether the vertical center line is truly in the middle or whether it tends to lean toward the right or left. If it is in the middle, this means that yin and yang are balanced. If the center line is too far on the right, which means that the right part of the spiral is also small, this indicates a blockage of the yang. Too far to the left means a yin blockage. Draw the appropriate card to find the cause of the blockage and proceed as described above.

Exercise 5: The Chakras in the CR Symbol

The gaps on the center line correspond with the number 7. This is also the number of the seven major chakras. Think of a topic and draw a CR Symbol at the same time. Compare the distances and check to see which chakras appear to be especially small and weak.

While you continue to think of the topic, use the Reiki Cloud Hands for this chakra. To do this, let your hands bob up and down lightly and move your fingers carefully without a gripping movement. This should resemble the movements of a jellyfish. Then write the symbol one more time.

Exercise 6: The Aura Fields in the CR Symbol

The spaces to the right and left of the center line each correspond with the number 4. This is also the number of the four aura fields. More detailed explanations about the aura fields can be found in the chapter on the Human Spiritual Energy System. The width and distances between the aura fields can also result in interesting conclusions, comparable to those of Exercise 4.

Writing in a Trance

Once you have learned to write correctly, as well as with *ki*, there is another form of calligraphy that you should also know about. This is writing in a trance, the roots of which can be traced back to Taoism in Chinese calligraphy. A very exciting article about this topic was written several years ago by Professor Ledderose of the University of Heidelberg, Department for East Asian Art. A summary of it follows below.

The period of the Six Dynasties (3rd-6th Century A.D.) was very significant for the development of Chinese calligraphy. In addition to the above-mentioned types of script development, there was an additional form of calligraphy in the *Mao shan* School of Taoism that is called sacred writing.

The written signs play an important role in the religious area throughout the entire history of calligraphy. Even the first characters on the oracle bones were used for religious purposes. The script is a medium for communication between human beings and the subtle world.

In a text called *Chen kao* (Explanation of the Perfected Ones) from the year 499, it says that *Yang Xi* (330-?) had visions in religious states of trance. One night, he was visited by various immortals who had come down from heaven to him. Most of the time, an enchantingly beautiful woman came and held his hand while he wrote sacred texts with the writing brush. The *Chen kao* also includes a text about how messages from the subtle world can be understood through the medium of calligraphy. It describes a hierarchy for the types of script. The highest type is called "The Script of the Three Origins and Eight Connections" (*san yuan ba hui* 三元八會). It exists in a timeless, primordial level and is used by heavenly beings of the highest ranks. There are many derivations of this type in lower realms that can be used for inscriptions on talismans. These sacred types cannot be easily understood by mortals. In even deeper realms, the script then assumes material form.

The beautiful women who visited *Yang Xi* at night never wrote themselves, neither with their hands nor with their feet. They wrote by using human beings as a medium. Their traces are what becomes visible.

Writing with a religious inspiration was widespread in China and is also still practiced today. A method that is still used today consists of the writer going into a trance and then writing in the sand with a wooden stick. In the process, he writes quite quickly and in complete ecstasy. He begins to sweat so vehemently that it far exceeds what is normally possible. The entire process lasts about 40 minutes. The surface of the sand is limited. As soon as the medium takes a short break, the sand is smoothed by a helper. Another helper reads the sign aloud so that the signs written in the sand can immediately be copied onto paper with the writing brush and Chinese ink. However, no breaks are planned. At any moment, the writing process can continue.

This method can be traced back to the Sixth Century in literary sources. However, it is presumed that it was already used in *Mao shan* Taoism.[196]

This method of calligraphy is a form of channeling. However, the channeling occurs here not through the spoken language but through the script. If you have already abundantly practiced calligraphy and at the

---

[196]   Ledderose, Lothar: *Some Taoist Elements in the Calligraphy of the Six Dynasties*. In: *T'oung Pao*. Vol. LXX. 1984, pages 246-278.

same time are also initiated into the Second Reiki Degree or plan to do so soon, then you can use the techniques of the Second Degree for the channeling of script.

Exercise 1: Writing Symbols with a Light Being

Select a light being according to the methods described above. After you have learned about the qualities that this light being has, establish the distant contact with it through Reiki. To do this, use your flat hand to write the HS Symbol vertically in the air in front of you and activate it by repeating the mantra three times. Now use the same approach to write and activate a CR Symbol. Think or say the name of the light being three times (for example: Archangel Gabriel, Archangel Gabriel, Archangel Gabriel) and greet it with respect. Tell the light being about your intention and send Reiki to it as compensation. Finally, pick up the writing brush and let the light being written the Reiki symbols through you.

Give thanks and take leave respectfully from the distant contact at the end, then enjoy the work of art.

Effect: The result is usually quite amazing since the signs look different than normally. This is simply because they have not been written by you but through you by the light being.

Exercise 2: Allowing a Light Being to Write Through You

As in Exercise 1, establish contact with a light being. This time, do not write any type of symbol but simply let it write through you—no matter how it comes out.

Effect: The result can be very different here. Images or even script may emerge. Generally, these are more or less understandable messages. If script emerges, you may also write signs that you do not recognize.

Exercise 3: Writing Script and Language with a Light Being

As in Exercise 1, establish contact with a light being. Agree upon which script you would like to write with the light being—letters, for example. Simply let it write through you, no matter what comes. You can also ask direct questions on topics that interest you.

Note: It is advisable to select a script and language that you understand so that you can also related to the channeled contents. When selecting the topic and asking questions, it is meaningful in the long run to formulate them in a way that is characterized by personal responsibility, love, and wisdom. This is also the approach that the light beings accept and how they respond. They always give answers that are for the highest good of the whole.

Effect: Individual letters, words, or even texts may appear. These are generally more or less understandable messages.

Copying the Sûtras

During the first 500 years of Buddhism, the teaching was mainly handed down in an oral manner. Even though King *Vittagâmini* of Ceylon permitted the sutras to be written down about 50 B.C., it still continued to be a custom for a long time in India and Southeast Asia to recite the texts by heart. Equal value was placed on the written and the spoken words only when Buddhism came to China, Japan, and Tibet.

Since the script and literature in China were already in full blossom when Buddhism was introduced, and also played an especially important role, it is no surprise that the Chinese collected the Buddhist sutras so eagerly and translated them into Chinese. In the city of Loyang, *Shigao* established the first center for the translation of the Buddhist sutras in 148 A.D. *Shigao* was primarily concerned with manuals for meditation. In 167, *Sythian Zhichan*, whose specialty was the *Prajna Paramita* Sûtra (The Sûtra of the Perfect Truth), arrived on the scene. Even better and more precise translations were created in the Third Century because of the expanded knowledge of the language.

Since the sutras were still far from complete, many Chinese monks traveled to India in order to find the missing texts. *Faxian* was the first to succeed in this and return to China. His pilgrimage and collecting journey lasted from 399-414. His biography states that the Indian masters recited the sutras to him from memory and had no recorded manuscripts. In a special type of training, they had learned to develop an incredible memory.

The arrival of *Kumarajiva* in the city of Changan in 401 set a new wave of translations of the sutras in motion that was also supported by the emperor's court. Chinese monks continued to travel to India time and again in order to expand their knowledge of Sanskrit or bring even more texts back to China. In the Seventh Century, the translations of the sutras reached a climax with the pilgrims *Xuanzang* and *Yi Ching*, who lived in India from 629-645 and 671-695.

In the translation studios, the old monks examined the accuracy of a Sanskrit text and, if necessary, compared it with other texts. Then the main translators began their work in that one of them orally recited the Indian texts and the other immediately wrote down what he had heard in Chinese. These written texts were subsequently examined by other specialists to ensure that the original and the translation really corresponded in terms of the content. Finally, the style of the texts was corrected before a calligrapher made fair copy.

Despite this, there were discrepancies in the translations since one person thought that everything must be translated very literally, independent of what type of style was the end result. Others believed that the texts should be adapted to the Chinese style and, if necessary, inappropriate sections should be shortened. *Kumarajiva* suggested the middle path by translating as literally as necessary and as freely as possible. A copy (a translation is also a copy) can never correspond 100% with the original. Something is always different and stands out when the two are compared. When you write the symbols, they always look somewhat different. But if the form remains the same, which means that no important parts are missing and the symbol can be clearly recognized, this copy can be accepted as a new original. This is also what *Kumarajiva* thought when he assumed that slight deviations are acceptable as long as the basic meaning has been transmitted in an easily understandable way in the translation without additional nuances.

As soon as the first translations appeared in China, the cult of the devoted practice of copying the sutras with the writing brush also started. Beginning with the emperor *Daowu,* a long line of sutra copying was initiated under the imperial commission.

Ritual Sûtra Writing

Devoted sutra writing is considered to be spiritual training in Buddhism. In Japan, this custom was first mentioned in the *Nihon shoki* from the year 720. It says that the court of the Tennô requested a copy of the *Daizôkyô* (*Tripitaka*), which was then prepared in the *Kawaradera* Temple in 673. During the *Nara* Period (710-794), entire offices were set up for copying sutras. When a person copies sutras in a ritual manner, he gathers merit as a result and can do much good for himself or deceased ancestors in this way within the framework of the ritual.

Depending upon which sûtra is written in a ritual way, some very different things can also be achieved. For example, it is possible to restore inner peace when a person has committed an evil deed through the copying and recitation of the Heart Sûtra.[197]

If a sûtra is simply just a text in which the teachings of the Buddha are imparted, a person can attain good karma through its duplication because this propagates the teachings of the Buddha as a path to happiness for everyone involved. If a sûtra additionally contains magical formulas such as mantras and symbols like the *Siddham*, these develop—especially on the basis of initiation—special powers for the person who uses them. As a result, writing the symbols is also very supportive of development.

Sutras are generally written with the Chinese writing brush and Chinese ink on a great variety of materials ranging from paper to roofing tiles. This also depends upon the purpose for which a sûtra is being copied. In the *Heian* Period, for example, there were many wars between the Samurai families. In order to finally achieve victory, in 1164 the then famous *Taira Kiyomori* ritually prepared several sutras, including the Lotus Sûtra and the Heart Sûtra, with paper decorated with gold and syllables. On one of the scrolls, a *Siddham* symbol also appears right at the beginning in order to invite the power of the light beings. But ultimately, the extinction of his entire family shows that it was ridiculous to perform rituals on the one hand and then burn down great temples and work against life in many areas on the other hand. This also shows quite clearly that the

---

[197] This can be seen very well in the Korean film *Spring, Summer, Fall, Winter and ...* when a young man uses a knife to carve out a sûtra painted on a bridge.

494

light beings help in particular when the situation truly serves the highest good of the whole.

Since the Chinese *Sung* Period in which the technique of woodblock printing was introduced, the copying of sutras by hand has become a pure form of spiritual training that continues to this day in all of East Asia.

Writing in Siddham—the SHK Symbol

As was extensively described in the chapter on the SHK Symbol, this is an Indian symbol of the *Siddham* script. Similar to the Chinese characters, the symbols for sacred rituals developed into a script for imparting information.

In India, the Chinese writing brush for calligraphy is unknown. It was customary there to write with a wooden brush, the tip of which is long like a thick stroke. When writing with such a wooden brush, the form of the Siddham symbols are the same but the type of lines are greatly varied.

With the introduction of the *Siddham* script to China, people also began writing these symbols with the Chinese writing brush. In Japan, there are still both variations to this day. In the West, where with the writing brush is rarely used and people almost never write with the wooden brush, other types of writing media are employed. Pencils and fountain pens work especially well for this purpose since they make a brush-like flow possible.

In terms of the pure handwriting, any type of writing tool will do. However, the writing brush is much more suitable for symbol calligraphy. Writing with it is a unique experience![198]

---

[198] In case this brief introduction has stimulated your interest, I (Mark) offer special calligraphy classes for Reiki practitioners (also in the USA). See my website for more information.

PART IV –

SPIRITUAL COSMOLOGY AND KNOWLEDGE OF ITS ESOTERIC BACKGROUND

CHAPTER 19

An Short Essay on Spiritual Cosmology

Blissful Yearning

Tell it no one but the wise,

The crowd will only jeer:

The living thing I praise,

That longs for death by fire.

Cooling, in those nights of love,

Conceiving as you were conceived,

A strange emotion fills you

While the quiet candle gleams.

You're no longer in the grasp

Of shadows, darkening,

A new desire lifts you up

On to a higher mating.

No distances can weigh you down,

Enchanted you come flying,

And greedy for the light, at last,

A moth, you burn in dying.

And as long as you lack this

True word: Die and Become!

You'll be but a dismal guest

In Earth's darkened room.

(From: *The West-Eastern Divan*, Johann Wolfgang von Goethe; translated by A.S. Kline)

The expression "spiritual cosmology"[199] characterizes an explanation of the structure and function of Creation in its entirety. Time and again, this book has referred to the concealed structures of the divine order and explained the related teachings of *Esoteric Buddhism,* Japanese *Shintoism,* and Chinese *Taoism.* However, these statements can ultimately only be understood when the appropriate, cross-cultural basic information on spiritual cosmology is available. Terms such as "love," "oneness," "light beings," "angels," "Creative Force," "free will," "healing," "personal responsibility," and "spiritual path" occur over and over again. But what *precisely* do these words mean within the spiritual context? How can they be applied in a *practical way?* Are there explanations of them that are valid for *all* spiritual paths?

In a practical sense, these topics can only be understood and sensibly integrated into everyday life when we can comprehend exactly what they mean on their own and within the context of life as a whole. The Japanese sage *Kûkai,* who has been mentioned time and again in this book, contributed to the further development of Esoteric Buddhism in a very special way by making it into a system that unproblematically offers recognition and space for every religion or spiritual philosophy—an important step to religious peace, which the Christian churches and Islam have unfortunately not always accomplished during the approximately 1,000 years since *Kûkai's* death. This is why it makes sense to include a coherent modern explanation of spiritual cosmology that is connected with the essential thoughts of this great spiritual teacher in this book. However, the cosmology explained in this chapter is not that of *Kûkai,* whose belief system was esoteric Buddhism. Yet, *Kûkai's* core thesis and convictions can be found here together with the basic teachings of Taoism and Shintoism.

In the system of Rainbow Reiki[200], which is taught throughout the world, this model has been used for many years with great results in order to receive practical explanations in response to the big questions of "from

[199] Definition: "*Cosmology* (Greek)—The teaching of the structure of the universe or the world order. *Kosmos* (Greek)—Order; universe; world order.

[200] As its foundation, Rainbow Reiki contains the car fully researched traditional Reiki of Dr. Usui and Dr. Hayashi. Based upon this, it has been expanded through powerful techniques of energy work that especially include symbols and mantras. Rainbow Reiki was founded at the beginning of the 1990s.

where?, "why", and "to where?" that can be understood and translated into everyday life. This is the first time that information about this is published in a written form.

This chapter describes what the "divine order" actually is and how this topic is useful in a *personal* way. Of course, it also provides a great many explanations about the bigger picture of life, within which we walk our own paths as individual beings.

The model described in the following text basically applies to all religions and all spiritual paths that see value in striving for *love, meaning, consciousness, personal responsibility, a lifetime filled with happiness in the material world and afterward,* as well as *constructive behavior in relation to the whole.*

This approach can help us—no matter which faith we currently follow—to see our path more clearly and better follow our vision that leads us to spiritual awakening, to the great, radiant light.

The Basic Assumptions of Spiritual Cosmology

As prerequisites for the following statements, we would like to assume that there is **one** Creative Force that has made everything that exists—from out of itself! If it had used a different source material that did not come from it, there would have to have been a second Creative Force because the other force had to have come from somewhere as well…

This essentially simple conclusion has important consequences! When we accept it, when we comprehend that there is just one divine order with just one Creative Force, there is no room for a "Second God," the Devil or whatever else the embodiment of evil may be called, as the great adversary. From where should he receive his power if all spiritual power, all consciousness, and all love only have the one source of the Creative Force? How can there be a being that can do powerful energy work—sometimes, for example, as claimed in the Christian churches, even in competition with the angels or other light beings—who is not connected with and close to the Creative Force? If there were a Devil—evil per se and in person—instead of just evil **behavior** on the basis of a meaningless use of free will in relation to the divine order—then this principle and the being that embodies it must be a special favorite of the Creative Force because it would otherwise be completely powerless.

On the other hand: What about the many goddesses and gods, angels, fairies, devas, power animals, and other light beings that are known in the great variety of esoteric traditions around the world? Where does evil actually come from? And where does good come from? Where do love and where do hate come from? Is the Creative Force indifferent to what the individual beings do or does it know and love each of its children? Are we truly taken care of or do we have to fend for ourselves? Is there some higher meaning in life and, if so, what does it consist of?

I hope to thoroughly answer these and other questions in this chapter.

Since the topic is quite extensive and at times complex, it may be helpful to read the various sections more than once. The individual sections of the chapters are related to each other—so the explanations for individual terms in one section may not be complete there but can be found in another section. The cross-references that are included from time to time will help locate the appropriate parts of the text.

Oneness

It is best to start where everything had its beginning and to which everything returns, as the saying goes: *oneness*[201]. A state of **true** oneness is quite boring, comparable to a free weekend in which there are a great many things that could be done but you simply cannot decide on anything. Everything is possible, but nothing happens at all if you cannot get dressed, call friends, and do something like going to the movies or inline skating with them—which means making a selection from the amount of possible alternatives for how you live your life and then consistently taking the appropriate actions. If you do not make a decision that is then translated into a practical action, you will just be killing time. Nothing happens.

---

[201] Incidentally, the mathematic symbol for true oneness is a point—without any expansion and, strictly speaking, without color or another specific quality. Something like this obviously cannot be drawn, so Illustration 1 is intended as a symbolic depiction.

In the state of *perfect* oneness, there is *no time* and *no space* since as soon as there is a course of events, a process of actions, the oneness would already be over. Actions occur through the changing relationships to a great variety of objects, beings, and parts of a being with each other (absorbing and emitting energy, metabolism; muscle and nerve activity), and situations. There is no such thing as time when nothing moves—in the literal sense and down to the subatomic regions. *For time to occur, something must also happen. On the other hand, nothing can happen without time.* Strictly speaking, the existence of space also necessitates the existence of the time and vice versa.

●

ILL. 193 – THE PERFECT ONENESS

The Meaning of the Quality of Time

Before the emergence of the patriarchal culture, people were basically accustomed to orienting their own lifestyle, thinking, decision-making, and actions upon the quality of time instead of a certain point in time. As a result, a strong positive resonance with nature, its energies, and potentials were built up. This attunement to the currently prevailing natural energies and processes made it easier to do what was necessary. This virtually resulted in a "tail wind from destiny." At that time, the Great Goddess was much more palpable in everyday life than today. Her help was directly perceived and integrated into everyday life by personally opening up to the natural qualities of time, such as those described by astrology or as are evident in the seasons. Human actions and natural processes were connected in this way and mutually supported each other.

Through the increasingly dominant patriarchal system in the societies, there was a constantly more distinctive countermovement away from the orientation toward nature. Instead of the surrendering to the natural time quality of the divine order, people now preferred to establish artificial systems of time-planning and order. The sense of human beings regarding "the right time" for a certain action, as well as the related attunement to the whole of life in the world, disappeared increasingly and must be awakened with much effort in most cases today. People now frequently tend to react in an annoyed or at least irritated and anxious way when their "orderly" scheduling is disrupted for whatever reasons by the natural course of life and they must remember that they can never rule over nature but at best must learn to understand it and use its gifts in a meaningful way. Many people are especially troubled by the process of aging and death.

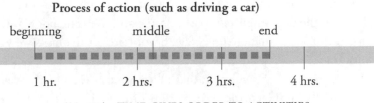

Process of action (such as driving a car)

| beginning | middle | end |

| 1 hr. | 2 hrs. | 3 hrs. | 4 hrs. |

ILL. 194 – TIME GIVES ORDER TO ACTIVITIES

The Spiritual Approach to the Aging Process

Aging is a natural process, as is *birth* and *death*. Through the pressure created by the process of aging, for example, human beings are constantly called upon to cultivate their inner values, to better understand the meaning of life, and to develop their ability to love through the challenge of their own shortcomings and those of others. Only aging beings have reasons for being committed and attending as effectively as possible to the realization of their life's meaning because their finiteness only allows them a limited amount of time for this purpose. Aging also challenges us to pay increasingly more attention to the inner values and to develop them. For example, an aging woman can recognize her inner beauty, which she has developed through an intensive process of character maturation, in the mirror of her beloved's eyes. This may even far outshine the splendor of physical beauty during her youth. The aging man may learn to perceive the emotional power that he has built up step-by-step through the challenges and ordeals of his life in the mirror of his beloved's eyes.

We are given the physical beauty of youth—but we must develop the inner beauty of age, the warm-heartedness, kindness, love, wisdom, naturalness, and grace. Then we can rightfully be proud of the latter as our own personal achievement.

Through aging, which actually represents an essential shortcoming, we must grapple with the world after death. This can also help us to see our fixation on material things in relative terms.

We can hate our wrinkles because we have not accepted the related experiences from the depths of our heart—or we can love our wrinkles because each and every one of them are connected with valuable experiences that have allowed us to more and more become beings filled with light and love.

Because of death, we have the possibility time and again to attune our body to the next important part of our path. We can endow it with all types of qualities that are precisely appropriate for the tasks we want to work on.

Through the great forgetting that takes place at each birth, we can also spiritually approach the next section of our life path in a largely unencumbered way and become familiar with truly new ways of looking at the world and have new experiences. Without this amnesia, most people would quickly become resigned and cynical, missing out on many wonderful opportunities.

For example, a great deal of emotional maturity is required to be open to the idea that this time the respective individual and the type of relationship can be completely different in a renewed encounter when we have complete memory of the experiences with a person.

Time as a Structuring Influence

Time organizes movements in the material world so that a sequence of cause and effect, together with a progressing, structuring development becomes possible on the generally applicable basis of structures created in the past.[202] However, in reality time is not a constant—it is not something that is solid. Depending upon the speed that a specific particle or being

---

[202] These explanations on the phenomenon of "time" only apply to the material world. Inside of the atoms, in the human mind, in the spiritual world, there are also rules related to time—but different ones! More on this topic later in this chapter.

has in relation to another, it runs slower (in relation to the other parts that move at a more leisurely pace) or quicker (in relation to the parts that move more rapidly).[203] The more closely the relative speed of a particle approaches the speed of light, the more slowly time passes. However, a material particle can never attain the speed of light. When it reaches the speed of light, it disappears from the material world. It completely changes its form of existence. The change of the "speed of time" docs not occur in a linear way but basically like an exponential curve. Why is this so? Through the increasing speed, the particle attains increasingly more energy of its own in relation to the other, slower particles. Absorbing this energy is only possible through an increasingly quicker oscillation between the states of "individuality" and "oneness." If the point is reached in which the state of existential truth is attained, as described more extensively in a subsequent section, the particle will only continue to exist as such when the appropriate method of study is selected. Otherwise, it is perceived as a wave. There will no longer be a differentiated appearance of one of the two states brought about by time in the sense of an "either-or." Strictly speaking, only light, pure energy, can be in the state of the speed of light—which is also completely logical in the sense of what has just been explained since a clear material state is always under the influence of time. This is because it only expresses one half of the existential truth of its being. So light is timeless. But just a moment! Doesn't light need time to get from one place to another—so how can it still be timeless? Well, now things get a bit complicated. The reason for why it seems that light needs time to go from one place to another actually depends upon the observer located in the material world, who is therefore bound to time. In quantum mechanics, there are fundamental theories and their related experiments proving that everything in the material world—meaning everything that moves at less than the speed of light—is equally distant from any given light particle. The interesting thing is also the fact that light always has the same speed, no matter how fast the movement of an observer measuring this speed may be.

---

[203] This was explained by Albert Einstein beginning of the 20th Century in his trailblazing theory of relativity, which has been more than adequately confirmed in this point in a practical way.

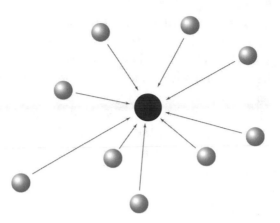

ILL. 195 – INDIVIDUALS STRIVE FOR ONENESS

When light begins to interact with a material surrounding, time has an effect upon it. However, light itself is not a component of the material space, which has also been demonstrated by modern quantum physics. It clearly displays behaviors that show its independence of the conditions of space. And it also possesses qualities that show it has a connection to space—and the matter. One example of this is that it can be diverted through gravity. Within this realm, its double nature also emerges. The appearance of light in the material world is always a result of the deep union of at least two previously separate parts.

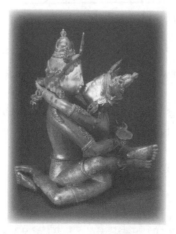

ILL. 196 – THE UNIFICATION OF OPPOSITES CREATES LIGHT

Wherever light appears, love has just been active and victorious by creating oneness. This can be seen, for example, in the chemical reaction of two elements, in the metabolic reactions within the body of a living organism (biophotons)[204]. In this respect, the expression of "light and love" that is frequently encountered in a spiritual context is totally justified. Light (enlightenment) occurs through union, and darkness arises through separation (isolation). Light experiences virtually always accompany the integration of our own divinity in the overall personality of a human being (enlightenment). When we strive toward the light, we can only do this by entering into continuously closer relationships to others, to opposites, and still remaining as closely connected as possible with our own path in order to finally dissolve the duality into complete union. Incidentally, this is the fundamental idea of Tantra, the spiritual path of the Great Goddess, which will be discussed in more detail later.

Space only exists when there are individual parts that are separate from each other in their nature. Examples of these are atoms, molecules, living organisms, and pebbles. Space is therefore related to the occurrence of matter. Energy only requires space in order for it to be able to interact with matter. Beyond[205] the speed of light, there is a type of beingness in which the currents of time in which individual objects or beings move behave in a way that is completely different than what we are accustomed to. Here, for example, two beings have the same kind of time, as long as their meaning in life is very similar in its essential qualities.[206] The course of time is not linear, but it exists. Consequently, time also takes place there, which is why there is also space. In and of itself, this space is just a result of the individual forms of existence moving through time. They

---

[204] The health-promoting quality of foods can be determined by means of modern technology through measuring the extent of their ability to store and emit light. A pioneer in this research work is the internationally known German scientist, Professor F. A. Popp (Max Planck Institute, Stuttgart, Germany).

[205] Please do not understand the term "beyond" in a literal way. In a certain sense, both forms of being exist—the one with a forward and linear orientation and the one that is oriented upon the common meaning—in a parallel manner and even within each other. The phenomenon of the double nature of existence also appears here.

[206] *see next page*

form the space by using time in a "meaningful" way. For abilities such as telepathy, clairvoyance, precognition, psychometrics, the reading of the Akashic Records, and magic of all types, the realm of meaning time-existence offers the suitable preconditions.

Even the spiritual beings, angels, goddesses and gods, power animals, and similar creatures that provide for a continuation and functioning of the divine order in the material world are at home here. The *Higher Self* of a being, a small part of which is found in the material level of existence, has a strong resonance with this meaning-time realm. Angels are also certainly not timeless creatures. They just experience time completely differently than we mortals and, because of their natural form of existence that is much closer to the divine in its state of oneness in some respects than ours could ever be, they have a much less restrained approach to it. For example, if a goddess[207] would like to establish contact with a human being, she places the focus of her attention upon his or her meaning in life and permits the part that shares this meaning to become dominant within herself.

Space and Oneness

The closer everything comes together, the less it is separate from each other, the more the state of these things approaches oneness.

The more things get closer to each other, the less space they assume and the tighter it gets. As a result, less freedom of movement exists and the group reacts more like a unit. This system is on a higher level of order than a group with members far removed from each other. An orientation of meaning in the material world is basically simpler through spatial proximity. But the closeness of the particle to each other is not necessary on a permanent basis! Once the mutual meaning has been created,

---

[206]   This is also a phenomenon that has already been familiar to quantum physics for decades. Of course, it has observed particles and waves instead of angels and gods. The corresponding research work shows without a doubt that subatomic particles cannot only travel forwards in time but also backwards. The process of entering into a relationship beyond the bounds of time and space, effected by a mutual reference system, has also been a scientific fact for decades. A list of literature for researching these topics has been included in the Commentated Bibliography in the appendix.

[207]   Also a type of angel.

many organizational structures can also have an effect over any arbitrary distance.

The phenomenon that groups of particles behave in many of their properties like an individual particle is known to physics. This applies to both the behavior of matter very close to the absolute zero point where— among other things—superconductor phenomena result, as well as in the ultra-high heated state that is not capable of expansion. An example of the latter is inside of suns where atoms of an element such as hydrogen fuse with each other and form a new element (helium) in this way. If the state of a particle comes close to complete immobility, increased qualities of oneness are demonstrated; if the state of a particle comes close to total movement (at the same time and everywhere), increased qualities of oneness are also demonstrated. However, while all the particles remain separate at the "cold end" of the temperature spectrum, even if they act in a unified manner in many respects as long as no heating takes place, at the "hot end" a true fusion with a lasting transformation of the participating partner occurs. This is a very important factor to consider when reflecting upon asceticism on the one hand and Tantra on the other in terms of their suitability as genuine, complete spiritual paths!

Oneness is related to timelessness. Wishes, longings, regrets, hope, and hatred are flickers of the mind that are related to time and direct the focus of attention to the past or future. Correctly employed, they are suited for approaching oneness, just like a ladder is used to climb up on the roof. However, when the ladder is not left at the end of the climb, the goal of reaching the roof cannot be attained. The *meaning* has not been fulfilled.

In these two types of approaches, increasingly less occurs *ultimately.* As a consequence for the spiritual practice, this means: Both self-contemplation and Tantric union with the soul partner result in a state of absorption into the divine oneness.

So far, so good. However, engaging in this together with another person is much more enjoyable from the start! However, there are some additional, very important reasons for clearly preferring the Tantric path to the ascetic way. Of course, like anything in life, there are probably exceptions that make it more suitable for certain people in special life situations to tend toward the path of asceticism. But if this were the norm, there soon would no longer be a human race. A more extensive discussion of this topic is included below.

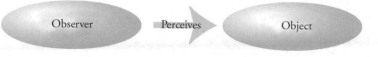

ILL. 197 – CONSCIOUSNESS REQUIRES SEPARATION

Incidentally, the motivation in striving for a state of oneness is called "love" in the current language of spirituality. Without the deep longing for fusion, for becoming totally absorbed in the other— the complete union and the overcoming of all boundaries of individuality—the entire material Creation would no longer function. Everything would dissolve into increasingly smaller individual components that refuse to have any relation to each. Correspondingly, *love is virtually the glue that holds the world together.* However, love is no longer present in the oneness (??!!). In order to be capable of loving, we need someone to desire. Once oneness has been achieved, the desire is dissolved—it no longer has a goal. This topic will be discussed in greater detail in the section on the path of the individual to the divine.

First, let us take a closer look at the matter of oneness! As already mentioned above, increasingly less occurs as the oneness takes over more and more. Consequently, there is increasingly less time and increasingly less space. In addition, individuality constantly decreases the more the fusion progresses, which means that consciousness also disappears. In order for us to be aware of "something," it must *somehow* be *separate* from us. Otherwise, we cannot perceive it. Anything that consciousness should grasp must inevitably exist **outside** of consciousness. The obvious conclusion that we can draw from this means that consciousness cannot directly perceive itself. This is comparable to how the eye cannot **directly** see itself without a mirror.

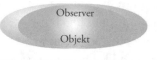

198 – WHEN THE OBSERVER AND THE OBJECT MERGE, ONENESS IS CREATED

However, it can do this quite well *indirectly* by observing the things and states that it has produced. If consciousness attempts to grasp itself "like an expert" directly, it falls back on itself and thereby creates a state of oneness that is called "enlightenment" in the language of spirituality. It unites with itself—releasing light in the process, as described above. Strictly speaking, light is love released through the perfect union that now seeks a new task in terms of uniting two separate partners!

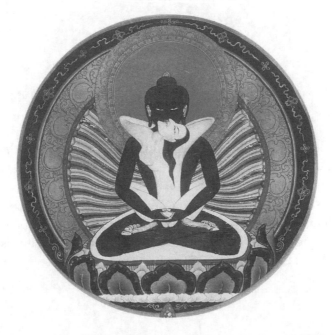

ILL. 199 – WITH INCREASED MERGING, ATTENTION IS DIRECTED MORE
AND MORE WITHIN

With increasing fusion, attention is directed more and more within—the others, the outside world is no longer important. This phenomenon can be observed in every couple that is head over heels in love.

In a state of **perfect (self-contained)** oneness, only "nothing" remains. What we are talking about here has no expansion and therefore cannot be perceived. It does not change, and it does not take action. It does not think, and it does not feel. Strictly speaking, it does not even "exist,"– at least not in the sense of the customary definitions of being.

511

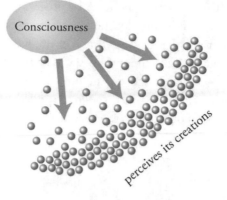

ILL. 200 – CONSCIOUSNESS CAN PERCEIVE ONLY ITS CREATIONS BUT
NOT ITSELF

It also does not love because there is nothing outside of itself with which it could come into contact. If it were to perceive something outside of itself and respond to it, the state of oneness would already be over since a reaction is only possible through some type of movement, and movement of individual parts of the whole leads to a distancing of these parts from the others. So all of this, as already mentioned in the beginning, is quite boring. There is absolutely no action in this scene!

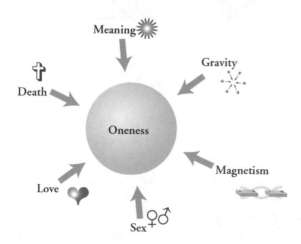

ILL. 201 – SOME OF THE FORCES THAT EFFECT A STATE OF ONENESS

However, things look completely different on the *path to oneness!* This is where it really gets wild…! Why? Because of love, desire, gravity, longings, lust, ecstasy, flirting, courting, excitement, enthusiasm, searching for meaning, magnetism, and many other strong forces that attempt to produce oneness. The typical reaction by beings to *approaching* a state of oneness is characterized by lust, desire, sensuality, feelings of happiness all the way to ecstasy on every level, the feeling of having a purpose, and fulfillment. It should be noted that this is a state shortly before the actual union. Once this has been completed, there is no longer anything that can be felt because now nothing exists on the outside as the object of the desire. In the practice, we can experience this with something like magnets. When a positive pole approaches a negative pole, the mutual attraction increases exponentially the closer the two come to each other. However, if both poles are together, the tension is dissolved. But this tends to function like a continual back-and-forth oscillation in everyday life. Once a state of oneness has been attained, this leads to a more or less intense balance of energy within a being—a harmonization. Yet, since the formation of a total (lasting) oneness does not function in the material world, an increasingly stronger polarity builds up; in turn, this produces the desire for a renewed experience of oneness.

The instinctual forces that press for oneness and union are so strong that they ultimately overcome even the most rigid moral, legal, and religious prohibitions and rules.[208] Among other things, this is how they secure the survival of humanity to this very day. If the major religions of the world would have their way, humanity would already have died out long ago.

After all, all of them ultimately preach that the worthy ideals are sexual abstinence, spiritualization, and the renunciation of partnership relationships and activities of a pleasurable, sexual nature. All of these systems allegedly inspired by the Creative Force see the ideal state to be the ascetic, completely disinterested in reproduction and sharing desire and union with a partner. Even during his lifetime, he cuts himself off from his body by practicing discipline and abstinence in order to never return to "life's vale of tears," "eternal suffering," and "indelible sin."

---

[208] In psychoanalysis (according to Sigmund Freud), these archetypal instinctual forces are called the *sexual instincts,* as opposed to the *death instincts.*

However, anyone who is celibate definitely makes no contribution to the preservation of humanity or the development of loving forms for living together in intimacy… He simply just shrinks away from the challenge of living spiritually with others in the material world.

This life- and happiness-negating trend in the religions is quite new, just about 5,000 years old.[209] It was brought into the world by the plundering and murdering Aryan nomadic hordes that had their essential ideals in conducting wars and keeping slaves, worshipping masculinity, and renouncing the body as a spiritually valuable form of existence. Before this era, in the so-called Age of the Great Goddess, there were much better conditions for living in a happy, spiritually meaningful way in this world and with a corresponding body. The great pre-Aryan cultures of the Indus Valley, cities like Catal Hüyük in Asia Minor, and the Vinca Culture in the region of the Danube and the Balkans were all part of this. The Commentated Bibliography in the appendix contains additional sources on this topic. In the Age of the Great Goddess, the body was considered to be a gift given by the Creative Force with which we can have experiences that are important and unique for the further development of the divine plan. These are experiences that are not possible in other, more astral forms of

[209] It began with the beginnings of the patriarchal cultural and religious currents, which then subjugated the previously dominating, highly civilized, and very peaceable culture of the Goddess through migrations of peoples and cruel wars of conquest. With the entry into the Age of Aquarius, a large-scale-countermovement has begun for the first time, supported by people who are committed to the environment and nature conservation, the well-being of animals, and a spiritual society in the broadest sense of the word. And the whole movement is still taking place in a way that corresponds with the characteristic of the Great Mother—in quite a peaceful and non-hierarchic manner. In Ancient Greece, the constellation of the "Water Bearer" was known as *Hydrokhoos* (Water Jug); in ancient Persia, it is called *Dul* (Water Jug); in the ancient Indian sacred language it was called *Khumba* (Jug); the Babylonians said it was *Gula* (Goddess) and the Romans used the word *Juno* (a name of the Great Goddess, the wife of Jupiter). *Aquarius* carries the water, the milk of the Great Goddess, to those who need it and pours it over them—like a horn of plenty that showers a human being with gifts. The term "Water Bearer" is still used to this day in the Orient for individuals who bring the cool liquid to human beings to saving them from dying of thirst. The Water Bearer carries the *Holy Grail*, which is another, well-known word for the Water Jug of the Great Goddess.

existence. But this will also be discussed in greater detail in the section on the meaning of the various existence forms for beings in the material world. We are sorry that this "stimulating" topic must be saved for later, but as we know, anticipation kindles desire (see above)…

Instead, the next section discusses the relationship between oneness and the many, the essence of the divine, and the material world of separation.

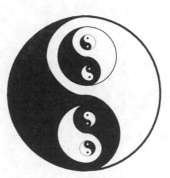

ILL. 202 – YIN AND YANG: THE COMPLEMENTARY OPPOSITES

Oneness and Separation– the Spiritual and the Material World

The process that leads to oneness has already been explained somewhat in the last section. However, this is just one part of the whole—after all, there is also separation, individualization, and isolation. Why and how does this happen?

We have all seen the above symbol that comes from the Asian region many times. It shows the two fundamental states of existence of the Creative Force—oneness and separation, energy and matter, idea and realization, man and woman, and yang and yin. However, it shows something else: Whenever one of the two states turns into an extreme, the other opposite—but also complementary quality of beingness—automatically develops! Yet, in addition to the above-mentioned qualities, the

515

symbol describes something else that is more personal: The Great Goddess *(Hou-t´u*[210] = Princess of the Earth) and the Great God *(T´ai-i*[211] = *the All-One or the Highest One)*, who are supported by the *Creative Force (Tai-chi* or *Tao)* at work in the background. Their perpetual Sacred Marriage allows life to continue on the material plane of existence. These two light beings will be discussed in greater detail below.

[210] The Great Goddess, the Queen of the Earth, who was worshipped by the *Wu* female shamans of ancient China, is the counterpart to the God of the Heavens. Everything on the earth is subject to her, and she brings the things into the world that have been conceived through her magic power with the God of the Heavens. The invocation of the sacred divine forces of heaven and earth played a central role in the initiation rituals and great healings performed by Dr. Usui and Dr. Hayashi. A direct connection to *Wu* shamanism can be recognized here through the old version of the Reiki characters that shows, among other things, a ritually dancing Wu female shaman asking for "rain" (symbol of a practical magic effect) with the help of her three spiritual *Hun* souls (three opened mouths). The Reiki system of healing also has its roots in shamanism, which joined with the Esoteric Buddhism in Asia at a number of opportunities.

[211] *T´ai-i* is also a god worshipped by *Wu* shamanism. Later, he was adopted by the Taoists and was often understood as the Tao itself. His hall for audiences is the square Chinese constellation *T´ai-wei* (Highest Mystery) and he resides in the round constellation *Tzu-kung* (Purple Palace). So he unites the divine feminine principle (the yin has the circle associated with it) and the divine masculine principle (the yang has the square associated with it) within himself. This is an important parallel to *Dainichi Nyorai*, who also bears both principles within himself, as expressed in the Master Symbol of the Reiki tradition through the signs for the sun and the moon. Furthermore, *T´ai-i* works through the feminine principle into earthly life in his circular palace, as *Dainichi Nyorai* also does this through the Great Goddess *Marishi*. It is said that *T´ai-i* "was already perfected before the Creation." This corresponds exactly with the structure of the Creation explained in this chapter: The Creative Force produces the Great God and the Great Goddess. In turn, these two create the material level of being together with everything that exists there. Incidentally, the sun and moon played an essential role as the deities associated with *T´ai-i* in ancient when the sacred offerings were made.

Tao has neither name nor form. It is the inner nature of being, the one primordial consciousness. The inner nature (essence) and life are invisible: They are contained, dwells, are maintained, and gathered in the light of heavens. We cannot see the light of heaven; it is contained; it is contained, dwells, is maintained, and gathered in the zenith[212] between the two eyes. The light is neither exclusively in the body nor outside of the body. Mountains and rivers, the Great Earth and, above it, the shining of the sun and moon—all of this is the light: rivers, the Great Earth, and above it, the radiance of the sun and moon—all of this is the light: So it is not just in the body alone. Good listening, sharp seeing, insight and intellect, and all movements also belong to this light. So is it also not just outside of the body. The garland of light from the heavens and the earth fills the entire, immeasurable universe. To the same extent, the abundance of light in the body also radiates through heaven and earth. Just as the light returns to its origin, heaven and earth, mountains and rivers, and all things return with it at the same time to the source. The life force of a human being streams upward to his eyes, in which the keys and looks of his body are kept. (From *Die Erfahrung der Goldenen Blüte,* by M. Miyuki, Munich 1984.)

---

[212] The "Zenith between the two eyes" refers to the 6th major chakra (Third Eye).

Examples of Correspondences with Yin and Yang

Yin	*Yang*
Water/earth/metal	Fire/wood
Body	Consciousness
Subtle matter	Mind
Matter	Spirituality
Kidneys	Heart
Moisture	Dryness
Evenness	Irregularity
Gathering/contracting	Scattering/expansion
Preservation	Change
Storing	Transformation
Sadness	Anger
Night	Day
Moon	Sun
Woman	Man
Shadow	Light
Passivity	Activity
Community	Aloneness
Chronic disease	Acute disease
Inside of the body	Outside of the body
Solid	Volatile
Round	Square
The right side of the body (strong)	The left side of the body (weak)

There are obviously many more equivalents, but this should clearly demonstrate the principle.

Today, the right side of the body is normally seen as yang and the left side as yin—for which there are many reasons, as well as other arguments that speak against it. Perhaps the following explanations will aid in understanding the overall picture.

Yin and yang are not fixed qualities. They always relate to each other on the one hand and to certain processes that take place between them on the other hand. As a result, the left side of the body (always seen from the perspective of the respective person) is yin in relation to actions because it tends to be more passive (in right-handers). However, at the same time it is yang because it is much weaker than the right side. The right side is yang because it is the more active (in right-handers) and yin because it is more powerful. The left is yin because it tends to be receptive while the right is yang because it tends to be more giving.

The situation is similar in terms of classifying the kidneys (yin) and the heart (yang). This is correct—however, as important energy organs of the spiritual element of water, the kidneys are vitally dependent upon the spiritual element of the heart's fire to warm them. Only warmed water moves and can therefore nourish life. Fire without an appropriate amount of water as an addition is only a flash in the pan that quickly flares up and burns out just as quickly. Only water has the power to keep fire on the earth and allow it to burn with calm, heart-nourishing warmth. (Also see the explanations on the two hexagrams No. 29 *K'an* and No. 30 *Li* from the I Ching, the Ancient Book of Changes, as well as other literature on this topic in the Commented Bibliography in the appendix.) So water cannot exist without fire and vice versa. Yin and yang is found in both organs, depending upon which of their qualities are considered at a certain moment.

So it is not that simple to understand yin and yang. However, since much of the Eastern wisdom teachings that have come to the West have only been translated in parts and incorrectly, or in a biased manner, many people have become accustomed to the more superficial, "simple" interpretation of yin and yang. However, this has the major disadvantage that it does not function in practice when viewed in more closely. But the above described, more complicated and simultaneously more exact approach does work.

And, in addition, yin and yang are always relative and refer to each other. This means, for example, that women are basically yin in comparison to men. However, a specific woman may be yang in relation to a certain man when dealing with a particular topic.

Yin and yang are states that complement each other in a perpetual state of change. As soon as one of the states finds itself at its peak—meaning that it shows its characteristics most distinctively and clearly—this results, without additional conditions, in the seed of the other state that then develops until it also passes into the previous quality at the peak of its realization.

If we apply this principle to the oneness, we can see that unity is always just a *temporary* state that results from separation—just as separation develops from a completed state of oneness! And a remnant of oneness also always remains within the most extreme state of separation, just as a remnant of separation is also maintained in the most extreme state of unity.[213] But if oneness is also a conditional state like separation, what is the Creative Force in this case?

Well, the Creative Force can *only be recognized on the basis of its effects:* The eternal change of yin and yang is based upon its inspiration.[214] We could call it the engine that drives the changes. Based on this, we can conclude that neither oneness nor separation can be divine per se. Both are just *manifestations* of the concealed principle behind the change that cannot be directly perceived or researched. It works, as it were, behind the scenes as the "Gray Eminence." Incidentally, this part of the spiritual philosophy has also been confirmed by quantum physics for quite some time now: Each of the subatomic particles in the entire universe stands in a direct relationship to all of the others. A change here gives rise to a change there. This even applies when there are a billion light years between "here" and "here"! And it occurs without any delays in time. Everything functions as a whole. Why? Quantum mechanics does not know. But it has long proved that this is the case in both theory and practice. Richard P. Feynman, who is probably the greatest theoretical physicist of the 20th Century, first described this in his pioneering quantum electrodynamics (QED). In it, he proved that the light covers absolutely every possible path from its "source" to its "goal." This should be understood literally and has actually been proved in experiments. Everywhere in the universe there is a probability of varying degrees that photons from one light source will appear at a specific place. Since this is not intended to be a book about

---

[213] Take a good look at the yin/yang diagram!

[214] In the Indian spiritual philosophy, the Creative Force in its function as the original source of all being is called *Akasha*. What triggers the effects that can be observed on the material level is called *Brahman*, the absolute consciousness in the sense of the word that literally encompasses **everything**.

quantum mechanics, interested readers can find the appropriate literature in the Commentated Bibliography of the appendix.

Back to the consequences of the yin/yang teaching…

We have now advanced quite a bit further in understanding spiritual cosmology. If we use what has been explained up to now as the foundation of spiritual development, we can conclude that *spiritualization as the definitive goal for the personal path to the divine,* which means merging into oneness, is just as meaningless as *making the material existence in individuality into an absolute* with its possibilities and practical constraints.

Enlightenment– a Preliminary Stage to Spiritual Perfection

Furthermore, the result of all this is that *enlightenment,* an elevation of consciousness to the state of the divine perspective of perception, is just a *preliminary stage of spiritual perfection*[215]. Actually, only a *complete* recognition and integration of *all* possible ways of being can lead to the realization of the divine in the individual. This is because the divine itself—the Creative Force—is also *everything!* We cannot unite with *everything* if we exclude *something.* This is clear—isn't it? Consequently, the development of the 7th major chakra (Crown Chakra) only occurs through the development of the lower six major chakras. The 7th Chakra has the special quality of unity. In order to achieve this, a human being must integrate the themes that occur on each of the levels of the lower six major chakras in a loving, practical, and constructive way. This state of oneness is characterized by the willingness to accept what is: The feelings, the separation, the oneness, the thoughts, the actions, the divine, the all-encompassing as well as the isolated, the individual parts separated from the rest of the whole, the weaknesses, the strengths, failure, success, bonds and dependence, power and surrender, pleasure and pain—simply everything! One important aspect of this way of being is self-evident and unreserved acceptance of what we are—because it is crystal-clear that we

---

[215] More information on this topic can be found in the chapter on "What Is Enlightenment?"

521

cannot do justice to our own divine responsibility to the whole if we deny our own self! Since awakened beings are completely aware of the sheer endlessness and boundlessness of their existence, they also accepts great difficulties that must be mastered on their path *if thoroughly confronting them is actually necessary in the sense of the divine order!* In itself, martyrdom to differing degrees is also not necessarily a sign of spiritual awakening but very frequently just an extremely disharmoniously expressed inclination to masochism[216].

This state of surrendering ourselves to the eternal change in its most meaningful form related to the whole is called *spiritual realization, great enlightenment,* or *spiritual awakening* in the language of spirituality.

As explained above, enlightenment is a preliminary stage to this. It is necessary and dangerous! Anyone who rushes into this without a good teacher—meaning someone who is already in a state of spiritual realization—often becomes useless to the world in the truest sense of the word. He can also suffer severe physical and mental damage to the point of a major psychosis. Anyone whose consciousness comes so close to the state of oneness that life in the material world appears meaningless will no longer want to take care of anything. The motivation for taking care of something, which means leaving the state of consciousness of oneness, is not very high. Anyone who takes action and accepts responsibility simply has to descend into the lower realm of matter. An exciting and insightful reader on this topic is the book *Siddharta* by Hermann Hesse.

Seen from enlightenment, everything is somehow divine and everything will ultimately be good. If not now, then in a million years from now on Alpha Centauri. Or it was already good at some time and place. And since time does not exist in the state of oneness, this is ultimately considered to be completely adequate. On the one hand, this is right. However, there is also the double nature of the divine and therefore, on the other hand, everything is not okay. And these two, inevitably complementary perspectives and ways of being are not yet integrated into the state of enlightenment.

---

[216] The masochist says to the sadist: "Hurt me! Hurt me!". The sadist responds: "No! No!"

The soul is truly not small but the luminous deity itself. In the West, this statement is either found to be very dubious, if not even reprehensible, or it simply adopts it without thinking twice and gains theosophical inflation in the process.

(Carl Gustav Jung in his foreword to the *Tibetan Book of the Dead*, Evans-Wentz, 1985)

Please keep in mind that the enlightenment described here is a spiritual state of consciousness that is *very close* to unity. If oneness were actually perfectly realized, the human being would spiritually dissolve into its nothingness! So what is generally called "enlightenment" is a state of consciousness quite close to oneness.[217] This is why people who have intensively experienced it also describe it as extremely joyful and absolutely ecstatic—if they dare to talk about it. And this description is totally understated. The state of enlightenment is mega-awesome! After all, it must be since it is just before complete union. Anyone who is not adequately prepared for this in terms of character, meaning that he has escaped from the swamp of moralizing petty-bourgeois concepts may blow some mental fuses and experience a more or less lasting black-out experience. Then this experience can obviously range from less nice to decidedly horrible. If it only takes place for a very short time, then moods of oneness in which everything is "perfect," peace, sacredness, and the like tend to prevail. The entire package needs a bit of time to manifest itself. But please do not assume that even these descriptions here are precise. The finger that points at the moon is not the moon. The descriptions are only intended to reveal a bit more of the atmosphere, the breadth of this type of experience. However, an experience of enlightenment can never

---

[217] Incidentally, enlightenment is not related to light experiences of any type, which almost everyone who meditates or does qi gong or yoga or similar methods will occasionally experience. However, during an experience of enlightenment some types of light experiences may occur.

523

truly be conveyed to other. There will always be a great deal that resonates with it, that is contradictory, that is impossible to describe because there is no word, no symbol for it. Yet, at the moment of the experience it is so true, so clear, and so genuine that every "normal" experience perceived with the five senses is like comparing the sound quality of the telephone and a Dolby THX system.

In my practice, I regularly take care of normal people who have had experiences of enlightenment and Kundalinî experiences and require help with the integration of their effects. I have never had the two of the same cases. In this sense, there is no checklist that I could include here to go through and evaluate afterward with a point system to find out what happened to someone when they had an impressive spiritual experience. Bioenergetic resolution processes, meaning when a great deal of the life forces that have been stuck spontaneously begin to flow, are often mistaken for spiritual experiences. The conscious experience of a partial personality with a great potential within a psychotherapeutic or spiritual practice can initially have a similar effect. The same applies to a psychotic episode, an energetic overloading or a too one-sided charging of the human energy system, or too much stress, or to an organic nervous disorder. Frequently, experiences of enlightenment also take place within totally everyday situations—especially when we are really not expecting them nor thinking about them. Then a freedom from prejudice, inner peace, and precise work is required to find out what really happened and how this has affected the respective person. Only then can suitable measures for integration be worked out and applied.

Enlightenment is definitely not a total absorption into the greater whole!

If the completely union with everything were to take place, all that would remain is absolute "nothingness." Possible practical consequences for a human being, in addition to many others, could be the death of the physical body or a state of the absence of the mind—the deepest coma. Anyone who gets lost in enlightenment has taken a drastic detour from his spiritual path since he (or she, obviously) prefers one of the divine states and shows the other state of existence a cold shoulder. This is extreme! This is pure separation, and separation is the precise opposite of oneness. And extreme separation makes people ill.

However, enlightenment as *a method of personality development* is quite okay in order to create an adequately strong counterbalance to everyday life with its more material life experiences and attitude toward life. In summary, we can accordingly say that only an unconditional acceptance of every possible state of being corresponds with the realization of the divine. And this means that renouncing life in a material embodiment with its possibilities and boundaries would be just as meaningless as an uncompromising attachment to physicality. This is an additional reason for not considering asceticism of any type to be a main means of pursuing the personal spiritual path to the divine. Asceticism turns away from what is right now the God-given, lived reality in a material embodiment and ardently demands a bodiless form of being, in relation to itself, as well as to the race and community of all beings. But self-denial prevents the creation of oneness because the self also part of the divine. Where would it otherwise come from if there is just one Creative Force? What should it be other than divine?

As long as we are in a body, there is no doubt that we have something to learn or experience in it. (Sri Aurobindo)

This is why Tantra[218]—the path of the Great Goddess—is the only, truly appropriate choice as the means to achieving divinity. Renouncing the acknowledgement of physicality leads to the destruction of the environ-

[218] The term *Tantra* comes from the ancient Indian language of Sanskrit. It literally means: fabric, context, continuum, or system. According to the spiritual philosophy of the *Vedas*, Tantra is one of the Eternal Religions. The central theme of Tantra is the opening and the proper approach of the individual to the divine energy and Creative Force (Devi/Shakti—the Great Goddess). Treatise on Tantra must contain the following five topics: 1. The creation of the world; 2. The dissolution or destruction of the world; 3. Worshipping the divine, both in the feminine and the masculine aspect; 4. How to attain supernatural (spiritual) abilities; 5. Various paths (practices/lifestyle) for merging with the highest spiritual principle. Because it fulfills these conditions, this book itself is a Tantra.

ment and the inner world. Anything that we do not love and basically want to get rid of because it only causes suffering is at best something we are indifferent to; in the worst case, we see it as an enemy to be fought with drastic means? And even by just taking a superficial look at historical reality, we can see that this is exactly what the patriarchal age has brought about.[219]

There is still much more to be said on this topic, but in a later section. The matter of oneness and separation still requires some additional explanations.

Everything changes—or, in the words of the classical Greek philosophy: *To panta rhei!*—Everything flows!

Various Forms of Change in Individuality and Oneness

These changes occur in various ways[220] and range from a very slowly to extremely fast pace. A very slow change is something like the formation and subsequent aging of our sun. At some point, it will suffer its own type of death, become a black hole, and disappear into itself. Or, if it cannot do this alone, it will be blessed by a larger sun that exists as a black hole and draws it into itself, thereby leading to oneness—in order to be changed into the form of the smallest particles and energy units and spit out again afterward by a so-called "white hole," a cosmic source of matter. And then it will once serve in many ways as the building material of planets, suns, and intergalactic nebulae, and obviously also the creatures that live there. This also makes new processes of individual self-realization possible.

A much quicker type of change is the process of the becoming and passing of human beings. This does not take billions of years but just a number of decades. This has its advantages and disadvantages. It is more difficult to continuously gather wisdom and competence but easier to

---

[219] An exciting and information reading tip on this is the novel *The Da Vinci Code* by Dan Brown. Well written and based on excellent research, it reveals much about the true originals of Christianity, what Jesus really taught—and to whom he was married.

[220] The ancient Chinese oracle and wisdom book, the *I Ching, The Book of Changes*, precisely describes the way and the archetypal stages of change

experience certain themes from a great variety of perspectives and grasp their essence.

A very quick type of transformation takes place in light. The change takes place so quickly here that time is transcended in the process—it no longer plays a role—since both states occur at the same time! This is a form of oneness with oneself, of spiritual realization, as described above. Quantum physics already discovered some decades ago that, depending with which experimental structure the nature of light is examined, it occurs either as a current of individual particles or as a connected wave. Put in somewhat simplified terms, this is like the space undergoing a local change in its state.

There is a rule of thumb rule for the process of change: Large systems change more slowly than small ones. The smaller the unit that is observed, the more quickly it changes its state, to the point that change can no longer be recorded as such but can only be determined as a "double nature" (wave/particle) by means of different forms of observation! However, there is still a small detail…

Large systems always consist of small systems—and while the big structures change slowly, the small ones transform themselves quickly. And the smallest only appear beyond temporal possibilities of determination as a double nature. So a large system also basically has such a double nature since it consists of small and smallest systems with precisely this property! Wow, now things are really getting complicated! This means that basically every large, slowly changing system—such as a human being—is already spiritually realized because on the smallest level he consists of structures whose nature can no longer be clearly determined and who is both of the following, depending upon how they are observed: individual and whole, matter and energy, particle and wave. Consequently, every being is already realized in the divine oneness. On the other hand, this is not true because the large system, which consists of the small systems, needs longer to change and therefore appears as individually manifested matter.

This is it, precisely! Human beings also have the double nature, just like the light. According to how we are seen, we are the Creative Force, the whole, or individuals in a state of separation and flawed with many weaknesses.

But we cannot just "shift" and be one way this time and the other way next time—or can we? Is it possible? Or should we not for some reason? The knots of these questions will soon unravel—and create a new, interesting form of confusion.

The Double Nature of Light

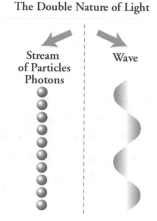

ILL. 203 – WHAT IS LIGHT?

The Creative Force basically appears in two completely different forms.

We can call these two states that constantly interact with each other everywhere the "duality of being." This topic will arise again later in various sections because the process known as "life" takes place in the tension field of these two forms of the divine in its infinite multiple manifestations. Similar to how light may appear as a stream of particles (corpuscles/photons) and then as a wave, depending upon the type of study, it has two contrary ways of being that exclude each other according to the rules of today's usual way of thinking. But "today's usual way of thinking" does not mean *quantum physics,* which has been accustomed to dealing with these types of themes for more than 40 years and has even been able to derive laws from its observations, as they have been formulated in precise scientific terms, among other things, in quantum electrodynamics, in quantum chromodynamics, and in the super-string theory.

As described above, there is a state of the Creative Force as oneness. No movement occurs at this point—time does not take place. It is not only unnecessary here but would even be disruptive. This state contains a boundless potential (non-realized possibilities; seeds of events) that just dozes on in a state of being devoid of space and time. *Absolutely nothing*—or *absolutely everything* occurs at the same time and in the same place, depending upon our outlook on it. Incidentally, both are the same from the spiritual perspective.

This boundless number of possibilities is reflected in the material state of being that expands infinitely in time and space with its number of individuals that is also immeasurable. If all of the things that have ever existed in a past that reaches into infinity, that are here at present, and that will exist in the future that reaches into infinity, summing up all of their relationships and experiences with each other would result in precisely the realized possibilities in the material universe. This is exactly what already exists in the boundless spiritual potential of the oneness!

Through the constantly occurring change of all things from oneness to individuality and back to unity, a perpetual exchange takes place between the two forms of being. As a result, the oneness is enriched with influences that are not available to it from within itself because a situation of separation is necessary and the material world of separation receives an influx of qualities of oneness that cannot be formed under the conditions of separateness.

In order to realize the boundless potential of the Creative Force in a state of oneness in the material world and make all of its qualities available there, various things are necessary. These will be explained in detail below.

As already described above, everything exists in the form of a type of double nature: individual – whole, matter – energy, profane – divine, and so forth. In order to make this double nature possible, everything that is present in the one outward form must also somewhat appear in the other manifestation. There can be no perfect oneness in the world of matter since it would then cease to exist—time and space would immediately end. So how does this quality become apparent here? This is basically all quite simple. Since time and space are infinite, have no beginning and no end, and everything here is constantly relating to the other, meeting and creating oneness with the other in various ways, then separating again and establishing unity with other participants in the grand scheme of the world, *perfect oneness is already present in the sum* of the whole. It is just organized in terms of time and distributed throughout space. But since time and space are just aids to facilitate relationships of boundless oneness with itself in a creative way, which is basically just illusions—called mâyâ in the Indian spiritual tradition—oneness is just as present in the material world as it is in the spiritual world. The state of oneness itself cannot show itself in its perfection—but it does manifest itself in the occasional union of living things and substances, atoms, molecules…

In this process, oneness is produced in a great variety of forms on three basic levels[221]:

ॐ Joy/desire/sex/conception of new life and new ideas – material level – 2nd major chakra

ॐ Emotional harmony/love/compassion/creation of new relationship structures between beings – emotional level – 4th major chakra

ॐ Constructive mutual work/purpose/vision/generation of structures of new life processes – spiritual level – 6th major chakras

Establishing oneness in the material realm of Creation requires more suitable material structures or actions, through which the power of unity can appear in a practical sense. In accordance with principle of similarities that says "as above, so below," a part of the infinite potential of the Creative Force, which is stored in the oneness, can only manifest itself through a symbolic similar appearance in matter (structure or action). Why does this principle exist? The answer can be found in the double nature of existence, as explained above. There is an infinite potential of possibilities within the "part" of each being that exists in oneness. Over time and through the actions of this being, this potential manifests itself completely. In order to show itself, it must be able to express itself on the material plane. This can always just occur in an incomplete way, just in "portions," since the

---

[221] Please also compare the information on the chakra teachings on pages 560 and 584.

perfect cannot show itself completely on the material plane because of the very limited possibilities. The expression of the perfect divine in the material world is inevitably always an *infinite process.*

This process must have an inner context of meaning so that different, actually not directly related, themes can be linked with each other. Otherwise, this would result in a chaos in which there are no connected strands of actions, the course of which offers the realization of the divine space. The appropriate type of manifestation for the divine in the material world is expressed by sacred geometry such as the golden mean and its translation into music and poetry. This is the divine structure in its material representation. In a narrower sense, divine action is characterized by desire, joy, creativity, love, compassion, reliable and constructive social structures, mutually realized visions of a great many different types on the basis of unique personal gifts. The central organizing element in this process is the spiritual meaning. Within this context, the spiritual meaning refers to whatever connects the particles and beings of all types with each other through the processes of events so that their imperfect qualities are supplemented at the right time in order to realize their divine potential—which means being able to enter into the current of the divine order. The divine meaning has a fine, patient little voice. It does not force anything but creates an inclination through love, joy, happiness, and desire.

All human beings carry unique gifts within themselves. When we realize these talents through appropriate activities in a way that makes us happy and have goals that bring benefit to others, as well as working together with people who meaningfully supplement our special qualities and share our visions, the divine order is expressed in the material world in practical terms.

When we live in this way, we contribute an important part to the great mandala of the divine plan. When we do not live our talents and spend our time with people who have completely different visions for their lives, we cannot follow our spiritual path of self-realization. Self-realization in the sense that has just been explained is simultaneously fulfillment of the divine plan for the highest good of the whole. For example, it has been my experience that those who suffer from constant fatigue, a lack of energy, and exhaustion will find an explanation for their state based on the fact

531

that they have blocked the practical translation of their potential. As soon as they make an effort to walk their own path and follow their purpose, the weakness and fatigue disappear because the 6th major chakra, which is responsible for the pursuit of the personal spiritual vision, now gives a green light for releasing energy to the 1st major chakra, with which it directly cooperates. In the 1st major chakra at the base of the spinal column, there is a tremendous energy that is still asleep in most people, the so-called Kundalinî energy. This spiritual power is directly associated with the Great Goddess, who allows the divine potential to be manifest in the material world. This power is released to the degree that we express our very own potential in a practical way. If we resist it and attempt to live according to the actual or supposed ways of other people, the Kundalinî force only appears in the organism as a type of "emergency power"!

Within the cosmic context, this principle manifests in the form of the so-called spiritual beings: the Great God and the Great Goddess. These two should not be confused with the goddesses and gods, with whom they work together as helpers!

During every epoch, these two light beings were known and are still known under a great variety of names. Here is a selection of them…

Familiar Names for the Great Goddess: Ishtar, Inanna, Freya, Hera, Shakti, Devi, Tara, Mârîcî, Dai Marishi Ten, Holy Spirit, *Shekina, Ashera,* and *Sandalphon.*

Familiar Names for the Great God: Tammuz, Frey, Odin, Wotan, Zeus, Jupiter, *Shiva, Dainichi Nyorai,* and Heavenly Father.

The task of the *Great God* is to bring the new out of the infinite potential of the Creative Force in the state of oneness into the material world and make it available everywhere. So he transforms something from out of the oneness into a —always still completely abstract, meaning that it has not yet manifested in the material realm—potential that is no longer in the state of oneness and therefore forms a type of energetic "grid" upon the occurrences can orient themselves as a component of the material world. For example, this may be an idea or even the spiritual "blueprint," the energetic manifestation structure of a sun or a "new" people.

The *Great Goddess* assumes the yang influences made available by the God from out of the oneness and gives them their due place within the framework of the material world. Consequently, the Creation is a continuous process in the material world that is constantly maintained through the sexual union of the God and the Goddess. In this process, the influence of the God is always of a the cyclical, rhythmic nature. He is so close to the oneness with his state that he cannot manifest in the material world without the help of the Goddess. In addition, he must be conceived and brought into the world with the potential to be realized through the Goddess, until he has fathered something new that is to be manifested in a specific cycle. So just as the Goddess also conceives and realizes other yang potentials, she also does this with the God who is at home in the extreme yang and thereby gives him the opportunity time and again to become directly involved in the material world. Yet, since he does not belong in it because of his nature, he must always leave again in order to do justice to his spiritual potential. Then he is born into the world once again through the Goddess in order to bring something new with him that is urgently needed so that the course of life can continue to move forward.

The Goddess has the unique power to make something concrete— things, substances, and beings—out of the seeds, ideas, and abstract potentials. If this all took place without a plan, the material plane would not have a meaningful structure. It could not continue to develop constructively, thereby reflecting the purpose, the love, joy, and beauty of the Creative Force. In order to appropriately realize the purpose, the Goddess has created a system of so-called "life nets". Each life net connects all beings from every type of biosphere, such as the planet Earth, with each other and harmonizes their activities on a very basic level. For example, among other things the life net of the Great Goddess ensures that the birth rate of men and women always fluctuates around one same average, that the temperature of the earth remains within a framework that is suitable for the living beings within it through the appropriate plant world and ocean currents, that the salt concentration of the world seas continually fluctuates around an average with only minor deviations, and that there are suitable food chains and living conditions for all beings.[222]

[222]   *see next page*

In ancient times before the introduction of the patriarchy, people consciously attuned themselves to the Great Goddess and her life net. In this way, they experienced important inspirations that helped them use their free will in accordance with the divine order. As a result, things were invented that shaped the society and used the personal talents in a way that was optimally connected with the rest of the life process on the earth. There was no environmental destruction and pollution, no major wars, no hostility toward the body and the resulting diseases of body and mind, and, of course, also no exploitation of the limited available natural resources.

This attunement was performed at the so-called power places, special places in nature. It used sacred rituals that gave the individual and the group an opportunity to harmonize themselves with the well-being of the whole. Songs and dances, meditation, and energy work were important components of these gatherings.[223]

By attuning ourselves to the life net of the Great Goddess, we receive a transmission of power from her that activates the 3rd eye (6th major chakra) and helps us to be intuitively guided by the Creative Force in order to better find our way in life. If we practice this on a regular basis, we will suddenly meet the "right" people, find the appropriate job, and live somewhere they makes us feel very good. Things fall into place and the mandala is perfected.

In my opinion, the technique for the fundamental attunement to the life net of the Great Goddess is so important that I would like to share it with you here. I hope you enjoy your experiences...

[222] For an in-depth understanding, please compare the following books: *Der Mensch und die Erde sind eins* by Rüdiger Dahlke, Heyne Verlag, Germany. *Gaia—A Biography of Our Living Earth*, James Lovelock, W.W. Norton & Co.

[223] Since the 1980s, there have been increasingly more people throughout the world who have begun, either consciously or intuitively, to revive this old art of attunement to the well-being of the whole. At seasonal festivals and other opportunities, individuals and groups who work in this sense can be found at many large and small power places. For the past few years, I have been practicing and teaching the rituals for healing the earth, which is an important part of this attunement work. If you would like to participate in it, please write me an e-mail and I will send you the corresponding information.

The Basic Attunement to the Life Net of the Great Goddess with Reiki

The precondition for applying this technique is training and initiation into the 2nd Degree of traditional Usui Reiki.

1. Draw the Distant Treatment Symbol and then say or think the mantra three times.

2. Draw the Power-Intensification Symbol and then say or think the mantra three times.

3. Say or think Great Goddess (add one of the above-listed names, if you like) three times

4. Draw some more Power-Intensification Symbols and activate each of them with the mantra three times.

5. Draw the Distant Treatment Symbol and then say or think the mantra three times.

6. Draw the Power-Intensification Symbol and then say or think the mantra three times.

7. Say or think your name three times while you imagine your face.

8. Imagine your entire body facing you with the head facing up.

9. On the area of the 1st major chakra (crotch), draw a Mental-Healing Symbol and a Power-Intensification Symbol. Activate each of them by saying its mantra three times. Then say or think: "First major chakra of …" and add your first and last names.

10. On the area of the 2nd major chakra (lower abdomen), draw a Mental-Healing Symbol and a Power-Intensification Symbol. Activate each of them by saying its mantra three times. Then say or think: "Second major chakra of…" and add your first and last names.

11. On the area of the 3rd major chakra (hollow of the stomach, two fingerwidths beneath the sternum), draw a Mental-Healing Symbol and a Power-Intensification Symbol. Activate each of them by saying its mantra three times. Then say or think: "Third major chakra of…" and add your first and last names.

12. On the area of the 4th major chakra (heart, center of chest), draw a Mental-Healing Symbol and a Power-Intensification Symbol. Activate each of these by saying its mantra three times. Then say or think: "Fourth major chakra of…" and add your first and last names.

13. On the area of the 5th major chakra (throat, at the center of the base of the neck), draw a Mental-Healing Symbol and a Power-Intensification Symbol. Activate each of them by saying its mantra three times. Then say or think: "Fifth major chakra of…" and add your first and last names.

14. On the area of the 6th major chakra (a fingerwidth above the line connecting the eyebrows, on the center line), draw a Mental-Healing Symbol and a Power-Intensification Symbol. Activate each of them by saying its name three times. Then say or think: "Sixth major chakra of…" and add your first and last names.

15. Draw several large Power-Intensification Symbols over the entire front side of the body and activate each symbol by saying or thinking its names three times.

16. Ask the Great Goddess to attune you to her life net so that your thoughts, feelings, decisions, and actions serve the highest good of the whole, to which you also belong.

17. Do not expect anything in particular. That allows more to happen! Be attentive and perceive what occurs. End both distant contacts after about 15 to 20 minutes. Give thanks to the Great Goddess.

❧❧❧

When you have performed this practice several times, you can also remain in the attunement longer. You will soon notice that you feel deeply relaxed physically, mentally and emotionally balanced, alert, and sensitive. With time, your intuition will clearly improve and favorable "coincidences" will happen. You will meet the "right" people and receive better opportunities in your work. If you have health problems, possibilities for healing will arise, as well as many other beautiful things.

❧❧❧

When we consider the consequences of the above-explained section, it becomes understandable why the attempt of a patriarchal religion or a corresponding path for awakening the spiritual potentials is doomed to failure from the start. Namely, this is because not the Great God is directly responsible for the organization of life on the material level but his companion, the Great Goddess. Since he is at home in very abstract realms that are distant from every biosphere and can only become active for the well-being of all creatures through the mediation of his companion, it is not possible to find and walk a path for spiritual awakening in the material world with his help. This is only possible with the specialist for life in the body, the Great Goddess. Through her, a very fruitful contact can also be established with the Great God and his realm. However, every true spiritual path does begin with her, the Divine Mother. Incidentally, this is something that all religions silently agree on because they would not function at all otherwise—even if they publicly depict the feminine as inferior, sinful, and negative. "Unfortunately," only a complete acceptance of the spiritual feminine principles makes the development of individuals toward the divine possible, the patriarchal religions that are most widespread today have not succeeded in helping people live in the sense of the divine order on earth. Instead, they directly or indirectly preach the eradication of people of other faiths, the primacy of the mind, and depict the body, which has also been given by the Creative Force,

537

with its essential functions as being false, a deplorable mistake, as evil itself that only causes suffering.

Now, at the beginning of the Age of Aquarius, the power of the Great Goddess is manifesting itself more clearly again. As a result, increasingly more people are coming to her on a great variety of paths in order to once again learn to understand her wisdom and build a new, natural way of life with the help of her spiritual power and all-embracing love. No wars or revolutions are required for this to happen. It occurs from below, from the people themselves and goes through all classes. One day, the old, life-despising system will be overcome and we will ask ourselves in astonishment how we could have ever put up with the earlier dreadful situation for so long.

*I am only now beginning to comprehend what it means to have a belief,
which means power and zeal. Yet, it is noteworthy that this feeling first
arose within me from the moment that religion was elucidated... and
enlivened for me through an individual standpoint and an individual
desire... It requires a special natural passion that is superimposed upon
the religion. This natural passion is the libido. The most alive thing of the
tangible world is the flesh. And for the man, it is the flesh of the woman.
Since my childhood I have been in the process of discovering the heart of the
material, so it was inevitable that I would one day find myself face to face
with the feminine. Seeking not the woman, but the feminine in all women
... without destroying the woman and without letting oneself be encircled
by her. ... We reach God through precisely that point of our soul that is
connected to the woman.*

*No, purity is not in the separation but in a deeper penetration of the
universe. ... It is in a chaste contact with what is the same in everything.
How beautiful is the mind since it elevates and decorates itself with all the
riches of the earth! Bathe in the material, Son of Man.- Immerse yourself
in it where it is the most violent and the deepest! Wrestle in its current and
drink its waters! Since time immemorial, it has rocked your subconscious—
it will carry you to God.*

(paraphrased from Teilhard de Chardin,
selected quotes from his journals and *Song of Praise*)

The Presence of the Great Goddess in the Various Religions

Here are some more examples of the concealed presence of the Great Goddess in the religions of the world.

Tara (Tibet/India), **Kuan Yin** (China), and **Kannon** (Japan) is the goddess of perfect love and all-embracing compassion. For many centuries, millions of people have prayed to her since experience has shown that she helps overcome difficult times, diseases, suffering, and pain. She provides powerful support for every type of spiritual healing. A story that tells of how she became divine says that she was an advanced student of a guru. One day, her teacher told her that she was now so developed that she just had to perform one ritual to ensure that she would be reborn as a man in her next life in order to have the necessary preconditions for enlightenment. *Tara* did not think about this very long and then performed a ritual with the goal of never being born as a man but always "only" as woman. She had the firm intention of proving that it was possible to be enlightened as a woman—or forgo enlightenment!

Odin, the Nordic main god, learned magic from *Freya*—one of the names of the Great Goddess. Since the beginning of time, magic has been seen everywhere in the world as a force belonging to the feminine. At the full moon, magical rituals have the most power and the moon is usually considered to be feminine in most cultures. With the rhythms that it triggers, it is connected with the archetypically feminine element of the water and the moon-bleeding (menses) of women. *Odin* received his initiation into the spiritual secrets from the Three Norns, the Nordic Goddesses of Fate, after he hung on the World Ash Tree *Yggdrasil* for nine days.

The Holy Spirit—which has only been given this name during a relatively recent period of time. The Biblical King Solomon still knew it under its original name: *Ashera* or also *Shekina*[224], a name for the Great Goddess that is derived from the Babylonian *Ishtar*. The Jewish spiritual literature says that her radiance nourishes the angels. In the Cabbalistic Tree of Life, *Malkuth* is in this form—the kingdom—in contrast to *Kether*, the crown, the Great God in his archetypal form.

[224] Also see the very interesting book *Yahwe's Wife*, Arthur Frederick Ide, Monument Press (Las Colinas).

The Cabbalistic Tree of Life describes the Creation and, like the Indian chakra teachings, builds upon the structure of six plus one level. The main channels of spiritual energy in the spinal column—*Îdâ, Sushumnâ*, and *Pingalâ*, as they are known from Indian yoga—are reflected in the three columns of the Tree of Life. In practical terms, very good chakra work (Cabbalistic Path Work) can actually be done on the basis of the individual *Sephirot* (stations that describe the archetypal powers and their effects and equivalents) and the paths that connect them.

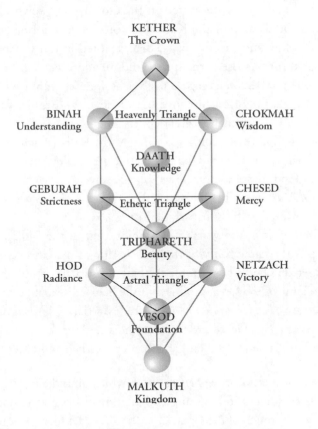

ILL. 204 – THE CABBALISTIC TREE OF LIFE

One of the animals that is particularly sacred to *Ashera* is the dove, which has been considered the symbol of the Holy Spirit since the time of Jesus and is exclusively connected with the Goddess throughout the entire Orient—but never with a god or other masculine principles. Jesus was baptized with water and water is probably, in addition to the earth, the typical feminine element. Baptism was also adopted from the Goddess culture. For thousands of years, it took place on the shores of the big rivers in Egypt, Mesopotamia, Asia Minor, and India in the name of the Goddess. Its purpose was to connect people with her milk, her blood, spiritually nourishing and linking them to the life net of the Great Goddess. The ritual of pouring water on the crown, the Crown Chakra, is a symbolic awakening of the Kundalinî force, a very strong archetypal spiritual energy known from yoga, that is stored in the 1st Chakra, the Root Chakra at the base of the spinal column and waits to be awakened. This happens when we accept ourselves as we are, embrace life in the material world fully from the love of our heart, and realize our divine potential on our spiritual path. Then this energy, which has been given by the Great Goddess (Shakti) according to the Indian teachings, rises to the 7th Chakra, the Crown Chakra. Here it persuades Shiva (a name of the Great God) to release his power in this way. The two then celebrate the *Sacred Marriage* in the body, mind, and soul of the respective person and thereby awaken his spiritual identity.

Moreover, it is also worth mentioning that in the Indian spiritual philosophy the name *Shakti* is the Tantric title of the Great Goddess. It is considered as both the term for the beloved sexual partner of the man and the name of the Great Goddess as the beloved sexual partner in the sacred creative act (*Hieros Gamos*—Sacred Marriage). Furthermore, it is the life-creating vital force and the innermost soul that animates the body of every human being, god and angel, every animal, and every plant.

The spiritual transmission of energy with which an Indian guru supports an advanced student in attaining enlightenment has always been called *Shaktipad*, the touch of the Great Goddess. In order for a guru to receive access to this force, he must practice a secret mantra of the Goddess *Sarasvatî* or of another suitable manifestation of the Great Goddess—that is only passed from mouth to ear until it completely fills him.

According to the Indian spiritual philosophy, *each mantra* attains its power solely from the Great Goddess since she created the entire material universe with "the Word."[225] In an ancient Vedic scripture it was determined that: "Only when Shiva unites with Shakti does he have the power to create." Today, most people associate the terms of "power" or "strength" with the masculine. However, in the spiritual tradition of India, Shakti, the Great Goddess, is seen as the dynamic, animating principle and Shiva, the Great God, as a resting potential that must be awakened by Shakti in order to show itself and become active. Even today, a powerful engine in India is described with the words "it has a lot of Shakti."

The manifestation of the Great Goddess that is particularly closely related with the power of the mantras is the Goddess *Sarasvatî*. She is customarily shown with a stringed instrument in one hand and a mâlâ (rosary for reciting mantras) in the other hand. In the oldest texts of the Vedic religion, *Sarasvatî* is given the name of *Vâc*, the Goddess of the Divine Primordial Language from which all the other languages that we know today arose. She has a close relationship with the 5th major chakra (located at the center of the nape of the neck, the area of the larynx) and the vowel "a." This is the sound of the love of the heart that is brought into the world in order to remind the beings that they are all ONE, the Creative Force, and to lead them to spiritual awakening in this way. After all, this sound also plays a central role in Esoteric Buddhism and the energy work with *Dainichi Nyorai*, the Transcendental Buddha and the source of Reiki. *Sarasvatî* watches over all the genuine religious and spiritual goals and promotes them. Through her, the mantras receive their power and gurus who want to initiate their students into mantras must turn to her. She is the source of *Shaktipad*, the spiritual force, through whose transmission a spiritual teacher helps a student in attaining enlightenment. Intellectual learning, teaching, understanding, and making things comprehensible is emphasized through her.

---

[225] The Bibliography in the appendix lists additional literature on this topic. In addition, it is possible to check my—unfortunately—brief explanations on this topic in the books listed there.

An important *Sarasvatî* mantra is:

OM Eim Sarasvatîyei svâhâ

Incidentally: If a mantra is transmitted per initiation to a student by a spiritual teacher, it has *Devi-Shakti*, the sacred power of the Goddess. As a result, it has an especially strong effect.

ILL. 205 – THE MANTRA OM IN A FORM THAT IS COMMON TODAY

OM–The Mantra Par Exellence

In the ancient Indian Upanishads, the mantra OM is called the "highest syllable" and "the mother of all sounds" (*matrikamantra*). This mantra is erroneously attributed to Sanskrit, meaning the Indo-Aryan culture. It is far older and cannot be traced back to Sanskrit letters. According to all of the existing information, it comes from the matriarchal Goddess culture that was conquered by the Aryan nomads.[226] Like many other spiritual concepts and tools of this culture, the OM also became a component of the new patriarchal Aryan-influenced society.[227] Without the Goddess, nothing functions on the spiritual level—it would all just be theory without her ability of transforming ideas into material manifestations and practical effects. In the Vedic text *Mahanirvanatantra*, it says: "…just as the birth also comes from the mother, the world arises from *matrika* or sound."

[226] Cf. with the above chapter on the Siddham Script and my (Mark) Master's thesis entitled "*Die Siddham-Schrift in der japanischen Kunst bis zum 14. Jahrhundert*" (The *Siddham* Script in Japanese Art Up to the 14th Century).

[227] The international renowned Monnier-Williams Dictionary of Sanskrit-English confirms that there was no trace of the word OM in Aryan texts that were written before the Upanishads. And the Aryans wrote these several centuries after they had conquered India!

The ancient Indian text *Chandogya Upanishad* says this about the OM:

> *The earth is the essence of all beings.*
> *Water is the essence of the earth.*
> *The plants are the essence of water.*
> *The human being is the essence of the plants.*
> *Language is the essence of the human being.*
> *Rigveda (sacred text) is the essence of the language.*
> *Samveda (sacred text) is the essence of the Rigveda,*
> *And the essence of Samveda is Udgith (another term for OM).*
> *Udgith is the finest of all essences, and it deserves the highest place.*

OM also represents the all-embracing cosmic consciousness[228]. The precise pronunciation of this mantra is not like the spelling of OM but AUM[229]. Like probably all mantras, this mantra has a great many different levels of meanings. Some of the important ones are worth explaining here.

Each of these letters has a spiritual meaning:

A **symbolizes** *Akar,* the form, the material structure, in its true, spiritual form. This means the Sacred Geometry and the material life that is lived in a spiritual way. This is the path to the divine in the earthly world as an important, indispensable part of the community of beings. This community is supported by the individuals with their unique potential and it supports the individuals with whatever they cannot provide for themselves on the basis of their limitations and weaknesses. *A* is also the waking state, the clear and subjective, meaning the individual consciousness. *Gyan Shakti*, as one of the three mystical main aspects of the Great Goddess, who brings the highest consciousness in the form of sound into the material world, belongs to this letter. She rules over the light that manifests, the clear knowledge that is rooted in the spiritual truth, and the deep wish for developing and unfolding our potential. The related masculine

---

[228] This all-encompassing cosmic consciousness is *not* the Creative Force in its entirety but the highest level of consciousness of the material universe formed by the Great God and the Great Goddess.

[229] The vowel *A* also assumes the first place here.

spiritual aspect is *Brahmâ,* the creative aspect of the Great God (not to be confused with *Brahman*, the Creative Force). The Great Goddess *Dai Marishi Ten* and the Great God (Transcendental Buddha) *Dainichi Nyorai* from Esoteric Buddhism can be classified here.

U symbolizes ***the dream state.*** This is where the individual consciousness dwells in the inner realm of desires, feelings, and thoughts. *U* represents the air element *Urdhagami*, whose movement is directed upwards toward heaven. It therefore rules over the powers of aggression, activity, and dynamics. The mystical main aspect of the Great Goddess is *Ichcha Shakti*, who governs the will. The related masculine spiritual aspect is *Vishnu,* who maintains the idea, the vision of the spiritual reality in the beings, and continually gives them new inspiration in terms of this.

M symbolizes ***the deepest state of sleep*** and simultaneously the consciousness of the perfect oneness. M shows the void, also called *Akasha*, the boundless potential from which everything comes and to which everything returns. Akasha is the foundation of the existence of all things and, from the perspective of being spiritually awake, is identical with what has been created.[230] The famous Buddhist *Heart Sûtra* says this about it: "Form is nothing but emptiness, and emptiness is nothing but form." At the same time, Akasha does not enter into mixing with the material forms of existence. It does not change, does not disappear, and can only be described through its effects but not directly. The mystical main aspect of the Great Goddess is *Kriyâ Shakti*, who rules over actions. The associated masculine spiritual aspect is *Shiva* (literally translated as "the Friendly One, the Kind One"), who dissolves and destroys what does not correspond with the spiritual reality and truth. He is also called the "Cosmic Dancer."

ILL. 206 – VERY ANCIENT, PRE-VEDIC WAY OF WRITING OM, AS IT WAS USED ON PALM LEAVES, FOR EXAMPLE

[230] Compare this with the comments on the double nature of existence.

The ancient Vedic text *Mandukya Upanishad* says the following about the function of the mantra OM:

> *Pranava (another name for OM) is a bow,*
> *The self (individual being) is the arrow,*
> *And Brahmâ (the Creative force) is the goal.*

As a result, practicing the mantra OM can lead to attaining spiritual awakening.

A type of half-moon with a point (small circle) can be seen above the written word OM in the traditional manner. This symbol is called *Candra-Bindu* or also *Nâda* (*Nita*) and *Bindu*[231]. These two Sanskrit words represent two important aspects of the Great Mother or Great Goddess (*Mahashakti*). *Nâda* is the tremendous radiating of the Goddess's power, which then gathers in the One point (*Bindu*), from which the material universe is created. It is no coincidence that the One point is associated with the Hara (Chin: *Dantien*). The Hara is where the original Water-Qi from the primary Qi of the kidneys—a power potential provided by the Great Goddess there to enable healthy cell division—is fed into the Small Energy Cycle, consisting of the Server Vessel and the Governor Vessel. In this way, the power of the water, the milk of the Great Goddess, is the element that nourishes the entire existence of a human being. As above, so below. As in the macrocosm, so in the microcosm…

From the One, the divine Creative Force pours into the half-moon, the lap of the Great Goddess, which she transforms into the three fundamental material qualities of existence, depicted by the three lower curves of the OM and manifests in the process. The participation of the Great God is concealed in the process. He only appears indirectly because he cannot show himself in the world without the help of the Great Goddess.

Consequently, *Nâda* and *Bindu* give rise to the basic three manifestations of the world in which inspired life is present: The dreamless sleep – the dream state – the waking state.

This also describes the highest spiritual power of a living thing as a trinity: *Sat* (being) – *Chit* (consciousness) – *Ânanda* (bliss).

---

[231] *Bindu* is associated with the 8th major chakra and *Nâda/Nita* with the 9th.

The original power of the Goddess, from whom everything is born, is called *Âdya-Shakti*. This is concealed behind the OM and cannot be perceived.

A – U – M also represent the process of life in its three parts and the divine beings who watch over them: Creation –Maintenance – Destruction.

OM is the root mantra of the 6th Chakra.

All spiritual goals can be achieved by practicing the mantra OM. OM is the mother of all mantras, the tangible presence of the absolute on the level of material existence.

A Special Practice with the Mantra OM

Sing the mantra in three parts: Ahhh—keep your attention on your navel and use your inner eye to see how a rose bud opens, radiating the light force of the mantra through its petals. Uhh—keep your attention on your heart and repeat the visualization in the preceding text. Mmm—keep your attention on the nape of the neck at the 5th chakra and repeat the visualization explained in the preceding text.

The Spiritual Path of the Individual in the Material World

So what exactly does the "from where?" and "to where?" of a human look like? In order to completely express the potential of the Creative Force in its state of the oneness, what is new from the realm of oneness must constantly flow into the material world. However, this new energy (yang) must be integrated by the already existing structures (yin). Because what comes from there is truly new, it requires much creativity[232] to incorporate

---

[232] Creativity is only possible through the use of the free will. However, the two are obviously not the same thing.

the "newcomer." The influx of these yang forces into the yin structures results in very complex rhythms. It is possible to depict and explain it, for example, on the basis of Western astrology and the transits[233] that it calculates and interprets or on the basis of a solar horoscope. However, Chinese or Indian astrology, as well as numerology, can also be consulted for understanding these sometimes very extensive processes.

The question may now arise as to how exactly we can imagine this.[234]

Here is an example of how this may occur in everyday life:

A young man has just strenuously worked his way through puberty and succeeded in becoming independent of his parents, learned to deal with the changes in his body, and has finally moved into his own apartment. How wonderful it is for him to do whatever he wants within his own four walls! Then he falls hopelessly in love and wants to move in with his beloved as soon as possible. Oh dear! How he has to be flexible! He must organize, make compromises, and learn tolerance and patience—otherwise "just the two of them" in one apartment will not work out. When they have finally worked things out, they may want to expand their love and together call a baby into this beautiful world. And as much as they love each other and the little being that comes from them and has very special, unique qualities, it once again requires much effort and a lot of creativity to integrate the new of this situation and to bring the whole thing once again into a pleasant, constructive functioning for everyone involved.

Similar processes take place for people starting out in their profession or children beginning school. The terror attack of September 11th,

---

[233]   At the time of a human being's birth, certain constellations of the astrological planets can be determined in the signs of the zodiac and houses. This is the so-called *birth horoscope.* For example, the sun is in the sign of Libra in the 2nd house and the moon is in Aries, and so forth. Of course, the planets do not remain in one place after the birth. If we follow their movements and put them into a relationship with the planet positions in the birth horoscope, this results in the *transits.* An example of this is that Mars moves through the birth sun or Saturn forms a square to the birth moon. An analysis of the cosmic forces affecting a human being within one year from birthday to birthday can be prepared as a summary of the forces, virtually a depiction of the themes for the year, in the form of a solar horoscope.

[234]   For some years now, this has become the standard question posed by journalists. But it is still quite useful at times.

the development of nuclear technology, and basically any invention—all of these things create new situations that we make compatible with the existing structures and for which we must find a meaningful response and appropriate reactions.

This should explain the eternally new yang influences and the efforts of the existing yin structures in integrating them…

There are some appropriate sayings on this topic: "Man proposes, God disposes!" and "Things work out differently than we think they will."

Every Being Is Unique

Every living thing is basically unmistakable and unique. Taken as a whole, all the beings that have ever lived, are currently alive, and will live in the future[235] show the infinite potential of the Creative Force in the conditional form of oneness. So every being and the path of every being is important—very important—because there is no substitute for it! Without a certain being and this being's path, an indispensable piece of the puzzle is missing to complete the great, multi-dimensional mandala of Creation.

An individual's various qualities in life are involved in a constant dance with each other. This is a matter of developing and appropriately applying a response to the processes that concern a person in the outside world, the demands for an attunement with his or her spiritual path, and the practical necessities (eating, sleeping, relationships, work, money, etc.), that affect all embodied beings.

The following factors determine the course of our path as a human being:

- ॐ Our distinctive characteristics

- ॐ Potentials

- ॐ Weaknesses

- ॐ The spiritual path depicted by the birth horoscope with the appropriate cosmic rhythms. The horoscope, of course, contains constitutional influences and karmic effects.

---

[235] This obviously means the past and the future that stretches into infinity on both sides, true to the motto of: "No beginning, no end!"

ॐ Our free will

ॐ Our dispositions

ॐ Our karma (on the one hand)

ॐ The decisions and actions of other people that directly or indirectly affect us (on the other hand)

ॐ The circumstances of the area and time in which we live

The Functions of the Free Will

If there were no free will, the universe would be like a big machine, a clockwork that—once wound up—will do its work at a certain time and then come to a standstill at some point. The future would be deadly boring because of this predestination. Every action of every material being and particle, every form of thinking and feeling would just occur according to the "big program."

However, in this case the material level would not be an exact reflection of the Creative Force in the state of oneness because there would be a beginning (the starting of the machine) and an end (machine comes to a stop). Of course, the whole thing could be started up again. But this would require a creative impulse—and this would cause everything to become thoroughly confused. Any predictable action cannot include creativity—because creativity only generates what is *truly* new. Yet, since an essential quality of the Creative Force is the creativity—after all, it has made everything (was creative) and the decision to do this was made without compelling preconditions[236] (free will), even though there are feasible alternatives (omnipotent Creative Force)—creativity must absolutely be part of the material level of existence. And a necessary precondition for creativity is the free will.

Free will arises from individuality. Because every being has its very own standpoint that results from the unique divine spark within it and its unique place in the process of the divine order, it requires and desires

---

[236] So how could the Creative Force be pressured into something? And by whom? After all, it is everything.

551

different things and experiences, for example, for its completion than *any other* being.

Free will is defined as such because it is, in its ideal form, in no way dependent in its decisions upon something or someone else. Turning its decisions into reality is obviously a different matter since, as we all know, the material world is not perfect.[237] In practice, this involves a larger or smaller degree of fee will. There are many, predominantly reciprocal dependencies in life. The driver needs the gasoline from the gas station, and the gas station needs the driver because it would otherwise have to close its doors.

Consequently, "I want this because I will otherwise not get that or must suffer that," is not an expression of free will in the narrower sense of the word. After all, a compulsion is at work here that only permits one decision. The decision without a condition is a divine quality in itself. Only with the help of the free will can the universe be truly filled with something truly new time and again and be enriched by it through its meaningfully integration into the existing life processes. Yet, all of this has a snag to it: Free will is free because it does not follow any rules. As soon as it were to do this, it would no longer be free. As a result, many things can also be created by the beings that disturb the Divine Plan[238] or could block it over time. Examples of these could be the pollution of the outer and inner worlds, the use of energy from nuclear fission and fusion on the earth, genetic engineering, the sprayed of poisons in agriculture, biological weaponry, demonization of our body and sexuality, and the like. The effects of these types of actions that do not fit in with the Divine Plan can have very complex and far-reaching lasting effects. If

[237] A person who is bothered by the blazing summer sun that I am enjoying as I write these lines on my beautiful terrace, can move to the shade, put on a hat, or set up garden umbrella. A dog can only trot out of the sun into the shade. A pebble must wait until it is night or someone with more possibilities carries it to a shady place. The beings with a less distinct free will (strictly speaking, one that works much slower in terms of time) stabilize the material universe so that the beings with a very strong free will cannot cause chaos with every decision they make. The inertia of one is the foundation of the other. The less free will a being has in the material world, the more it appears to be inanimate to other beings with a more strongly pronounced free will.

[238] *see next page*

there were not any correction possibilities in the material Creation, there would soon be no practical possibilities for the fulfillment of personal vision because of the lacking preconditions and increasingly stronger "senseless" influences and

But it is obvious that a provision has been made for this situation. After all, the Creative Force is not foolish.

ॐ On the one hand, it has created the light beings, gods, angels, power animals, and many others for this purpose. With their direct and indirect work, they attempt to correct the disharmonies.

ॐ On the other hand, it gave humans and other beings capable of consciousness the spiritual toolbox of magic.

ॐ And, as the most important counterbalance to free will, it has given us love.

The two complement each other like yin and yang. The more choices we consciously perceive, the more free will comes into play. Free will should not be viewed in digital terms of whether it is there or not there. An on/off mentality never does justice to the life process.

The more we free ourselves of fears, prejudices, greed, and other limitations, the more we perceive everything that occurs within us and around

---

[238] We can imagine the Divine Plan to be like a plant pole that gives a beautiful flower the support it needs in order to develop. The Divine Plan does not prescribe what exactly an individual should do at what time, where, and with whom, or what the result will then be. However, it contains visions for each individual being. The fulfillment of these offers optimal preconditions for the fulfillment of the visions of the other beings. So this is a classic win-win and dovetailing situation. If we follow our own vision, we create what another person needs in order to have the required resources available for the practical fulfillment of his vision. In turn, we then use what others, who have translated their visions into practical terms, have made available to us. Among other things, the Divine Plan includes the laws of nature (which essentially apply absolutely only in the gross material plane) and the cosmic rhythms affecting a being that can be tracked by the birth chart and the resulting transits. In a fixed sequence, these confront the respective person with specific themes. However, the astrological influences do not apply to someone who is in the state of spiritual awakening.

us, the more our free will can develop and create our life path in this way. This is obviously a wonderful way to live out our individuality.

This quality is a necessary precondition for the Creative Force to manifest at all in the material, realized form. Every particle of the concrete Creation is absolutely unique and contains a spark of unique divinity.

But without a suitable counterpart, the individual parts of the material Creation would increasingly drift apart. The application of the free will generates increasingly more personal freedom, which is used in turn by the free will. This creates even more personal freedom in the process. Absolute *personal freedom* is the *total lack of commitment!*[239] However, this would mean that there is no possibility for creating oneness between the endless consecutive encounters of the individual parts with each other and the resulting relationships that include the appropriate new experiences. There would be no room to live love because it only occurs within relationships. And this would mean the end of the two aspects of the Creative Force that are equal to each other and yet appear to be completely different.

Incidentally, the free will is the basis for the ego's existence since it sees itself as independent of others and not connected with them. As a result, it keeps on trying to satisfy its own needs and assert its views so that other people comply with it and it is therefore more secure—or this is what it believes. However, the free will develops out of the constant influx of yang qualities from the infinite potential of the Creative Force in its state of oneness. This takes place in the microcosm, such as on the cell level (cell division), as well as in the macrocosm (creation of new matter in the cosmos). Urged on by the influence of what is new and unique, the individual strives for new ways of integrating these qualities into the accustomed, the yin structures that have already been solidified by the more or less interlinked life processes.

[239] So this involves the theme of freedom from something versus freedom for something. Only the latter is truly compatible with love, desire, and meaning—in other words, the divine order.

Free Will and Love

As already stated, the counterbalance to this is love. It is an additional effect of the Creative Force's infinite potential in the state of oneness within the world of matter. Only in the union with the other sparks can our individual divine spark experience for one moment our great longing for unity. This is why there is love—so that individuality and the related free will do not lead to a complete disconnectedness of the material Creation in which each of us just follows our own interests and is therefore no longer capable of any encounters, ultimately even losing the necessary space and the playmates because of our interests.

This whole thing could also be divided into two basically different natural endeavors that are both focused on the same goal:

ॐ The urge for oneness with ourselves, finding unity within ourselves—and increasingly ridding ourselves of the obstructing "foreign factors". This ultimately leads to disappearing into nothingness—the associated spiritual path is asceticism.

ॐ The urge to find our way out of loneliness through union with the "other" and once again experience oneness. When this occurs, oneness can only be felt in the moment just before union and just after separation because there is no possibility for perceiving it within the unity. To do so, we must first come out of the unity in order to observe it from the outside as it were.

Love is the natural tendency to unite with the other in order to return to the original state of the Creative Force in oneness. In order for the whole thing to be organized in a meaningful way, allowing it to take its course in accordance with the divine order, there are rules for the functioning of love:

ॐ We can love everything and everyone to the degree that it or they are in resonance with our spiritual path.

ॐ We cannot love anyone and anything that is not in resonance with our spiritual path.

555

Time and again, people appear in my consulting practice who are virtually desperate in their efforts to love a partner or work that has very little in common with their path. Since they are continuously confronted with their inability to open their hearts, they believe at some point that they cannot love at all. And their hearts actually do close more and more because of the traumatic effects of the many wrong relationships. The best "medicine" against this is once again opening up to our personal path in life. Then there are more than enough opportunities for experiencing and developing our own ability to love.

> ॐ Love, consciousness, meaning, and personal responsibility belong inseparably together.

> ॐ We can only love what we can also perceive and what we are capable of being conscious of.

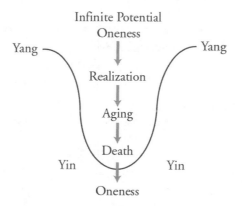

ILL. 207 – INFINITE POTENTIAL

As simple and obvious as this may sound—it has tremendous consequences! What do we know about ourselves? What can we perceive of ourselves? How about our friends, children, parents, and partner? How much of them can we grasp with our consciousness and through our senses? The response shows us the momentary boundaries of our ability to love! If we

556

would like to open our hearts further, an expansion of consciousness is necessary.[240] As already explained in the last paragraph, there are limits set for the ability of people in the embodied state to love. These boundaries result from the divine meaning and the divine order.[241]

A spiritual rule related to this theme says: "Love is the whole law, love under the divine will (meaning)!"

When we notice that it is totally easy for us to include a place, a job, or a person in our hearts, then we know that we are on our path. If it is difficult for us to love or we cannot do this in relation to a certain environment, this shows us that we have drifted quite far off our path. Of course, this rule only applies if—and to what extent—we have learned to feel the stirrings of our heart.

Love is not the relief you feel when you believe that you no longer need to be afraid.

Love is guaranteed not to be when you assume that you can satisfy a craving

As long as our main motivation is to escape from fear, suffering, the negative, the threatening, the lack, we take exactly this with us in some form. This is because life energy—our life energy!— flows to where our attention is focused. Only when our main motivation for an action consists of attaining love, good, joy, and meaning will the flow of our life force also move toward these beautiful things.

Love is ultimately also the reason for gravitation. Every definable particle in the material world attempts to achieve a state of oneness with others. It desires to once again feel the oneness that is experienced when it was formed.[242] The particle has a very pragmatic approach in achieving this. They prefer to move toward another particle that has already

---

[240] In this context, the heart is synonymous with the 4th major chakra. Consciousness is one of the essential functions of the 3rd major chakras (Solar-Plexus Center).

[241] Meaning as a spiritual function, the orientation upon and toward the divine order, is the main function of the 6th major chakra, also called the Forehead Chakra or Third Eye.

[242] If we follow the thoughts introduced in this sentence to their logical conclusion, the result will be some surprises and a better understanding of the world and what happens in it.

attained a higher form of unity, which means a greater mass/density ratio and therefore has more power. If there is no such particle close by, two or more approximately equal particles first build a system. If the opportunity arises, they will unite in a cataclysm[243] of passion.

Love constantly attempts to produce a higher degree of unity. As it does this, it forms more stable yin structures that are complete within themselves. This applies to atoms and molecules, but also to beings like humans as they form couple relationships, families, circles of friends, town and city communities, states, and so forth. The extremes in the universe are the black holes.[244] They are suns that have collapsed almost to a mathematical point. Strictly speaking, they are the size of a subatomic string. With their immense gravitation, they draw increasingly more other matter into themselves. They collapse into a spiral of extreme energy density that disassembles everything that gets caught in their wake into its individual components so that it can be easily integrated into every creation process in the material universe when it rises in one of the matter source. Astrophysicists have recently proved that these are the "white holes," which only open themselves for extremely short periods of time to transport new building material to the different regions of the universe. Every creation—and therefore every loving encounter that leads to union—moves in the shape of a counterclockwise-turning double spiral that, when a certain degree of closeness and therefore energetic density is achieved, is blessed by a third power, a pure yang influence, from the infinite potential of the Creative Force in the existence form of oneness. After this extremely brief—but also tremendously meaningful moment—the double spiral separates again in a clockwise movement. The relationship

---

243 A cataclysm of passion is a catastrophe—but a very, very beautiful one. "And is a moment of the highest, loving bliss not worth a thousand deaths?!"

244 These statements about love may help us better understand why the color black symbolizes the all-embracing love, one of the essential qualities of the Great Goddess. Topsoil, which lets so many plants thrive and grow, is black. The Black Madonnas lose their healing powers if they are painted in a different color. A black wall that has the sun shining on it will warm up much more quickly than a white one because black does not reflect anything back. Of course, the pull of absolute love can be very dangerous for those who would prefer to remain in separation from others, who want to remain in absolute individuality and total asceticism instead of pleasurably and ecstatically merging in union with the other.

partners separate but they may again turn to the loving union with each other or another at a later point in time in a counterclockwise spiral…

This process takes place within every time frame. In very long-term time frames, these are the movements of the stars and the star families in the universe. In more short-term time frames, this is two human beings forming a couple. In a very short-term time frame, these are energetic structures that vibrate so quickly in this process that they appear to show the qualities of solid matter. Consequently, when they come together they form electrons, photons, protons, neutrons, and other subatomic particles that in turn come together to become atoms, and then these make up molecules. Yet, matter is ultimately pure, highly vibrating energy: $E = mc^2$, superstrings, and particle waves. An airplane propeller displays two, three, or four blades when it is at rest or turning slowly. When it moves very quickly, it looks like and mechanically behaves like a disk—which it certainly is not while at rest. DNA, carrier of the biological genetic make-up, shows this process with its form. Water also reflects the principle very well in the way it forms vortexes. With the appropriate technology, even energy can be created through the systematic use of the 3rd ray.[245] Nature does this constantly, and some researchers have already copied important things from her. Incidentally, the above-explained principle of the three archetypical creative forces is used in the energy-work tradition of the Three Rays Meditation in a direct manner for spiritual healing and personality development.

If the effect of love did not have the counterbalance of the free will, everything would eventually find its way back to absolute oneness with all through the power of the love. But then there also would no longer be a material world and the Creative Force would be sad because it would have lost such a beautiful toy—or something like that…

Love is the longing to return to the state of oneness. Through the encounter and occasional union with the other, this longing will always be fulfilled a bit, the divine becomes tangible. This is why sexual energy, the desire for physical-spiritual union with the complementary other that cannot truly be controlled by the mind—and love, the longing to form

[245]   Compare this with the following literature: *The Energy Evolution* by Viktor Schauberger and Callum Coats, Gateway. *Living Water* by Olof Alexandersson, New Leaf.

a stable unity with the complementary other—and meaning—the kind of union, the oneness with other beings, places, situations of the divine order—all belong inseparably together.

Love and the Chakra Teachings

The ability to love is created through the series of yin chakras, which are the 2nd, 4th, and 6th chakras. It develops in the 2nd chakra, which is the energy source, in the form of a pleasurable sensation during physical closeness or within the context of physicality, or through the appropriate mental images, for example—but the two are obviously not the equivalent of each other! If this pleasurable sensation continues, it results in the wish to also establish mental and social closeness that is more lasting than the encounter that takes place in the 2nd chakra. So this turns into a relationship in the 4th chakra. If this social, mental closeness continues, if it is stable and the previously described physical closeness and the pleasurable, joyful aspects are maintained, then the energy for supplying the 6th chakra results from it. This is a matter of taking a mutual path in life together, which means entering into a spiritual relationship and linking the individual visions into a mutual vision as a couple—making space for meaning in the life together.

The sensation of pleasure or joy in the 2nd chakra does not necessarily have to be of a direct sexual nature. This is simply a matter of the one body feeling sensually good with the other body. So the 2nd chakra can also provide the starting point of the relationship for the foundation when it concerns a plant, an animal, a friend, or a child. The erotic, sexual closeness is a special form of this but it also provides an absolutely essential foundation for the other expressions. In principle, the entire series of yin chakras participates in love in this way.

Some frequently encountered difficulties are based on the emphasis of the relationship on just one or two of the three chakras because of unconscious reservations or even conscious convictions. For example, an overemphasis on the 2nd chakra can lead to difficulties in entering into lasting commitments of any type. In the same way, an overemphasis on the 6th chakra can lead to sharing a common interest in relation to the personal visions; however, a simultaneous practical translation of these visions into everyday life and into the everyday companionship hardly occurs. For example, this may be manifested in the way that two people frequently enjoy fantasizing together about how they would like to live together or do projects together, but there are almost no practical results.

An overemphasis on the heart chakra results in seeing the companionship as the most important thing and allowing the physicality or even the vision, for example, to suffer as a result. When the companionship is seen as the most important thing, this means that one partner cannot separate from the other at family celebrations, parties attended together, and mutual activities, for example. There is also no inclusion of higher values (6th chakra), long-term visions that are important for the personality development, or playing with the partner and having fun (2nd chakra) or experiencing sexuality and eroticism.

In my experience, the various facets of love are the most frequent topics in life-coaching sessions. One very important factor of this is taking into consideration that human beings who do not experience their own physical nature as basically sensual, who cannot accept themselves in this way, basically also have a just a very weak energy supply to the upper chakras. This can lead to tensions in the emotional area, as well as physical difficulties. Of course, these difficulties may also only appear in certain life themes. We should not be too quick to generalize in this respect.

The various facets of love should play a role in the life of a human being and have their appropriate place.

Every long-lasting form of one-sidedness also leads to disharmonies in other energy organs and/or in the entire life structure.

Love Can Only Exist When the Reign of Fear Is Broken

Living in love means refusing to fear. It means shaking off the yoke of its dictatorship and opening up to the truth. Personal responsibility, love, and consciousness (truth) are conditional upon each other. They cannot exist without each other and cannot have an effect without each other. When we try to live in personal responsibility and consciousness (truth), love cannot be far away.

Love helps build closeness, peace, joy, desire, and understanding. However, love must be conquered because our fear builds walls against it. If we are not prepared to fight for love to the end, we will not capture the stronghold of our fears—and will continue to dwell in the illusion of separation without hope, in despair, and lonely. Where there is love, there is life, meaning, healing, desire, togetherness, and happiness. Where there is fear—no, this is not where death is because death belongs to life and can also be deeply permeated by love.

Where we find fear, we also find coldness, isolation, lies, meaningless-ness, brutality, hatred, and finiteness.

In order to live in love, we must decide time and again in favor of it instead of fear. The methods presented in this book support this goal.

What Love Is ...

Love is what is left when fear has gone away and taken greed with it.

We should not put too much effort into defining love in a personal way for ourselves. If we turn away from fear, we will almost automati-cally experience it. It is guaranteed to clear away all doubt. Love is a natural quality of the Great Goddess, and therefore of life in the material world. Where love is, life happens. Through relationships with other be-ings, oneness and—as a result—divinity can be experienced individually. Relationships are only possible through love, sex, and meaning in all of their varieties.

   ॐ Love makes us curious about encounters and relationships with the other participants in the big game that we call "life."

   ॐ Love opens us so that the other person can come into us in his or her way.

   ॐ Love is joy. Love is desire. Love is hope. Love is forgiving. Love is peace. Love is fighting for life.

   ॐ Love is the essence of truth.

   ॐ Love is the heart of justice.

   ॐ Love is living softness.

   ॐ Love is meaningful tolerance.

ॐ Love is surrender to what truly suits us.

ॐ Love is the constructive togetherness that makes more out of all of the involved resources than we as individuals could ever have had available to us.

ॐ Love is ecstasy, the rejoicing joy on the certain path to divine oneness.

In oneness, there is no love. All that is there is nothingness, the absolute. Love has fulfilled its purpose when perfect unity is achieved. Then it sleeps, prepared to once again fulfill its task if a separation should occur once again.

The Soul Family

In order to follow our spiritual path in a good way, we make an agreement before our conception—even while we are still dwelling in the light worlds close to the angels—with others who also want to "come down" again for the mutual project. Together with them, we form a so-called *soul family*. In the course of an incarnation, we will encounter one or the other from this group time and again. And we will have exciting adventures together with them! People who fit especially well with us and wonderfully complement our strengths, weaknesses, idiosyncrasies, and learning themes are called *dual souls*. Yes, there are several of them—and they do not necessarily always have to be our partner. Our dual souls may be relationship partners, such as in a marriage. But they can also be very good friends. Or they may be someone who we just briefly encounter, but with whom we share a tremendous experience that enriches our view of the world and our self-image in a lasting and profound way for both people. They may be children, parents, superiors—as well as animals, the so-called *familiars*. These animals are special! They can perform spiritual energy work, often perhaps even better than we can! They understand us in a very deep, unique way like a very good friend. So, is it any wonder that familiars are *very* good friends! They enrich our path in a way that a human being cannot in many respects. And vice versa.

We rarely are involved for an entire incarnation with the same representatives of our soul family or dual souls. Our "friends from above" usually come and go, depending upon how certain life phases occur for us. We should be happy when we once again meet an old friend and not be too sad when he disappears from our life for a while. We are certain to see each other again. Those to whom our hearts are close will be led to us again by the mutual spiritual meaning. And then new, exciting adventures and beautiful experiences will be waiting for us!

Reincarnation

The process of life is infinite, without beginning and without end. The teaching of reincarnation is very extensive—explaining it in a more or less complete way would require an extensive book of its own. So it will only be discussed briefly here in relation to the themes that are important within this context.

When we the in the material world, we first enters into the so-called *Bardo*. This is a Tibetan word that roughly means "the twilight realm." This is where we process our last life, make peace with ourselves in relation to the associated experiences and increasingly detach from our self-image as an embodied human being until we "turn around" and perceive the waiting angels and other members of our soul family who are already dwelling "above." Accompanied by our friends, we then enter into a form of existence—by means of a type of light column with a transforming effect—that is basically different from living as an embodied human being. Here we are no longer accessible—not even through paranormal mediums. A medium can only establish contact with the deceased who are still in the *Bardo*. Normally, we separate from the *Bardo* after about three months and then continue on to "above." However, if we are very strongly attached to the material world because we want power, sex, food, an addictive substance, activity for our helper syndrome, admiration, or the fulfillment of a task related to an earlier incarnation—or have died under a great shock—it may take decades or centuries for the "ascent" to occur. This is not because we are prevented from "ascending" before this time, but because we are still too attached to the embodiment for a great variety of individual reasons.

Such a case is then a task for shamans or appropriately trained light-workers. A special training in Rainbow Reiki, for example, involves this topic. With the appropriate knowledge and abilities, the person stuck in the *Bardo* can usually still be lead into the light realm, unless they have un-compromisingly decided against it on the basis of their own free will.

Ascended Masters and Spirits of the Ancestors

An exception to this are people who have reached a high level of develop-ment in one incarnation and who, for reasons of personal responsibility in relation to a spiritual tradition, decide to leave their Higher Self at a level that is still medially accessible for the living even after their death. The other two parts of their personality (Inner Child and Middle Self), which determine the everyday personality in a narrower sense, then wan-der on "up" into the light realm until the next incarnation. The Higher Self remains accessible to the students of the tradition. When the spiritual lineage is called upon in the Reiki initiations, then the Higher Selves of the deceased masters are called upon in order to provide support for the important ritual of the initiation.

Jesus, *Gautama Buddha*, *Lao Tse*, and *Kûkai* are examples of this theme.

Meta-Incarnations, Young Souls, and Old Souls

Each incarnation has a specific, connected group of themes that are to be worked through. But depending upon the precondition and interactions with others, this may happen more or less successfully. Several incarnations that are thematically related make up the so-called *meta-incarnation*.

An "old soul" is someone who has already gathered abundant ex-periences within the scope of a meta-incarnation and has meaningfully integrated them. A "young soul" is someone who may be in the first incarnation of a meta-incarnation cycle and still hardly knows the way. Yet, when we begin a new meta-incarnation cycle, we must have already learned a great deal in the preceding meta-incarnation cycle. We had already existed as an old, wise soul since otherwise we could not have "switched." Now we are starting anew again, with fresh themes and usually also with a different soul family—a new game and new happiness!

Because of negative karmic burdens, meaning the effects of non-meaningful actions of past lives, the effectiveness of the learning and the ability to love in an existing incarnation can become very limited. If it is determined that this is the case, appropriate measures such as reincarnation therapy, mantra work, rituals, or the Rainbow Reiki karma-clearing techniques should be applied in order to once again free the path for spiritual self-realization.

Disharmonious karma must not be suffered until the bitter end. It can—and should—be healed with holistic methods such as those also used for other disorders.

What Is the Purpose of Magic?

As already mentioned above, magic—also called witchcraft—is an important means for correcting lasting disharmonious consequences of the free will.

By means of magic, certain tendencies in the life processes of beings can be strengthened or weakened. Magic does not work without the appropriate practical efforts.[246] Magic also does not make decisions for anyone. We also still need our hands for manual work, our head for thinking, and our heart for feeling so that the good preconditions created by the magic will bring about something good. It cannot save truly shattered partnerships or sick people who do not want to become healthy. And if a certain path is simply totally wrong for us, magic will not make it right. If we do not whole heartedly wish to be happy or successful or reject an otherwise positive change in our lives—because of fears, greed, or prejudices—we will be exposed to even greater tension through the energy influx of magic, which means we will subjectively suffer even more than before. *Ora et Labora!*[247] Magic can make life much easier, but it cannot relieve anyone of life. It also cannot be used to change or invalidate the laws of the universe established by the divine order. The rise and fall of the yin and yang forces, the interplay of the cosmic rhythms are maintained,

[246] Rituals for fertility do not replace sowing, fertilizing, watering, and harvesting.

[247] Latin: Pray and work!

just like our own constitution. However, magic helps develop the best from all of this in a holistic sense.

There is a certain flexibility in the state of lasting spiritual awakening. In this state, we are no longer subject to our birth chart with its patterns that are determining for a certain incarnation. However, this does not mean that we can literally do *anything* that we want. On the basis of the spiritual awakening, a new karmic path can be derived from the old without having to the beforehand. The selection is large. However, as long as we are in the embodiment, we cannot be omnipotent. This would also not make any sense because the purpose of our life, which basically always consists of loving and learning, could no longer be fulfilled in that case. There would no longer be a path. Everything would immediately be "here" and "perfect." But particularly *the walking of the path* makes the wonderful and very essential important experiences of the material level of existence possible. In the narrower sense of the word, magic always functions only through the support of light beings such as angels, gods, and power animals. Our human abilities to take magical action in a direct way are conceivably limited. However, with the assistance of the spirits—as light beings are also called—even greater magical works can be performed in a relatively simple way.

In the narrower sense, the magical work that we can do begins with the transmission of energy from spiritual sources outside of ourselves through the laying on of hands[248] and ends somewhere beyond influencing the life-structure processes of an entire continent's population. The latter is obviously somewhat more difficult than the laying on of hands and not very many human beings have attained such extensive competence during the course of human history.

Magic is the art and science of changing the tendency of the life process in terms of quality and quantity through energetic or spiritual interventions. Examples of this are having different "coincidences" occur than before, creating additional types of opportunities and encounters, and giving the thoughts and feelings encouragement for new directions.

---

[248] In keeping with this, the Usui System of Natural Healing is also and especially a system of magic. This is true particularly when the verifiably existing shamanic roots of this tradition and the possibilities of energy work resulting from this understanding are taken into account.

This can change decisions based on the potential of the free will as little as the fundamental conditions of the birth chart can be altered.

Personal wish fulfillment[249] is also part of this, but only makes sense (meaning that it only functions under the condition) when the fulfillment of the wishes helps us move forward on our spiritual path. It is also best if others who are associated with the theme and with whom we feel connected from the heart, are appropriately supported by the magical work that we do, whereby direct interventions are obviously only permitted with the express permission of the respective person. Under these preconditions, the fulfillment of personal wishes in a magical way is most powerful.

Magic *always* only becomes effective through the contact with light beings (such as angels, etc.). The so-called "black magic" is not magic in this sense because its results are very limited and work through throwing the victim's personality off balance by charging split-off parts of the personality with normal *Ki* and not through changes in the life-structure processes. In addition, it is certain that light beings do not participate in black magic. And neither does the devil, who does not exist! (See below.)

Light Beings and Magic

So nothing works without the spirits. This is why good relationships with the light beings are decisive for effective magic work. Angels and other inhabitants of the astral worlds basically like to help in magic work in the above-explained sense. After all, magic was given to the beings in order to direct the destructive effects of free will into constructive channels—also and especially when the effects have already become very crass, complex, and lasting. This means that they are too complicated to be straightened out through with contemplation, diplomacy, and manual work.

In principle, all of us can do magic as long as we have acquired the necessary knowledge and abilities by means of training. However, it is necessary to observe the following preconditions:

---

[249] There is a rule for this in witch circles: "Do what thou wilt, an'it harm none!"—Do what you want and harm no one (including yourself). This is simple, clear, and loving.

1. Do not perform magic out of fear or a lust for power, a drive for recognition, anger, or other acute surges of emotion, or a motivation based essentially on the wishes of the ego. This does not work.

2. Spirits are neither slaves nor servants. Even if they work modestly in the background, we should behave respectfully, ask, request, and thank them. It is also absolutely necessary to come to an agreement with them, both basically as well as also regarding the details in relation to complex practices works of magic that extend beyond the transmission of direct healing spiritual powers (for example, Reiki) to people who consent to it. Oracles are a good help in communicating with them and in the development of a holistic understanding of the respective themes. We should not be too quick to assume that we have understood everything correctly when we are channeling, doing astral traveling, or using the pendulum and that all messages come from one light being. The more ego-related themes and views are involved and the less we want to question our opinions and plans, the more certain we can be that the messages do not come from the spirits but from deep within our frequently prejudiced subconscious mind.

3. It is better to scrutinize the meaning and purpose of the planned work, our own motives and attitudes once too often than not enough.

4. Spirits are very loving and powerful beings. The more closely we can approach them, the more we can participate in their power. However, in order to be able to approach them, we must learn to question our own moral limitations, doubts of self-value, megalomania, and certain behaviors that are essentially founded on feelings or the ego and basically make peace with the major questions of life and death. Being in the direct presence of an angel would kill us if we do not love who we are—and this is meant literally. However, light beings are wise and loving. They do not permit unprepared people to be that close to them so that no harm can occur.

5. There are gardens, temples, power places, and other sacred sites in the astral realms. The more we fulfill the above-mentioned criteria, the more access we have to them. In addition, there must be a necessity for going to such places and doing something important there that cannot be completed equally as well somewhere else.

6. The more we want to approach astral power places and light beings and have magical power, the more such things will evade us. They would be too dangerous in the hands of an uncontrolled, neurotic, and fear-motivated person. Whenever we come across a new source of genuine magical power on our path, the guardians will ask us the question: "Why do you want to attain access to this power?" And if we do not respond from the bottom of our heart: "In order to better serve the divine order!" the door will remain closed to us until our ability to love, our humility, and our wisdom have developed appropriately. We are the Creative Force. If we wish to enter into our legacy, this also includes assuming the related responsibility and opening up to the wisdom required for this purpose.

7. In order to work successfully with magic, we need the closest possible personal, positive connection to the theme and the person—which also means to ourselves! The less personally we approach magic, the less it will work. Magical work "in passing" has virtually no effect. If we open up to it, then the divine power of serving life will flow to us.

8. This is not a matter of magically asserting our personal views but freeing the path for the fulfillment and continued development of the divine order, to which the magical also belongs, when magic is performed. The light beings are only interested in philosophical motives, as noble as they may appear to be, religious projects, the implementation of moralistic rules when they serve the realization of the divine order—and therefore life.

9. Implements such as magic wands, incense, magical times, incantations, power objects, candles, symbols, mantras, stones, technically correct rituals, and the like contribute essential factors to magical work. Under certain conditions! At the same time, when they are correctly used, letters, words, and sentences in an archaic, holistic language can express the contents that words cannot—or just inadequately—convey. We must know how to use the magical tools of the trade in a meaningful way. The objects that we use must truly hold power, and it must be available to us through initiation, for example.

10. A clear focus of the will is necessary for effective magical work. The more "ifs or buts" within us, the less power there will be. However, goals that we have not carefully scrutinized also obstruct the magic in just the same way! A lack of clarity blocks the will. In the fog of trances, it becomes difficult to orient ourselves.

11. Ultimately: We cannot magically influence what we do not love! The more we love something or someone (and this means genuine love in the sense of the above statements!), the more magical power we can use with respect to this person or thing. This is why we should always try to design magical actions on the basis of promoting our own development toward the divine in a loving and not in a confrontational or even compulsive or violent way. Then they have a better effect or even an effect at all.

What Is "Black Magic"?

"Black magic" is the attempt to create advantages through energy work with personal energies or spirits forced into service[250] at the expense of other beings or to achieve power over others in order to attain material advantages. *The black magician always acts out of fear* and the conviction that there is either no God, the Creator, or that this God is not there for him—or even against him. He believes that the structure of the divine order is threatening or does not take his needs into consideration. As a result, he must learn to force it to do his will. Correspondingly, the feeling of security within the divine plan, the primal sense of trust, the spiritual power of the heart, is not present in a black magician.

People who attract black magic on a regular basis are *guaranteed* to escape this influence when they are prepared to apply God's law of love to themselves and their relationship to the surrounding world without any "ifs or buts."

---

[250] Strictly speaking, this is simply a case of split-off parts of the black magician's own persona since angels, gods, and comparable beings do not let allow themselves to be forced into anything—especially not by human beings since we only receive the magic power from their hands as a loan when we have a compatible attitude toward the divine order.

Problems with disharmonious influences *always* are somehow related to the person who suffers from them. According to the ancient universal law of the Egyptian sage Hermes Trismegistos, which among other things is one of the essential foundations of the Tarot and astrology, we attract what we most fear or secretly desire in the subconscious mind, even though our consciousness acts like this is repugnant or means nothing to it. So this is the hook-and-eye principle, which always applies.

If we do not clarify and cleanse the fields and structures of attraction in the affected person when working with extreme disharmonies, there will always be new difficulties. For example, because I know this, I do not protect myself against black-magic influences, even though I work on a regular basis in countries where such practices are part of everyday life. Why should I? When life energy is sent into suppressed parts of my personality and I can consciously perceive them as a result, this saves me the many hours of therapy. Since my basic attitude is oriented toward consciousness, love, and purpose, I can only say a hearty "thank you!" for the nice service. If love really is the greatest power, then we should trust in it and use it!

What Is Evil?

These are the decisions and actions that are senseless from the perspective of spiritual understanding. The desire to harm another in order to satisfy one's own ego is motivated by fear, greed, or religious-moral dogmas. This is also wanting to use others as instruments of one's own desire for power, in whatever form this may take.

We can *act* evil but not *be* evil. Each of us is essentially divine—even if we forget this at times. Yin and yang do not exist in the realm of the spirits in the same sense as these two polarities manifest in the material world—spirits are much closer than human beings to the Creative Force and therefore to light and love. This is why they have so much more magical power. The ability to structure life is a divine power. The closer a being comes to the center of love and oneness, the more access it has to this power. This is why an angel cannot be evil. If it were, it would lose its entire power and become equivalent to or less than a human being.

What Are Angels?

This book frequently mentions light beings, angels, and other heavenly creatures. This section is devoted to explaining what these terms mean by using angels, who are the best-known example in the West. However, the explanations given for them equally apply to other light beings of all types such as devas, power animals, and gods.

The word "angel" is derived from the Greek term *aggelos*, which means something like "messenger." This also describes the essential characteristic of the angel race: They are servants, helpers of the Creative Force. They deliver not only news but also heavenly powers, inspirations, and development-promoting influences of all types. They weave nets of energies, information, moods, inspirations, dreams, occurrences, encounters, and coincidences that help the human beings, animals, plants, and the earth take their individual paths and connect them into a meaningful whole. Their light-filled nature makes the closer encounter with them into a very special experience that can change an entire life. Angels like to help people take their own path, become whole, develop themselves, and fulfill their true needs.

Like all of the "spirits," the angels also do not have the kind of material appearance to which we are accustomed. They basically also do not have names in the human sense. They recognize themselves and other beings through the perception of individual energetic information patterns and currents of power. People have given them names and other attributes in order to make the etheric beings easier to understand and comprehend as a vis-à-vis who can be addressed and directly perceived. However, angels are very much individual beings with their own themes of development and their very own character traits. At the same time, their freedom to make decisions (free will) is considerably more limited because they are much more directly connected with the divine order than human beings.

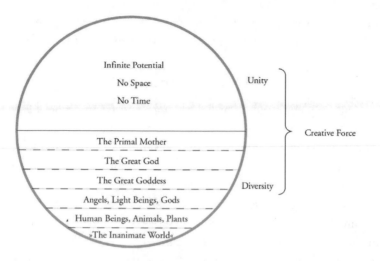

ILL. 208 – THE CREATIVE FORCE ENCOMPASSES UNITY AND DIVERSITY

A great many angel races have a gender; the Archangel Gabriel, for example, is even depicted in some church paintings as a clearly feminine being. Since there is a tremendously great number of angels with very different qualities and fields of activity, many qualities are basically not the same for all angels. As mentioned above, angels are individuals.

In the Jewish Tradition, the names of the angels, who usually have quite simple everyday names of human beings, have the suffix "el" added to them. This means "God" or "Lord" and shows that the bearer of the name is "one with divine qualities." This tradition stems from the ancient cultures of Mesopotamia, Sumeria, Akkad, and Babylon that were already ancient in Biblical times. The word *El* was used there to generally mean deities of both genders. The plural is *Elohim*[251], a word that has also become well known through the Biblical language. In Phoenicia, a country that was approximately located in the regions of the current nations of Lebanon, Syria, and Israel, the word *El* described the highest god of their pantheon, the "Heavenly Bull," spouse of the highest Goddess

---

[251]   In a precise translation, the Hebraic word *Elohim* means: "goddesses and gods." This only became the one, masculine god in the Christian churches because the entire patriarchal religious doctrine would understandably not have been valid otherwise.

Ashera (Ishtar). The Phoenician *El* was often depicted as a human being with bull's horns. Some sources suggest that the horns later became the well-known halo. However, it is quite likely that the symbol of the bull's horns was based in the crescent of the moon. Together with Venus, the Morning and Evening Star, this had a special meaning in relation to the Great Goddess, the mother of all life, in all of the cultures of the antiquity in the Orient.

The Great Goddess, the Pentagram, and the Course of the Planet Venus

An interesting explanation of certain numbers and symbols can be derived from the following: If we imagine the signs of the Zodiac arranged in a circle and use a line to connect the points in which Venus is in conjunction with the Sun in the sequence of its course within eight years, the result is a five-pointed star—the famous *pentagram*—in the signs of Virgo, Taurus, Sagittarius, Cancer, and Aquarius. Scorpio also occasionally takes the place of Sagittarius. The numbers *five* and *eight*[252] are therefore especially associated with the Great Goddess. The Olympic Games, which are taking place in Athens again as I write these lines, take place every four years, which is the "halftime" of the transit of Venus through the pentagram in the sky. Originally dedicated to the Goddess Aphrodite—the Greek version of Venus—the pentagram was intended to become the symbol of the Olympic Games. Then they ultimately became the five (!) rings in order to highlight the idea of connection between the participants.

It is basically not possible to completely define the beings of the subtle worlds in terms of our own time/space-oriented, analytical thinking. However, they can be comprehended more though *process-related* qualities and analogies. Depending upon our culture and the spiritual tradition when we see angels or related beings, as well as which personal experiences, preferences, and aversions we may have, we will perceive them in a different way. This is why there are many different names and descriptions of angels, their stories and mythologies, even though the spiritual beings

---

[252] The sum of five and eight is 13, the number of moon months in a year and the maximal number of members in a witches' coven. The number 13 is sacred to the Great Goddess. Of course, it has been and still is thoroughly damned by the Christian churches, just like other wisdom that has been derived from nature.

to which they refer are always the same and fulfill the same functions in Creation. People have invented a great variety of religions and fight over them. In the meantime, the spiritual beings take care of maintaining the foundations of life for all of us and supporting the material beings on their individual paths to the light. So shouldn't we orient ourselves upon them and their wisdom?

It is therefore quite unnecessary to argue about what the personal guardian angels are *really* called and how they *actually* look. After all, these are actually just analogies that correspond with the personal concepts and cultural structures of the respective people. However, it is important to find a name and a description that fits our personal spiritual companion and also works for both of us when we have contact with each other and work on mutual projects. The most important thing is a good understanding with the guardian angel.

Even though it may now perhaps sound like everything is oneness "up there" with the light beings—this is not really the case. The distinctions are only quite unaccustomed for human beings. Once we have been in contact with an angel or directly experienced a power animal and an elf, we know quite clearly that these are very different creatures. Despite this, it is quite correct to speak of power animals as the "angels of the Native Americans," for example. However, this comparison is obviously weak and a modern-day Native American has no problem working with both types of spirits.

In summary, angels can be described as personified, individual spiritual beings who mediate between the incomprehensible something, the Creative Force, and human beings and other occupants of the material levels of existence or help attune the structures of the material level of Creation with the forming-giving ideas of the Creative Force, the Divine Order.

There are basically three types of spirits, angels who are directly connected with the material world. These are spiritual beings who have the following functions:

a. building

b. maintaining

c. destroying

For people not trained in the spiritual sense, the spirits with destructive tasks often appear to be evil—which they are not in any respect! Without them, the cycle of life would function just as little as it would without the building or maintaining spiritual forces. Examples of these include: digestion, the immune system of the human body and the compost heap that turns into good garden soil.

Yin and yang does not exist for the spirits in the human sense. Their metabolism vibrates so fast that the boundaries of these two qualities appear to blur from the human perspective. Angels have a much finer perception in relation to this, unless an angel would like to stay in a certain quality for a while. Angels also relate differently to time than the occupants of the material world. Time does not run in a linear and unidirectional way as for the occupants of the material world. This is something I had to learn to deal with when I came into closer contact with these beings.[253] Angels orient themselves upon the spiritual meaning in order to move through time. If they would like to make contact with another being, they form close resonances with the life-purpose structures of the appropriate being and then find themselves in the same time with him or her.

Light beings belong to the material plane and are inseparably connected with it. Without it and its diverse occupants, the light beings would not have a mission. So, the light beings are also material in a certain sense. They consist of something that interacts with others and is different from them in terms of its nature. They are very intelligent and have unique talents—however, they also have their boundaries, as do all creatures. They are wise—and there is much that the individual angel does not know. For example, if an angel essentially looks after the sun of a spherical star cluster, it has little knowledge about the everyday routine of a Northern Irish machine fitter or a Brazilian saleswoman. Angels are neither omnipotent nor all-knowing or equipped with unlimited wisdom. However, in comparison to the most human beings they have an unbelievable additional amount of possibilities of all types. Since angels are specialized, it is worth turning to the suitable "experts" among them for the fulfillment of a certain task. Other chapters of this book describe the

[253] My first encounter with an angel took place at the tender age of about three years as I played in the summer. It has shaped my life from the very beginning.

many light beings with their special talents who have a close resonance with the spiritual lineage of Usui Reiki. When we connect with them, we can have our own individual experiences. They do not bite and are very nice—above all, when we treat them with respect, love, sincerity, and gratitude.

Magic and Energy Exchange

When we perform magic, there must always be an energy exchange between the various levels of existence in order to maintain balance. This process is called spiritual offering. Whatever is given—this should be done from the heart and dedicated beforehand to the appropriate spirit. It should not be something that we urgently need ourselves but something that we either have an abundance of or what obstructs us in our spiritual self-realization. In the human sense, it does not have to be valuable. Value is defined differently by angels in comparison to human beings. It is more closely related to love, meaning, and joy…

Examples of spiritual offerings are: songs, dances, a celebration, a good deed brought about by the magic in the sense of the divine order that does not directly benefit the person performing the magic; consecrated tobacco, flowers, sex, Reiki, incense, or candles. However, it can also be anger, hatred, sadness, envy, greed, or fear. Everything is energy for the angels. They transform whatever is given into something that is useful for them and their tasks with the immense power of their divine love.

Everyday Life as a Spiritual Offering

As nice as the above-mentioned offerings are, they are still just the preliminary stages. The more we consciously strive for the realization of the divine order, the more power flows to us from the angels with whom we work. A type of "magical reservoir" forms and we can draw upon it in case of need. Methods like Reiki are similar in a certain way. Reiki, the spiritual life energy, is absolutely necessary in the material world in the sense of the divine plan's organizing force. When we use it here, we offer a suitable return favor to the light worlds. As people initiated into Reiki, the more consciously and extensively we used the abilities given to us per initiation and training as co-creators of the divine plan, the more a "magical reservoir" will be formed for us in the light worlds. This is the reason why many people who intensively practice Reiki gradually also attain access to other magical and mystical abilities. When used correctly, Reiki is virtually the catalyst for the development of practical spiritual abilities. This is one more reason to use and spread the knowledge about the spiritual life energy.

The Special Characteristics of the Goddess and the God

The conclusion of this chapter will be a somewhat closer look at an important special characteristic of the two "head angels," the Goddess and the God. These two beings assume a special position among all of the light beings since they are closest to the Creative Force in their state of oneness. The Goddess and the God work very closely together, much closer than the other angels. The other light beings become active receiving instructions from them.

The Goddess and the God exist in various ways on a great variety of levels in the world of separation. They must be present everywhere in order to equally animate and organize all things. On the highest level, which is closest to oneness, it is the Goddess, who as the mother of all life brings the God and his potential into this world with the sacred word, the origin of all mantras. This is a mystical realm that is never directly accessible to the great majority of human beings. In the levels beneath it, they are so closely connected with each other that they are almost one. In Esoteric Buddhism, the two of them together are then called *Dainichi Nyorai*. In their form of manifestation on a somewhat lower level, the God is directly perceivable and the Goddess just indirectly. Somewhat lower than this level, the Goddess appears in the forefront. She is called *Dai Marishi Ten* in Esoteric Buddhism.

In a certain way, the Great Goddess and the Great God are in everything. Yes, and even more: They are everything! This is another paradox. In Esoteric Buddhism, *Dainichi Nyorai* in his most spiritual manifestation, the pure light body, is seen in such a way that many tiny little *Dainichi Nyorais* fly out of the "pores" of his "body" into the universe. This means that they actually create the universe since they are the core of every material being, every particle, and every object. In Taoism, there is the ancient teaching that all 36,000 deities of the universe are also in the body of every human being at the same time and each of them looks after a precisely specified part of it. This is easier to understand when we consider the above statements on the double nature of Creation.

Everything is the Goddess and the God—and is the Creative Force in the state of unity—and is an individual being, a particle disassociated from the others. This brings us back to the archetypal trinity of existence!

When we turn to the Great God, the Great Goddess, then we attempt in a certain way to establish contact with one facet of our beingness (as the Creative Force). Yet, the Goddess and the God should not be confused with the facets of our human form of existence, the partial personalities with which we are familiar from modern psychology and psychotherapy.

In order to make all of this somewhat more complicated: Human beings also have a light body and an angel-like form of existence. Important information on this topic is included in the next chapter on the teachings about the chakras and the light body. But very extensive explanations of this would totally go beyond the scope of this book, which is already a heavy tome. The Rainbow Reiki seminars on the topic of light-body work, which are offered throughout the world, can provide more information for anyone who is interested.

CHAPTER 20

The Spiritual Energy System of the Human Being

In this chapter I (Walter)'d like to provide an overview of the most important areas of the human energy system. The spiritual energy system completes the material components of the organism and establishes its connection with the rest of Creation on planes that resonate at a higher frequency. A profound knowledge of these energy systems is absolutely necessary in theory and practice for holistic healing and personality development.

The Functions of the Aura

The aura is an energy field[254] around the human body that can only be proved indirectly with conventional methods of scientific measurement. This energy originates largely in the crown area, flows in a clockwise spiral around the body and moves downward to the feet, as well as the arms and hands. Mainly at these end points, the energies and information that are to be communicated to others or simply eliminated from the body system are released into the surrounding world. The energy of the aura itself then enters the body once again through the palms or the center of the soles of the feet. It rises from there upward to the crown, where it exits and the cycle begins anew.

In addition to this "large" energy cycle of the aura, there is also a series of additional, smaller types of energy cycles, which are produced by the major and secondary chakras, as well as the acupuncture points. The aura contains a complex system of fine energy channels, as well as special chakras. This also allows it to support the harmonious organization of the processes in the body, particularly the formation of new tissue.

---

[254] For example, with Kirlian photography.

The aura around the human body basically fulfills the following purposes:

ॐ Energetic detoxification

ॐ All types of communication processes

ॐ Temporary storage of energy and information that A) either
   will be passed on from the body system to the surrounding
   world at a later point in time or B) will be received from the
   surrounding world and integrated into the body system at a
   later point in time.

ॐ Protection against disharmonious influences of incompatible
   energies and forms of information. This function is closely
   related to the element of *metal*, known through Traditional
   Chinese Medicine.

ॐ Supporting the energetic body structure and the formation of
   new tissue.

If, for some reason, too much information or too many energies become
temporarily stored in the entire aura or in parts of it, we will have problems
with perception. We easily fall into trances, and perception becomes very
selective or responds only to crude stimuli. In the application of therapies,
especially those oriented upon energy, this *reduction of resonance*[255] blocks
the body's ability to respond to subtle healing stimuli.

Most of the energies and information from the body system are
channeled into the aura through the 5th major chakra (Throat Chakra).
Through the 3rd chakra (Solar-Plexus Chakra), most of the energies and
information from the surrounding world are absorbed into the body
system.

I essentially work with four fields of the aura in my system of spiritual
energy work and personality development:

---

[255] Compare this with the chapter on Reiki Resonance Therapy in my book
Reiki—Way of the Heart , Lotus Press. Translated by Christine M. Grimm

1. The Etheric Body: This part of the aura borders directly on the physical body. This is where the largest portion of the communication related directly to the physical body takes place and is, if necessary, temporarily stored. Information about the physical structure is contained here; nourishing energies from the surrounding world are absorbed here and distributed in the body. The etheric body is also involved with access to the energetic abilities to feel and act. The etheric body has a strong resonance with the muscular system and especially the seven muscle-armor rings familiar to us from bioenergetics—a somatic form of psychotherapy.

2. The Emotional Body: This area of the aura connects to the outside of the etheric body. This is where emotional and instinctual energies of all types are communicated, temporarily stored, partially organized, and sent to the various areas of the body.

3. The Mental Body: This area of the aura connects to the outside of the emotional body. This is where the conscious and unconscious functions and factual thought processes are communicated, temporarily stored, and partially organized. This also includes the habitual ways of thinking such as evaluations, and ethical and moral concepts.

4. The Spiritual Body: This area of the aura connects to the outside of the mental body. This is where spiritual themes—as well as larger groups of extensive projects that are important for a great many people, together with their corresponding energies and information—are communicated, temporarily stored, and partially organized. This aura field connects us with the Creative Force and its helpers, such as angels or gods. This is where spiritual energy currents are perceived and absorbed and the sensation of unity with everything becomes possible. Prayers, medial perception, and many forms of healing and magical energy work are put into effect here.

The Major Chakras

1st Energy Center (Root Chakra)

Location: Base of the coccyx. The 1st chakra radiates downward into the earth from the perineum.

Basic Polarization: Yang

Spiritual Element: Earth

Functions: This energy center contains the blueprint of our physical existence. Its themes are survival and self-preservation in the broadest sense; preservation of the species; structure; grounding; dealing with material practical necessities; fight and flight; sexual vitality and physical potency; capacity to work; primal sense of trust; resilience/ability to cope with pressure. It is the source of vital power for the entire organism and the energy system. It is the center for the will, energy for short-term activities, and the manifestation of all types of life circumstances.

Associated Organs and Organ Functions: Everything solid within the body; bones; blood formation, blood vessels, and formation of new cells; teeth; adrenal glands; rectum, anus, lower spinal column, and legs; vitality of the blood. This is where we have continual feedback about our organic condition.

Healing Experiences and Behaviors: A happy nursing period as a baby; honorable behavior; self-esteem; respecting and honoring the personal and spiritual roots; giving respectful thanks for food and money; thanking Mother Earth for her gifts and treating her respectfully; success through a meaningful and joyful expression of our own potential in being together with members of the soul family; being greeted in a cheerful and warm way; developing team spirit. Acknowledging the good in changes and learning to use it; enjoying the new and systematically integrating it into our lifestyle; tolerance; letting go of what is no longer appropriate; letting ourselves be helped by loving fellow human beings; letting others treat us when we are ill; being an accepted member of a group; ignoring our work when we are tired and recovering instead; understanding failures and rejections as guidance and help in learning for a better orientation on our own path; baptism as a ritual of being accepted into the community of beings of this world and into the life net of the Great Goddess; and a conscious decision for constructive thoughts and good nutrition.

Problematic Experiences and Behaviors: Continual struggle for survival (subjective or objective); continually calling to mind difficult times that have long passed and acting, thinking, and feeling correspondingly; feelings of guilt; fears; long-term or shock-like occurrence of a lacking sense of security; fear of changes in the life situation; (fear of) humiliation or rejection by others; pettiness; pedantry; stinginess; clinging too much to social, religious, and moral rules, values, and standards; shame; out-of-control self-criticism; overemphasis on structure, discipline, and organization; abuse of authority; narrow-mindedness and obstinacy; pathological compulsion for perfection; getting stuck in formality and superficiality; predominately superficial formation of opinions; alone against the rest of the world; failure; being rejected; and being disparaged by others.

2nd Energy Center (Sexual Chakra)

Location: About two fingerwidths above the pubic bone at the centerline of the body. The 2nd chakra radiates to the front.

Basic Polarization: Yin

Spiritual Element: Water

Functions: Joy in life; directly flowing, unreflected feelings; (physical) encounters; sensuality in general; eroticism; distribution of the life forces; instinctive perception; flexibility; astonishment; relationship to the body; desire; creativity; enthusiasm; energy for long-term activities; bridging function for spiritual (medial) perception of every type. Instinctively finding the right path in life that brings joy and good things time and again.

Associated Organs and Organ Functions: The urogenital system; kidneys; appendix; intestines in general; large intestine; small intestine; skin; pelvic area; bladder; arms; all fluids in the body (blood, interstitial fluid, lymph, mucous; sexual secretions; saliva; sweat, urine, secretions of the mucous membranes; tears); absorption of nutrients and vital substances in the metabolism; the breasts; prostate gland; ovaries; uterus; motivation for sexual activity and ability to feel sexual sensations.

Healing Experiences and Behaviors: Happy playing with no purpose; curiously and joyfully exploring something; pampering our body; acceptance and creative, constructive expression of feelings; being emotionally oriented upon the here and now; forgiving; enjoying our feelings and dealing with them in a constructive way; assuming responsibility for our own feelings in ways such as spiritual practices for the positive orientation of the feelings or consciously focusing our attention on what is beautiful, true, and good in order to create a positive basic mood (but not denying the problems!); pleasurable, satisfying sexuality with a partner for whom we have strong positive feelings; pleasant, tender body contact; stroking; gentle massages; beautiful fragrances; nourishing cosmetics; healthy common sense and practical thinking; union with the divine, such as in the form of Tantric rituals—during which the man asks the God within and the woman asks the Goddess within to permeate him and her with their sacred power and open them on a higher level for union.

Problematic Experiences and Behaviors: Inner and outer conflicts related to the topics of money, power, and sex; too many frustrations in everyday life; forced or voluntary sexual abstinence; moral concepts that have the consequence of suppressing joy, sexuality, enjoyment, beauty, desire, and play, judging them as negative. Work situations and relationships that are the source of constant frustration. Compulsively wanting to control others and ourselves; fearing a loss of authority, esteem, status, and control; intoxicating drugs; compulsive eating; chocolate; essentially doing something because of the money or the related esteem or power (prostitution); being a victim; sexual and emotional abuse; being dominated by our feelings; pathological dependency; addictions; jealousy; prejudices; over-excitability of every type; obsessively relating the behavior and the conversations of other people to ourselves; strong rejection or "worship" of teachers and gurus; being a groupie or a fan; aggressive territorial behavior; acting like a macho or a vamp; always desiring to have some type of remedy (medicine, supplements), meditation, other spiritual practices, astral journeys, and the like as a substitute for everyday life (flight response).

3rd Energy Center (Solar-Plexus Chakra)

Location: About two fingerwidths beneath the sternum at the centerline of the body. The 3rd chakra radiates to the front.

Basic Polarization: Yang

Spiritual Element: Fire

Functions: Power; fear; organizational abilities; dominance; karma; separation; analytical, relevant thinking and intellectual understanding; boundaries; moods; saying "no"; ego function of the personality; intellectual wisdom; free will; self-confidence and self-esteem; contentment and discontent; transferences in the psychological sense; transformation of matter into energy.

Associated Organs and Organ Functions: Digestive system; transformation of the gross into the more subtle; energy metabolism; excitability; temperament; detoxification through elimination, transformation, or encapsulation; liver; stomach; the middle section of the spinal column; digestive functions of the pancreas; solar neuroplexus, autonomic nervous system; joints; tension of the muscular system; balance between the building and decomposing processes in body and mind.

Healing Experiences and Behaviors: Allowing self-confidence and systematically cultivating it by being open to the appropriate demands, legitimate praise, and constructive criticism; assuming personal responsibility; consciously making decisions and taking the appropriate actions; understanding that effortlessness is not necessarily contentment; achieving contentment through meaningful accomplishments; healthy sense of achievement; not only joyfully accepting meaningful challenges but also looking for them if they do not appear on their own; eating quietly and consciously; deliberately selecting what is to be let into our personal life and what is to be removed from it; taking inventory time and again; consciously rewarding ourselves for what has been achieved; decreasing the distance between the mind and the feelings through a conscious involvement with poetry, music, and art in general; balancing the brain hemispheres through Applied Kinesiology or Reiki techniques; chakra-balancing; attaining clarity with ourselves; not demanding more from ourselves than we can achieve; consciously choosing challenges that correspond with our own talents; and knowing and respecting our own boundaries.

Problematic Experiences and Behaviors: Not listening to our own feelings; always just remaining in the pleasant comfort zone and not allowing ourselves to be confronted or challenged; destructive, haphazard use of our will that does not consider our own true needs; wanting to achieve everything with the will; doing things for the sake of doing them without considering the meaning, purpose, and lasting effects of these actions; perceiving the questioning of our personal opinions as an attack on ourselves; not being able to tolerate criticism; lies; taking action and forming opinions on the basis of beliefs[256]; negative self-image that says we are all sinners; communicating what is not desired instead of clearly expressing

---

[256] In the narrower sense, belief is a nice name for a lie. Belief does not mean knowledge… And in the Christian churches, it is unfortunately even customary to quite consciously judge the desire for scrutiny as negative behavior and punish it, if possible. When we orient ourselves upon belief, we remain emotionally and mentally stuck at the level of a toddler.

wishes; "love" that is attached to conditions; blackmail behavior; pathological self-denial; criticizing others in a hard and uncompromising matter; being stuck in the intellect, wanting to control and evaluate everything from the perspective of the mind alone; intellectual coolness and aloofness; the fixation of wanting to analyze everything; pedantry; obsessive egoism and egocentricity; always thinking and talking in an abstract manner and abstract categories; major problem in concretely saying what we want, what we do not want, and what has happened; passive, fatalistic acceptance of occurrences: "this is how it is meant to be…, I am incapable of…, others want me to…"

4th Energy Center (Heart Chakra)

Location: About two handwidths beneath the nape of the neck (heart area). The 4th chakra radiates to the front.

Basic Polarization: Yin

Spiritual Element: Air

Functions: Love (with the expectation of also receiving love in return); tolerance; compassion; gratitude; diplomacy; harmony; the feeling of belonging to a group; empathy; romance; silent joy; oneness; family; self-love; integration of various parts of the personality; working for the benefit of family; being able to say "yes" and also mean it; meaningfully connecting the spiritual and the material.

Associated Organs and Organ Functions: Heart, lungs; endocrine portions of the pancreas; thymus gland; the body's own defense system; detoxification through storage in fatty deposits; blood circulation; arms and hands; relaxed state of the muscular system.

Healing Experiences and Behaviors: Sitting in a circle and holding hands; eating together in the circle of the family; family celebrations; doing something for the community; loving and being loved; forgiveness out of love (instead of a sense of obligation or insight); cheerful serenity in dealing with ourselves and the world; accuracy as the result of inner peace, loving surrender, and objectivity; accepting ourselves and others as they are—without the urge to want to change ourselves or the others; experiences of happiness; knowing why and what we are living for; loving ourselves in order to also be willing to love others from the abundance of our heart's power; understanding for the idiosyncrasies of other people.

Problematic Experiences and Behaviors: Sorrow; embitterment; abandoning and being abandoned by the other person, even though the relationship is still meaningful; loneliness; co-dependency; everything has to revolve around us; steadiness; committing to a relationship, even in stormy times; excessive day-dreaming; overemphasis on self-protection on all levels; inability to be down-to-earth and objective; never being able to relax because what we have or where we are at the moment is not good enough, could always be better; higher, faster, further, greater, and more beautiful; constant regret at what we believe we have missed or have actually missed; regretting time and again that we cannot be with a certain person or at another, "ideal" place; betrayal and being betrayed; being habitually non-committal; over-sensitivity; always wanting to do things that make others happy and meet their expectations.

5th Energy Center (Throat Chakra)

Location: In the body centerline at the base of the neck. The 5th chakra radiates to the front.

Basic Polarization: Yang

Spiritual Element: Ether

Functions: Individuality; the developed personality (the original); self-expression; inspiration; mental expansiveness; mental clarity and wisdom;

transformation of fear and other oppressive feelings into appropriate, constructive actions; practical creativity; communication; charisma; clairvoyance; artistic understanding and the respective talents; voice; facial expressions and gestures; inner peace (meditative calm), physic talents.

Associated Organs and Organ Functions: Vocal cords; respiratory organs; throat and nape of neck; thyroid and parathyroid gland; jaw area; mouth; teeth and gums; windpipe; neck; hypothalamus; speed of metabolism; coordination of physical and emotional/mental growth.

Healing Experiences and Behaviors: Showing ourselves with our innate potential; standing up for the truth and expressing it appropriately. A good, harmonious conversation in which all participants show who they really are and we get to the bottom of things; fairness; conducting ourselves with dignity; publicly representing an institution in a proper way; singing, dancing, sculpting, carving, painting, making music, or reciting a poem; conscious, clear communication; standing up for ourselves in front of others; deciding upon "your will be done" in the way we live our lives, which means surrender to the personal spiritual path that automatically brings us the highest degree of happiness, success, fulfillment, love, and joy; singing overtones and playing instruments rich in overtones; flexible approach to our personal creativity; continuously looking for new, beautiful forms of self-expression and refining the old ones that fit us.

Problematic Experiences and Behaviors: Far-reaching tensions between our feelings and the rational mind; showing ourselves to others in a way that is not authentic; constant rejection of our own artistic talents; not acting within our own rhythm; letting ourselves be controlled too much by others in the things we do; saying things that we do not believe; forcing ourselves to perform (or letting ourselves be forced); absent-minded behavior; withholding important information; lies; being a workaholic; not coming to rest because the activity we are engaged in does not truly satisfy us; constant fear of hurting someone else; shutting down, acting dead, not showing anything of ourselves, having a poker face; primarily carrying on conversations with empty words and clichés; always vacationing in the same place and eating at the same restaurant; not attuning the outer life circumstances to our own process of change on a regular basis.

6th Energy Center (Forehead Chakra/3rd Eye)

Location: About two fingerwidths above the root of the nose. The 6th chakra radiates to the front.

Basic Polarization: Yin

Spiritual Element: The energetic quality of the Divine Spirit that is connected with everything and yet is still aware of itself (the Light of the Universal Mind).

Functions: Perception of our own path within the cosmic context; meaningful cooperation of the body's organs and systems; the ability to find the individually appropriate place in life; intuitive, holistic thinking and insights; the transmitting and controlling of spiritual energies; creating reality through the power of thought; having visions; clairvoyance ("seeing" energies); access to Akashic Records; intuition; working for the benefit of the perceptible surrounding world; understanding our own divine power for shaping our life.

Associated Organs and Organ Functions: Eyes; ears; nose; nasal sinuses; frontal sinuses; cerebellum; control over the central nervous system; pituitary gland; memory.

Healing Experiences and Behaviors: Being able to be a witness (neutral observer); uniting feelings and mind with spiritual consciousness; consciously requesting situations and life circumstances that help advance the personal learning process in the best possible way; letting the waters of the mind come to rest in the stillness and observing what happens then; expecting nothing so that everything can happen; meditation in the narrower sense (this does not include fantasizing); creative, constructive visualization; listening to the intuition and learning to separate it from the feelings, moods, associations, and messages of the personal unconscious; becoming a member of a spiritual community or spiritual tradition; oracle work and involvement with wisdom teachings; setting out on the path and being happy without any conditions because we increasingly feel our own divinity, which means that we no longer feel we lack something or have awakened out of the illusion of deficiencies and loneliness.

Problematic Experiences and Behaviors: Not having any distance to occurrences, perceptions, feelings, and opinions; not being able to come to rest or not wanting to; wanting to cling to things, people, and experiences; always insisting on a direct exchange; always wanting more knowledge without being clear about the reason for it; being greedy and living with poverty and victim consciousness; everything must have a direct benefit; rejection of spiritual things; not having a higher goal in life beyond money, status, power, and the appeasement of fears.

7th Energy Center (Crown Chakra)

Location: Crown area and fontanel. The 7th chakra radiates upward toward heaven.

Basic Polarization: None

Spiritual Element: Spiritual existence

Functions: Integrates the states of the lower six major chakras within itself and organizes how they work together; opening for the divine; working for the benefit of the entire Creation; realizing our own divinity; oracle work; insight into the cosmic plan; natural magic (creation of constructive reality, healing, teachings without the necessary techniques, direct contact, appreciable effort, or decisions of the will; effortlessly flowing along with the current of life); free approach with karmic structures of all types, social dispositions; being completely in the here and now; supernatural abilities; being in the state of bliss (*Ânanda*); the occurrence of meaningful

593

coincidences; teachers appears to their students in lucid dreams—healing through their presence, their image, or objects blessed by them. They bring experiences of enlightenment through their presence.

Associated Organs and Organ Functions: pineal gland; skull; cerebrum.

The Light Body, Its Organs and Functions

The light body is an important part of our spiritual energy system.[257] It has a relationship to the major and secondary chakras, as well as the auric fields, but is in no way identical with them. With its extremely high-frequency structures, it forms the connecting link to what is our spiritual existence form in the narrower sense of the word. The following text explains what occurs within it.

An Overview of the Human Energy System

ॐ Nerves

ॐ Meridians

ॐ Secondary chakras and meridians/*nâdis* that connect the secondary chakras with each other and then with the major chakras.

ॐ The *major chakras* [a total of nine, beginning with the Root Chakra; above the Crown Chakra (7th) are the *Bindu* Chakra (8th) and the *Nita* Chakra (9th)]. However, the position of the latter two is just an approximation. They exist at such a high vibration that an exact determination of the positions—such as for the lower seven major chakras—is not possible. This is why they are treated and contacted through the six lower major chakras.

[257] Rainbow Reiki offers a series of special seminars that focus exclusively on work with the light body. These seminars include special initiations and the symbols and mantras taught in them, in addition to many effective techniques of spiritual energy work. Training in Rainbow Reiki Light-Body Work is available from qualified teachers throughout the world.

ॐ The *sacred mountains,* especially *Meru:* This spiritual energy structure represents a type of blueprint for our individual material existence and its spiritual meaning.

ॐ The *light body:* This spiritual energy structure mediates between our individual material existence on the one hand and our individual angelic existence on the other hand. The light body has no specific, spatially definable position. It can be reached through the aura chakras and the centers of the major chakras.

ॐ The *gates of heaven* are strongly protected accesses to our personal angel existence. They cannot be reached or passed through using just any method of energy work.

The *major chakras* constantly organize the flow of the life forces, which are directly connected with matter.

They receive their instructions and the energy flow from the level of the *sacred mountains* with the center of *Meru.*

These well-concealed spiritual structures, which cannot be located spatially, are organized in many respects to correspond with our astrological patterns in our incarnation or contain these patterns.

Yet, they also hold many types of information about our meta-incarnation process, as well as aspects of our spiritual vision in an incarnation. When we die, most of the spiritual structures connected with our material existence are stored in the sacred mountains so that they can serve as a basis in the next incarnation.

From the sacred mountains, four tremendously currents of the sacred life water flow in a variety of qualities—those of the four spiritual elements of earth, water, fire, and air—into the material existence. These are guarded by special angels, the light dragons, so that they cannot be influenced by human beings. As already mentioned, these four currents are connected—among other things—with the four elements, our astrological constitution, and the spiritual assignment that we are to fulfill in a respective existence.

The light body is connected with the spiritual center at the core of the Heart Chakra (4th), with the personal guru in the spiritual core of the

6th chakra, as well as with the flame of secret desire in the core of the 2nd chakra. It channels the non-polar energies such as Reiki.

The *light body* is constantly concerned with creating a relationship among our material and spiritual parts, structures, and needs and harmoniously balancing them. Lasting spiritual development, enlightenment, and awakening are only possible by means of a comprehensive integration of the light body.

The spiritual core structures of the 4th and 6th major chakras are nourished and protected by the divine flame of the secret desire in the spiritual core of the 2nd chakra.

There are many so-called *aura-chakras* that are not components of the human aura in the narrower sense but still influence it. These energy organs belong to the outer areas of the light body.

The Bindu Chakra and the Nita Chakra

These two chakras have a very high natural frequency. This is why they are as good as meaningless for most people in everyday life. Their themes have little in common with customary everyday life.

Some Functions of the Bindu Chakra: Understanding the truth behind the ONE and the material world, integrating this perception into everyday life in a spiritual manner; understanding the spiritual consequences of certain actions; performing magic in the divine sense through pure presence; understanding the magic of animals and their effects on nature and human beings; the ability of helping others through dreams; creating situations in everyday life that open up opportunities for spiritual healing; grasping our personal responsibility for the life net of the Goddess and learning to take the appropriate actions; opening up the access to our personal spiritual legacy; stabilizing the material body in the work with the light body and during its development.

The Functions of the Nita Chakra: Understanding how karmic burdens can be healed through everyday actions; understanding how to be connected with parallel lives and receive useful information from them;

harmoniously integrating the influences of astrological rhythms into everyday life; the direct perception of the spiritual nature of human beings, animals, and plants.

The Most Important Aura-Chakras and Their Various Functions for Healing and Personality Development

The aura-chakras are *not located at a certain place* in the aura. They constantly move in an oscillating way on the circular channels around the body. Some can be reached more easily from the front side and others from the back side of the body. The sketched positions are the so-called access zones, through which the aura-chakras can best be reached by means of energy work.

The aura-chakras are numbered from top to bottom and divided into aura-chakras in front (ACF) and aura-chakras in back (ACB).

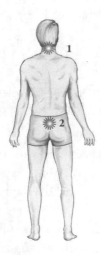

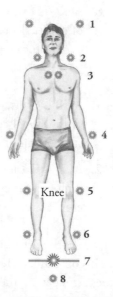

ILL. 209 – AURA-CHAKRAS BACK   ILL. 210 – AURA-CHAKRAS FRONT

Some of the important functions of the aura-chakras within this context are:

1. ACF – Direct communication with light beings.

2. ACF – Using communication in a spiritual way; integrating spiritual powers of healing in the voice and body movements.

3. ACF – Loving and embracing existence for itself; producing strong grounding; loving the polarities of life and approaching them in a spiritual manner.

4. ACF – The ability to create our own path in a magical way.

5. ACF – Connecting with spiritual teachers, living or dead.

6. ACF – Using the process of giving and taking for the promotion of spiritual development; connecting with the personal spiritual traditions of past lives.

7. ACF – Directly using the power of the Great Goddess for healing; connecting with power places and connecting them with each other.

8. ACF – Learning wisdom from Mother Earth; creating an area of spiritual protection and stability around us; being able to communicate with crystal angels.

1. ACB – Conscious control of the three major energy channels of the spinal column; connection to the divine powers of the sun and moon.

2. ACB – Creates stability when a direct encounter with strong, high-frequency spiritual powers has occurred; using sexual energy consciously for the promotion of personal development.

When we work with the aura-chakras on a regular basis, our spiritual visions become much clearer and our dedication to spiritual assignments becomes stronger. At the same time, our everyday life with its demands becomes more closely attuned to our spiritual needs and visions.

Furthermore, our powers of healing, spiritual talents in general, and ability to listen to light beings improves considerably. One very important function of the work on these energy organs is stabilizing the material body on all of its levels as a precondition for light-body work in the narrower sense.

In the light core of the 2nd chakra is the access to the divine flame of the secret desire.

In the light core of the 4th chakra is the access to a balanced oneness.

In the light core of the 6th chakra is the access to the Crystal Path.

Special Rainbow Reiki Affirmations for the Light-Body Work with the Mental-Healing Technique of the 2nd Degree

The following affirmations can be used within the scope of the mental-healing technique from the 2nd Degree of the traditional Usui Reiki in a very effective way to begin creating the preconditions for integrating our light body. For example, they can be used within the framework of a practice series by applying one of the affirmations for seven days in a row for at least 10 minutes within the scope of a mental-healing session. It is also possible to select one of the affirmations intuitively or with the pendulum to find out which affirmation is most appropriate right now.

Words of Light for Awakening Your Soul

1. *I am the pure light of the eternal flame of divine love.*

2. *Whatever may come to me and happens to me is the direct effect of the perfect love of the Creative Force.*

3. *Especially today I understand myself as a pure, divine being.*

4. *The precious jewel that I am sends brightly shining sparks of light to everything and everyone around me and within me.*

5. *Whatever happens to me is a valuable lesson in perfect love and divine wisdom.*

6. *My material existence is my prayer.*

7. *I am the One and the One is me.*

8. *No cause, no effect; no beginning, no end; no injury, no pain.*

9. *I play seriously and create joy in the way that nourishes my divine soul.*

CHAPTER 21

What Is Enlightenment and Spiritual Realization?

First, I (Walter) would like to ascertain that enlightenment is basically a natural state, as is spiritual awakening. In other words: It costs much energy, time, and creativity to not be in these states, which can lead to something the Chronic Fatigue Syndrome! The precondition for corrupting ourselves in such a way is the denial of the spiritual meaning of physical existence and its natural needs, as well as the denial of the meaning of life related to these two themes. This decision, which is usually made through social pressure in various ways—and sometimes as a result of individual traumatic experiences, results in the development of many unnatural fears, of all types of neuroses and dogma. In turn, these give rise to self-denial, a sense of guilt, shame, and repulsion at the form of the current existence given by the Creative Force.

Enlightenment and the ensuing spiritual awakening, is also a return to the original, healthy way of being that is appropriate for the nature of human beings and our path! Okay—this may sound simpler than it actually is in the practice. But this is no surprise considering that our society has already been in an extremely sick state for many centuries now. Despite this, there are feasible ways for us to once again return to our original, natural state of being.

The divine state of being is not somewhere *outside* of us. It is already present within our mind and in what we are! It absolutely permeates everything that we are! The beingness—another expression for the divine state—is within our own body. It expresses itself in every moment through the continuation of our life. Once we understand that we have already arrived, are already spiritually awakened—and that there is nothing to achieve, nothing to develop, nothing to let go of, nothing to accept, nothing to transform, and that it is very important to strive, to change, to grow, to let go of what is unsuitable, to not place attention upon our fears and tremble in dread, to love from our whole hearts, and to try to open our closed heart through forgiveness—then it is accomplished.

601

Then everything is completely new and breathtakingly different—and just as drab and ordinary as before. Before the spiritual awakening: eating, drinking, working, mastering conflicts, sleeping, loving, and striving. After the spiritual awakening: eating, drinking, working, mastering conflicts, loving, sleeping, and striving.

And yet—when we experience it, it descends upon us and bursts out of us like a landslide in the form of a delicate, translucent rainbow of unknown, fascinating colors filled with a contemplative, quiet roar. Images and poetry are required to be able to describe it a bit—but each statement about it is stifled in its triviality in comparison to the truth that we experience. And if we believe that we have consciously perceived it, it evades us with a roguish laugh and leaves us with our hands full of quickly fading, sweetly smelling smoke. The awakening is an absolutely radical change of our existence. It is as if we were turned inside out and our mind does a complete turn-about—yet, at the same time it is just the roaring silence making us so speechless that we could fill volumes with it. This is what leaves us without speech and thought. It makes us a part of the whole, less than a speck of dust, and like the Himalayas that celebrates their birth and their death at the same moment as their non-existence.

Spiritual awakening does not truly solve any of our problems or heal our neuroses; fears do not disappear and feelings do not become transformed into light—and why should they since *everything already perfectly expresses the divine.* It is so perfect that there is nothing and everything to change. The desire to change something or to change ourselves is identical with blocking the awakening and its absolutely necessary preconditions! Yet, unless the entire theme is not completely unimportant to us, we will never find the way.

If you are surprised about my approach to language here: It is not possible to express the divine of itself in a one-sided way. Strictly speaking, it cannot be communicated at all. However, the completely unnecessary attempt to smother the indescribable with words is just as important and right as the refusal to even attempt to take the whole thing seriously.

It is! I am It—It is I. "It" is called *Tat Twam Asi* in the form of an ancient Indian mantra.

The trial attempt to not judge in conversations that are intended to awaken the spiritual consciousness is doomed to failure from the start since language itself is an act of judging and can be nothing else. Yet, the attempt is helpful under certain circumstances because it show the boundaries and conquers new territory, which helps expand consciousness. Even just the attempt to have a more flexible approach to language and leave behind the accustomed valuation structures can affect much healing time and again.

Conversations during *Satsang*[258] are often held with speech patterns like those in above texts or something similar in order to attune the consciousness of the students with their beingness and promote spiritual awakening. Speaking like this in everyday life is not just strange but also nonsense—but it can also be very amusing in the company of the right people…

Sanctify what is! When it comes to doing a job or sharing an intensive, intimate experience with someone we love, it is in keeping with the

[258] *Satsanga* or *Satsang* is composed of the Sanskrit syllables *Sat*, which means "good" or "genuine," and *Sanga*, which means "contact/relations." The term basically means being together with holy (spiritually awakened) people. When we come together with a spiritual teacher, the spark of understanding the divine truth can jump from him or her to us and inspire our willingness to open up to the adventure of spiritual awakening. Spiritual teachers pass on their teachings on various levels that include language, non-language, energetic and spiritual ways. However, they primarily share their way of state of beingness with their students. Among other things, this can produce vehement physical, emotional, energetic, or mental crises. Students often spontaneously fall into a state of sleep or trance (states with very limited attentiveness), become aggressive for practically no reason at all, or become afraid. The latter occurs because the protection programs that defend the supremacy of the ego—a partial personality formed in attunement with the social environment during the childhood and teenage years—sees its "King" threatened when consciousness drinks at a true source and washes away the mud of ignorance and lack of love with the clear water of the Great Goddess so that the natural state of beingness, spiritual awakening, can emerge. Spiritual teachers hope and worry with their students, giving help that is uncompromising and individually attuned to each of them. At the same time, they speak through their behavior about various matters without being obvious to those who are not involved in the topic. Their behavior is not motivated by psychological identification with the students or because they are controlled by their helper syndrome. They are completely conscious of the fact that they are also students because they are everything and because they are the Creative Force. It may sound somewhat psychotic, but it actually works quite well.

divine truth to behave in a way that serves the situation and best does justice to its specific characteristics. Be in the world, but not of the world! We should enjoy what is, and let it go when our journey continues and it would be unhappy in our suitcase. But only then—and not from the misunderstood idea that non-attachment means never getting involved. When we do not get involved, we also cannot let go. Unfortunately, if we have not developed an ego there also will be none to transform. This means that we miss out on wonderful hours of intensive learning, both alone and with other spiritual seekers, and the intoxicating feeling of occasionally freeing ourselves from the straitjacket of the ego. Relationships make half of the Creation possible in the first place. So what could be wrong with them?

Being able to do everything, being invulnerable, and no longer having any serious challenges ahead of us makes life into one big boring yawn. This is why the Creative Force in its wisdom has also built imperfection into the material existence and every superhero in the comic book series has his or her own Achilles' heel.

Your own consciousness, which has not been formed into anything and is empty in reality, and the perceiving mind, radiant and blissful—these two are inseparable. The union of the two is the Dharmakaya state of perfect enlightenment. Your own consciousness, radiant, empty, and inseparable from the great light body, has neither birth nor death and is the unchanging light.

(paraphrased from *The Tibetan Book of the Dead*, Evans-Wentz, Oxford University Press, 1974)

As mentioned above, it is normal to be enlightened. If we sit on a park bench and look up into the sky, are "gone" for a moment without daydreaming, we *are* simply just *with everything*. This is enlightenment. Then we notice it, become afraid that this could last, and begin to think about it. But we do not realize it because we believed that it required decades of meditating like crazy and strictly resisting the cravings of the flesh in order to experience something like this. And then so easily? So that cannot be it… and what if it is?

We can also experience similar states while having sex when we are so utterly one with the desire and the beloved that we no longer think, no longer reflect, no longer feel—but are simply are immersed in bliss.

This can also happen the first time we look into the eyes of our newborn child. Or at the moment when we fall madly in love.

Or this may occur while doing some type of work that flows out of us so naturally and easily that we no longer notice that we are actually doing something. We "are" the work, become one with it, are completely connected with the theme in the process of the action. The doer and the object therefore merge into one. In modern management training, this is called the Flow State. I think this is a beautiful choice of words. It aptly points to non-attachment, the surrender to the life current and the divine order.

We may experience spiritual awakening as a result of a deep conviction that we have to do something, as a moment of totally being with our feelings, and for once not avoiding the confrontation with ourselves. It is difficult to perceive this precious state and take it seriously. It slips away from the unpracticed person even more quickly than enlightenment. We feel that it is right to embrace suffering, to truly taste it and let it enrich us, and to let our heart be opened by it. This does not mean the desire to suffer exhibited by masochists or the pseudo-philosophical indifference of the stoics. The same applies to happiness, desire, joy, and success. It means simply doing something in order to integrate these qualities within ourselves, to feel them flood through us—to integrate another facet of life, without really having the motive of gain, of being acclaimed, of becoming famous—and still embracing all of this and more because it is necessarily a part of the whole and has already been a part of us since the beginning of time.

Spiritual awakening is a paradox. The Greek word *para* means "beyond" and *dokein* is translated as "thinking," as in "logical, conceptual understanding." In order to truly understand spiritual awakening, we must move beyond thinking to another level of being and consciousness.

As the great scholar Albert Einstein, who was very interested in spiritual philosophy, so beautifully said: "Problems cannot be solved on the same level that they were created." This also applies to the problems that life places at our feet on the material level.

A beautiful story about striving for the meaning of enlightenment and spiritual awakening comes from the Greek philosopher Plato. It is called "The Allegory of the Cave."

Plato's[259] cave allegory is a very popular didactic play in philosophy classes. It can be found at the beginning of the 7th Book of the treatise *The Republic*, which the philosopher wrote in about 380 B.C.. The dialog on the allegory of the cave takes place between Plato's teacher Socrates and Glaucon, his partner in the conversation. Socrates talks about how the mental state of many people can be described as if they had had been chained since birth to the rear wall of a cave with their backs to the entrance and facing the rear wall. As a result, they can always just see the rock wall that is slightly illuminated by light penetrating from outside. So they can only perceive whatever takes place behind their backs through the diffuse shadows that the occurrences throw on the wall. Because they do not know any different, they believe that the shadows are the reality. And they insist upon this conviction even when one of them, who was able to untie himself and spend some time outside of the cave, tells them about the world beyond it. They do not believe him since they have not shared his experience.

In this allegory, the human being who was able to escape the prison of the cave represents the awakened one to the philosophers; the people chained to the cave are imprisoned by their everyday consciousness. There were and always are hefty communication problems between the two parties. Only when one who was chained to the cave also frees himself and goes outside can he truly understand the stories of the other person who was already there. *C'est la vie...*

---

[259] Plato was a Greek philosopher who was born in Athens in 427 B.C. and died in Athens in 347 B.C. He began his career as a poet, but then turned to philosophy through the influence of his teacher Socrates. He established the Academy of Athens. In his teachings, the visible world is a constant process of becoming the actual, indescribable existence.

The Rising of the Kundalinî

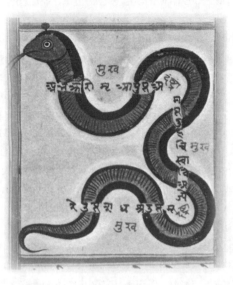

ILL. 211 – KUNDALINI DEPICTED AS A SNAKE

The word *Kundalinî* comes from the ancient Indian sacred language of Sanskrit and literally means "snake."

It is essentially the power of the Great Goddess (*Kundalinî Shakti*), usually stored as a resting potential in most people at the lower end of the spinal column. If it is awakened, it rises through the six major chakras to the seventh, the Crown Chakra and seat of Shiva, the Great God. He sleeps here as he waits for the kiss of his consort, the Great Goddess. It awakens his desire to unite with her, to conceive and bring life into the world. Since each individual is also the divine itself the Great Goddess and the Great God are present in every being as a potential. However, this fact should not be confused with teachings about partial personalities. The psychological perspective fails here because the Goddess and the God are completely independent beings and simultaneously the spiritual potential of every human being, comparable to the double nature of the light. Partial personalities do not require spiritual explanations. They are components of the human system and are neither encountered nor do they function as independent beings outside of and above it (in the astral plane).

607

Awakening the Kundalinî within the scope of spiritual personality development is possible in various ways. However, this is ultimately always related to accepting and realizing ourselves in particular and life in general in the thematic areas of each chakra in a loving and constructive way in everyday life. Meditation, yoga, Tantric practices, Qi Gong, the Reiki practice, Tai Chi, as well as simply living a life that is rich in meaning and experiences, can effect the rising of the Kundalinî. This process requires—as always applies when we walk the spiritual path—patience and perseverance, flexibility, creativity, and a prominent fun factor—for its success. Discipline, strength of will, and concentration are like the starter of a car engine—they are good to get things moving but completely unsuitable for taking a trip! This requires the engine—and this is what is fun. When we try to artificially force the Kundalinî to rise– out of fear, a drive for power or recognition, to become healthy, to be loved, to put an end to suffering, or to please someone else—through willful effort, discipline, and a systematic overloading of the 1st chakra using the respective techniques, there will be no result in the best case and a disaster in the form of serious illnesses of body and mind in the worst case.

Under certain circumstances, a rising of the Kundalinî into parts of the chakra systems can be forced for a short period of time. But I will not describe this approach here because it is truly unnecessary. The path explained above is the only one that is guaranteed to bring good and lasting results.

When the rising of the Kundalinî is forced—either through particular practices or under unfavorable circumstances such as an accident, an anesthesia shock, a traumatic experience, terrible hardships, or torture—the major chakras are usually not prepared. Their themes have not been lovingly and practically integrated into the overall personality. The Kundalinî then clears a path through these blockages on its way and the organism exerts itself in order to stop it because it has not yet learned to trust in the divine. This enormous expenditure of resources usually leads to lasting harm for the body and mind in the unhappy victims. Despite this, people who have been harmed in this way may still possess for some time much charisma and abilities (*Siddhis*) that are impressive to people without spiritual training as a result of this experience since they are extremely charged with yang energies. However, this in no way means that they have become spiritual teachers. They cannot lead anyone to the light because they are still dwelling in the darkness of ignorance and non-loving through the power of their own decisions. In addition, through the very strong, non-integrated yang energy, they are no longer centered and normally also have all types of major grounding problems. Wisdom cannot be forced but attained only through surrender to the fine vibration of the heart.

How the Kundalinî Rises

The Kundalinî rises naturally in five basically different ways, which individually obviously still have various qualities of experience inherent once we explore the details.

1. The rising of the snake force can occur in a leisurely way, over months or years and hardly perceptible in the moment. Sometimes this process is accompanied by a tingling sensation in the entire body or just parts of it and small spiritual leaps of consciousness, visionary dreams, and the slow manifestation of spiritual powers (*Siddhis*). In my opinion, this is the most pleasant path and most suitable for everyday life. It can be compared to how a plant grows, then stabilizes itself before it sends the new shoots to the sun, the great light. In this case, it is not necessary to withdraw in order to integrate the experience. This happens practically in passing. This is why I strive for this process with my students, giving them the appropriate accompaniment. In the East, this process is compared with the creeping of an ant.

2. A pleasant but considerably more dramatic rising of the Kundalinî takes place when we immerse ourselves in divine ecstasy, sometimes for a very brief time (a few minutes to several weeks). Laughter becomes our language and joy and desires our state of being. Drunken with happiness, we are very inspiring for the people around us, in as far as they are not shocked by so much charisma and such a relaxed nature. Over time, we integrate all the happiness. A spiritual teacher is recommended as a helper and companion for this process. We may not be useful for human matters for some time—except perhaps as a special type of clown—but we respond more amused than irritated

by this fact. In the East, this type of process is comparable with the happy swimming of a fish in the ocean of bliss.

3. When the Kundalinî "catches" us from one moment to the next, we must apply all of our energy for some time in order to integrate the experience, the possibilities, and the new state of being. A spiritual teacher is absolutely necessary in this case. In the East, this type of process is compared with the leap of an ape from the ground to the crown of the respective person. This can definitely bring us out of balance.

4. Another type of rising of the Kundalinî is the ascent of the snake force to one major chakra or a part of it, or to different portions of the various major chakras. Then nothing seems to happen for a while, sometimes for hours, months, or years. And then the next area of the energy system enjoys the power of the Great Goddess, followed again by a period in which everything is quiet. After each of these "Kundalinî bouts," it takes a while to meaningfully integrate what has been experienced and the awakened potential. Then it is necessary to get to know ourselves again in this new state. In the East, this process is compared with the hopping of a bird from one branch to another.

5. Last but not least, it may be that we feel a more or less even rising of the snake force over a longer period of time (weeks, but usually months or years). It flows from one energy center, from one area of the body to the next, collecting itself here and there. Sometimes it moves quickly, and sometimes more leisurely, until it has reached the crown and all five natural processes of the rising snake force have mutually triggered a fine trickling of Shiva's power from the Crown Chakra through the entire body. At first this trickling is felt clearly, perhaps like the prickling of champagne, and then it is intoxicating, electrifying, eroticizing… Later it becomes normal, but as soon as we consciously tune into ourselves, it is there again—enlivening, refreshing, enticing, and producing a state of fulfillment in the peace of being connected with the whole. In the East, this process is compared with the snake that winds back and forth through the body to the crown.

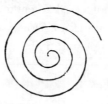

ILL. 212 – THE CREATIVE SPIRAL OF THE KUNDALINI

The healthy, natural rising of the Kundalinî brings about more or less profound experiences of enlightenment. Enlightenment is dwelling in the divine state of consciousness. This is where oneness is perceived—but strictly speaking, this is not the case: When we are far into it with our consciousness, we do not perceive it. However, whenever we are just about to attain it, to enter into this state, or to come out of it, we feel this overpowering unity, this sense of being "whole" and "one." The rising of the Kundalinî alone rarely brings about permanent enlightenment. It is usually a recurring, occasional, deliberate or even unplanned immersion in the divine consciousness—which is not consciousness in the human sense. Yes, these annoying paradoxes. In any case, this is usually quite nice…

Very intense feelings are often suddenly present. The body may assume difficult asanas (yoga postures that move spiritual energies and meaningfully organize them) and mudrâs (hand positions that move spiritual energies and meaningfully organize them) even without much effort. Various light experiences, the feeling of energy tickling or flowing through the body may take place, as well as a tension headache, a state of detached observation, a change in thought processes in the sense of slowing down or speeding up, a state of trance that is more or less deep, confusion, and changes in vision. In addition to the perceptions and states listed here, there are still many others—and all of them may just as well also be a sign of a mental disorder or physical illness! There is no inevitable connection between one of the symptoms and the rising of the Kundalinî. There is no doubt that only someone who is spiritually awakened can properly diagnose the rising of the Kundalinî. Otherwise, there are only more or less qualified speculations.

As already mentioned further above, even attaining this state does not at all mean that we have arrived. This requires spiritual awakening, the conscious, loving, and practical acceptance of all forms of existence with its possibilities and boundaries. Otherwise, the enlightened person becomes more or less incompetent in life.

The truth is understood through sudden enlightenment, but the complete realization must be practiced step by step.

(Zen proverb)

The following section discusses this proverb and how we can progress on the path!

Incidentally, it is not absolutely necessary for the Kundalinî to rise in order for us to have experiences of enlightenment. The latter can also occur without it. However, the constant—not the temporary, short lasting—state of spiritual awakening does absolutely require an ascended Kundalinî. Otherwise, the necessary balance between the everyday surroundings with their influences and experiences and this constantly equalizing spiritual light within does not exist.

Types of Experiences of Enlightenment and Awakening

Enlightenment as a One-Time Experience

As already described above, experiences of enlightenment can take place in everyday life but still not be grasped in their meaning and spiritual sense. As always in life, the quality of an experience—meaning the valuable aspects that we ultimately learn from it on the rational level, enjoy emotionally, and integrate into our personality as an enrichment—comes from the attention that we pay to it. So this is related to the intensity, the orientation, and the breadth and the depth of our perception. In addition, an essential point is the meaning that we ascribe to the experience—which is a creative act of consciousness that drives the search for meaning in order for it to be meaningful. The path to the divine ultimately results from our devotion to this search for meaning. Life not only appears to be pointless, it is definitely meaningless when we avoid the effort to make sense of what we have experienced in a way that corresponds with our special nature and our path.

It is also completely possible for an experience of enlightenment to be recognized as such—but afterward, obviously. It may be pleasant, frightening, confusing, or strange. However it may be experienced, the protection programs of the unconscious—which have been essentially imprinted during childhood by social patterns of adaptation such as: dogmas; opinions about ourselves and the world; neurotic fears; feelings of shame, guilt, and repulsion; moral rules and religious convictions intended to protect against change, in order to remain an accepted member of the family of origin and its related social reference group—will not at all like this "glimpse over the garden fence of the ego" and react appropriately. This automatic protective mechanism is more or less necessary for the child for survival. But for adults, it is crucial to be able to change these often extremely limiting ideas or be able to put them into perspective in order to become or remain healthy, happy, and holistically successful.

The protection programs must also learn to clear the way for the growth of the personality, expansion of consciousness, and the healing of neurotic feelings and patterns of adaptation. This plan requires a great deal of commitment, patience, and strength. Fears and anger, states of trance, fatigue, exhaustion, and deficient emotional motivation, as well as unpleasant physical symptoms, are just some the weapons with which the protection programs prevent progress on the spiritual path and attempt to maintain the adaptation program of childhood.

Correspondingly, the state of enlightenment—even if it has been more or less clearly recognized as such—is not necessarily accepted. On the contrary, we can usually observe an averting of whatever could produce such an experience. A client once described this type of reaction to me. She told me about a wonderful, very powerful state of enlightenment that arose during a breathing exercise. Afterward, she decided that she never wanted to experience something like that again because it was too beautiful.

Making experiences of enlightenment conscious and understandable in their meaning, requires some practice in developing the sensory and spiritual perception, as well as adequate information about this state. Once it has occurred, it is almost always absolutely necessary to work with an experienced teacher on the integration and acceptance of what has been experienced. Otherwise, the activated protection programs will prevent or strongly restrict an appropriate lasting development toward spiritual consciousness.

If enlightenment just occurs one time, its effect on the personality can become increasingly weaker after a while. Its subtle power must be carefully cultivated and spread into the mind and body, as well as everyday life, in order to have a lasting effect.

Enlightenment as a State Not Produced per Conscious Decision but Continually Occurring

In this case, there are powerful parts of our personality that exert themselves for the progress on the path to the divine. The occurrence of such processes is usually supported by the appropriate transits of planets in our horoscope that are important for spiritual development. Without the help of an experienced teacher, strong emotional and mental states of tension and psychosomatic symptoms will usually occur until the constructive integration of the experiences has been completed.

Enlightenment as a State Produced by a Conscious Decision

When we have consciously decided to accept experiences of enlightenment and learn how to integrate their meaning into our lives in a practical way, we can discover how to consciously produce this state after a transitional period that may individually range from days to years , depending upon the extent of the resistance to be overcome and the possible support from a teacher. This is an extremely important additional step in order to come closer to the divine within ourselves.

People sometimes ask me: "Sokei-an, you have experienced the transcendental world and are still there. How do you feel?" I respond: "Because I entered into the transcendental world in my twenties and have lived there ever since, I have had few experiences with the other world."

How did I enter it? I will tell you the truth: One day I wiped all of the concepts out of my mind. I gave up all desires. I put away all the words with which I thought and remained in silence. I felt somewhat strange—as if I had been carried into something or as if an unknown power had touched me. I had already been close before, and had already experienced this a number of times, but each time I shook my head and ran away from it. This time I decided to not run from it and quickly—entered it. I lost the limitations of my physical body. I still had my skin, quite obviously, but my body extended to the edge of the universe.

I walked another two, three, four yards, but I stood at the center of the cosmos. I spoke, but my words had lost their meaning. I saw people approaching me, but all of them were the same person, all of them were me! I had believed that I had been created, but now I had to change my opinion: I was never created. I am the cosmos. There is no individual Mr. Sasaki.

I went to my teacher. He looked at me and said: "Tell me about your new experience, your entering into the transcendental world." Did I respond to him? Had I said a single word, I would have left the new world that I had just entered. I looked at my teacher. He smiled. He also did not say a word... There is just one key that can open the door to the new, transcendental world. I cannot find one word in your language, but I can perhaps intimate this through two words: "radiant trance." In this clear crystallized trance we quickly enter into the transcendental world. We can enter it in one moment, and in a moment our perspective becomes completely different. Then we understand why people build churches, sing hymns, and do strange things.

(Paraphrased from *Zen Pivot: Lectures on Buddhism and Zen* by Shigetsu Sasaki Sokei-an Roshi, Weatherhill, 1998).

Enlightenment as a Constant State

In a state of lasting enlightenment, we would not be capable of living everyday lives. As explained above, the "normal" does not make any sense from the perspective of oneness and it only appears meaningful to do "nothing" because "everything" occurs on its own anyway. From this point of view, this type of consciousness is dangerous because it can become a dead end. The acceptance of accompaniment by an experienced teacher is usually the only way to prevent becoming stuck in the oneness. If we only accept half of the divine, we cannot unite with the divine. Of course, anyone who has not yet had an experience of awakening (see below) easily believes that this is "it." Outfitted with the sometimes-impressive charisma of the enlightened, this person can easily pass on the confusion to students who are even less experienced. Entire esoteric schools and venerable teaching structures have been created through the course of the millennia on the basis of these types of misunderstandings. A permanent feeling of uncertainty about turning the interpretations of experiences of enlightenment into absolutes and a constructive confrontation with everyday life in the sense of work oriented upon a practical, strenuous, and meaningful goal are some of the most important aids in this stage of spiritual development.

Spiritual Awakening as a One-Time Experience

In each of the various types of experiences of enlightenment it is basically possible—with or without conscious work and guidance by a suitable teacher—to experience a spiritual awakening. In rare cases, there is also an experience of awakening without previous enlightenment. In this case as well, the statements in the above section on "Enlightenment as a One-Time Experience" basically apply. The protection programs of the subconscious mind will dislike this state as much as that of enlightenment and attempt to appropriately block it.

Spiritual Awakening as a Recurring, but Not Consciously Producible Experience

When an experience of enlightenment results in the inner pressure that supports partial personalities that are interested in spiritual progress, situations of awakening will occur over and over again. In my experience, these will initially not be taken seriously in their meaning or even emotionally rejected. The awakening is characterized by peculiar states. We are completely human—we suffer, are happy, strive, are impatient, blocked, limited, and talented— yet, at the same time, we are simply just the witness of what is happening, the observer. And this is not a split personality and not a schizoid state in which we have no genuine access to our physical nature and our feelings. When we lack the appropriate information, mistakes can easily occur. Then the necessary recognition of the personal spiritual awakening as a precondition for an integration process obviously cannot take place.

Through the appropriate support, as explained above, we can learn in time to consciously produce the state of spiritual awakening.

Spiritual Awakening as a State that We Can Consciously Choose to Create

As soon as we have acquired the ability to consciously enter into this state, this is an excellent precondition for experimenting with it. This is important because the lasting integration of the spiritual awakening requires some creativity. In the state of enlightenment, we can hardly be part of everyday life—we simply are not of this world. In the spiritual awakening, we are "here" and "there," either at the same time or alternating between them. Those who are "not awakened" generally find it to be annoying, unintelligible, threatening, non-authentic, inhuman, cold, and irritating if we have not succeeded in finding the appropriate "interfaces," meaning socially tolerable behaviors, that make our state at least slightly bearable or—at best—acceptable.

Why do other people have a hard time dealing with those in a state of spiritual awakening? Well, the protection programs of the others feel the unbelievably intense emanation of freedom, boundlessness, and employ

617

their possibilities against others in the same way that they deal with their own state.

One of the frequently encountered effects of the presence of someone who is spiritually awakened is spontaneous fatigue, more or less deep states of trance, and fears and aggressions inappropriate to the respective situation.

The emanations of someone who is spiritually awakened are obviously very healing. But someone who is still intensely preventing themselves from being in their own divinity will tend to see them as very threatening. Each of us has the right to have our own path, as well as being however we want to be at the moment. Just as it is not in keeping with the divine order to do direct energy work with people who have not expressly requested it, it also is not correct to want to force someone who is not awakened to wake up or to not want to be responsible for the respective effects of our own personal charisma.

So even the spiritually awakened also still have a few things to learn. It may take many years for us to recognize our own awakening as such and be able to understand and accept ourselves as a result. It may take additional years for us to learn to do something truly useful with the immense potential. And the learning never ends…

After all, it is wonderful to dwell in the divine security. But how can we impart this state to others so that they recognize its importance and can easily learn to attain it? Being spiritually awakened does not make us geniuses at communication! Any advice that we give may be completely correct, true, and valuable from our perspective—but is it also acceptable and translatable under consideration of our client's existing ego structures? Reading an individual's karma and Akashic Records like the daily newspaper is sometimes very useful as an aid. However, we must find continually find ways to serve the respective person with these insights packed in appropriate portions and bite-sized pieces. Otherwise, it is very easy for stress, rejection, and misunderstandings to occur.

Many of our attitudes will be completely unintelligible to others if we do not express them in an appropriate manner. Since we are everything—everyone and nothing—and are one-hundred percent sure of this, life, suffering, death, birth, success, failure, disease, feelings, sex, relationships, partnership, friendship, time, health, play, and happiness (just to mention a few points) have a completely different, multi-dimensional meaning for us than for others. It takes a great deal of time and effort to even begin to convey this perspective to those who are not awakened, even when they would like to open up to it.

At this stage, where it becomes increasingly possible for us to deal with the state of awakening in a meaningful way, a progressive rise of the Kundalinî force can frequently be observed as well. Although it can already become active at a much earlier time, this occurs here with particular frequency. An important symptom of this can be the tremendous power that flows to us in this way. This power is extremely closely connected with the spiritual meaning that we live. It becomes available to us in an increasing degree the more we do what corresponds with our spiritual potential. This happens because the 1st major chakra (Root Center), where the Kundalinî is stored and rests in the passive state, is connected with the 6th major chakra (Third Eye). So the 6th major chakra virtually clears the path when actions of all types fit us and our aptitude and visions in the spiritual sense.

In practice, it may be that we are ill, that we feel very bad, that we are weak and exhausted but as soon as there is something to do that is closely connected with our path we can act with unbelievable energy and are alert and responsive. If the situation changes, we more or less fall back into the lethargy—the Kundalinî power is mostly gone again.

This can be annoying, but it helps greatly in orienting ourselves correctly in terms of our path. However, it usually takes a while until we learn to truly stand up for this type of energy supply and its consequences for our private lives.

The heart of the great Tao is contained in the four words: "Wu-Wei-Erh-Wei" (Not doing and yet doing.)... So the secret of the elixir for achieving this consists of attaining non-doing (Wu-Wei) through doing (Yu-Wei)... One must not skip everything and want to penetrate directly.

(paraphrased from *The Secret of the Golden Flower,* Tung-Pin Lu, Harvest/ HBJ, 1962).

Spiritual Awakening as a Constant State

If we are constantly in the divinity, then we live "our film" (our life), as I call it. This film is deeply moving and sometimes banal. It has its own rules, its special dramaturgy and actors with specific roles and character-istics. There are stories within the stories, and it is good to occasionally take the film so seriously that the divine reality steps back. Yet, we still know—at any time—just like in the "genuine" cinema that the film will be over at some point and the real life will continue. At latest in the lasting awakening, our Kundalinî will be "above"—so we will not have any energy problems as long as we act within the closer field of our vision. And when this does not fit at times—such scenes are also part of the film—then you know exactly why. It is a good life—a divine life in the truest sense of the word. In my opinion, the type of life that each of us should have is summed up beautifully in the phrase "living to the max!"

One problem can result if for some reason the spiritual awakening befalls us without any "prior notice" and a preceding process of enlighten-ment or the rising of the Kundalinî. This is also possible, although it occurs rarely—seen in terms of the statistics—and regularly. When this happens, it may be decades until we find a way to learn how to live with it in a sensible way and use the immense possibilities in a meaningful manner. This occurs much more quickly if we put our trust in a competent spiritual teacher in such a situation. Even then, getting used to this state is still a rough ride. But then we constantly receive a good orientation and the necessary support for mastering difficult processes of integration and adaptation.

Spiritual awakening is the whole of life—as the Creative Force and human being, universe and individual, speck of dust, galaxy, vacuum, and Himalayas. It is the consciously lived and applied double nature that is inherent to every being.

Summary

A spiritual experience must first happen at some point and be recognized as such by the mind and the feelings. Blockages against this experience and their consequences for everyday life, the development of the personality, and the social life must be harmonized. Ultimately, lastingly functioning life and personality structures must be set up that offer the appropriate space for the progressing integration and practical translation of the spiritual experience.

All of the above-described experiences are ultimately the same in their essence—the difference lies in the degree of depth in our resonance and the degree of truth that has been accepted per our decision and actions in our personal life and work. Light, love, and divinity all require time in order to flow through the human organism that is bound to them. Much work, care, and commitment are necessary in order to transform the structures of thinking, feeling, perceiving, acting, surrendering, and decision-making that are oriented upon deeply rooted dualistic, ego-oriented, and social adaptation patterns and habits through the divine truth. This will allow us to lead a holistic life on earth in the true sense of the word—with the recognition of every state of being!

Strictly speaking, this is obviously also not the end of the story since the life process of the individual is infinite. The same ascent will take place over and over again from a great variety of directions. Each time that it has succeeded again in a completely new way, the rejoicing of the angels and gods echoes through the wide universe. Because this one is that one, is everything, and is nothing!

The Bodhisattva Vow

When a person who is not constantly or intentionally in the state of spiritual awakening seriously takes the Bodhisattva Vow, then he or she will naturally move toward the ability (way of being) to permanently live in the state of spiritual awakeness from then on. The gist of the vow is to commitment of our own free will to help other beings who have not yet attained this state until the very last beings in the material world have realized their own divinity. This is the alternative to leaving the cycle of reincarnation and spiritualization and entering into the pure and constant spiritualization in the sense of dissolving into the Great Void of Akasha. As explained in this chapter, since Creation is unlimited in time and space and there is an infinite number of individuals, the practice of this vow means the acceptance of what is: The eternal cycle of existence.

621

So the true spiritually realized person is not the Buddha who attempts to flee from one part of the Creation into Nirvana—which is ultimately not even possible in practice—but the Bodhisattva, who understands the divine whole and has responsibly accepted it from the heart as an important part of Creation.

The Ego

Time and again, people talk about how the ego is detrimental to spiritual development and must be dissolved, transformed, or destroyed. The bad news is that we cannot live without the ego. The good news is that seen in spiritual terms, there is no problem with the ego because it does not even exist!

So let's take a closer look at this matter.

The story of our life—our past life—is ultimately a burden as long as we identify with what we have experienced, in the sense of: I am what I have experienced. As long as we, just as we are today, see ourselves as a type of product of past occurrences, influences from the outside, of our genetic make-up, and social and karmic dispositions[260], we cannot realize our divinity. This is because the Creative Force is free! It cannot be trained or forced by "society" to achieve things that it does not at all want to do.

The ego develops through an identification with what we experience and the desire for us to deal with it in a way that is successful for us. It is a part of our "operating system" that should and can more or less facilitate

---

260   Karma: The law of cause and effect. If we do something, it has consequences. On the one hand, this is true. But on the other hand—think of the double nature of existence. Time and again, there are situations where we decide anew, where we can drop out of the karmic loop. We do not constantly have to suffer from the decisions of our past. The more we accept our divinity, the more we will be freed from karma. However, karma also has many advantages. For example, through karmic structures, we can reliably and without much reflection clarify the important questions for our development and have experiences with the consequences of our actions, let our personality mature, and give ourselves wisdom when we approach it in the correct way. In addition, there is also quite definitely positive karma—in the direct sense of nourishing, supportive influences from our deeds in the past.

automatically coping with the challenges that we face because of life in a society with certain dogmas, opinions, and rules, as well as existence in general within the material world, together with its restrictions, practical necessities, our individual needs, weaknesses, and strengths. The role that the ego assumes for us—more or less successfully depending on the level of development—is how we can best get along with the people around us who represent society per se to us: how we assert the fulfillment of our needs against the resistance of limited resources and the demands of others, conceal and protect our weakness, draw so much attention to our talents and successes that others consider us as a partner for their projects and secure our existence and help extend our resources as a result.

The ego is an interface of the soul with the respective environment. It must change when the life situation has changed. As an aid of the soul, the ego must orient itself upon it and its wishes.

So far, so good! However, in order to attain a better understanding of our true being, we should identify with our ego and its many masks, judgments, fears, and programs for greed and worry. It is important to learn to use the ego as an aid and advisor in dealing meaningfully with the appropriate themes. For example, if a guru does not have a well-functioning ego, he will one day be the only one left in his ashram. If he spends the whole day without any interest in self-promotion and marketing (even though there is certainly a tremendous range of possibilities for doing this), potential students will not even know that he exists. His teachings will not be spread if he does not hold public speeches and does not publish anything so people go to others who do not shy away from making themselves well-known. An example of this are the enormous marketing efforts by Lao Tse, Osho, Satya Sai Baba, Yogananda, Rudolf Steiner, Confucius, Jesus, Gautama Buddha, Mohammed, and the Sufis. No matter what we call it, the function of public-relations work is marketing. The ego is responsible for this—this is its domain. However, this also entails a major problem that must continuously be coped with anew. A busy ego that is intensively integrated into everyday life comes up time and again with the idea that it is terribly important and actually the one that can and should master the shaping of life. Nothing is more wrong than this! The ego is solely a tool. If it gets out of control, it must be thoroughly

623

cut down to size. If it begins to do things in order to justify its fears, greed, worries, and its other motives instead of serving the purpose, the personal responsibility, the development of consciousness, the love, and the personal manifestation of the divine plan, it must be rigorously called to order and its activity once again oriented upon the genuine spiritual goals. Otherwise, we will sink in the mire of our own grand delusions. And that can happen *to any of us at any time.*

Why am I emphasizing this so strongly? There are a great many ideas about how people who are enlightened and spiritually awakened should be. For example: They are never sick, always nice, always successful, always loving, devoid of certain feelings (anger, sorrow, sexual desire, etc.), they understand everything, always have the right answer, never have weight problems, everyone likes them, they have nothing more to learn and if they do, it just costs them a snap of their fingers at best. They can immediately heal anyone of any disease and solve any problem on the spot. They know everything and do not need a partner—but if they have one, their partnership is always completely harmonious. They never have money problems or legal difficulties, and they are always well-rested…

This should be quite clear by now. Nothing on this list corresponds with the facts, as a quick look through the biographies of such people will affirm. Despite this, these types of ideals are still stubbornly upheld in the circles of people with esoteric interests. All of us can have every single problem as long as we live because as long as we are in the physical form, we also have something to learn. So even gurus keep learning—for example, how to be a guru, but certainly not just that. The ego is always present in a human being. It must be because this is how we can appropriately adapt to our individual experience and our life. This enables important learning processes, without which a distinct individuality would not be possible.

Incidentally, the basis of the ego is the free will. As a result of it, each of us shapes our path in a way completely different from the others—it is individual and therefore unmistakable. See above for the extra section that has already been included on this topic.

The ego is always present and is needed more sometimes and less at other times. It must be employed differently time and again because of our constantly changing and transforming life. Consequently, it may well be that the previously reliable control mechanisms—which ensure that the ego serves the divine purpose and its related themes instead of setting itself up as the ruler—suddenly are no longer effective. Then more development is once again required and the creative part of the personality must find new, safe, and meaningful ways to integrate the ego into the overall personality. For example, someone who says: "I have completely transformed my ego!" has just been taken for quite a ride by it. As I mentioned, this can happen to any of us at some point.

An important blockage created by the ego is clinging to certain memories. We once experienced something wonderful and now long so much to "have" it again! Unfortunately, this is impossible. We can never enter into the same river twice and never truly experience the same delights in the same way twice. However, as long as we do not truly want to understand this, the path to happiness available at any time in the here and now is completely blocked. We do not want the chocolate that life holds directly in front of our mouth because we insist upon having exactly the same one we had last night for dessert. That is not possible because we already ate it, which made it change as a result—and we have also changed in the meantime. We have both been changed through the relationship that we entered into with each other. If our paths crossed again, it may be that we no longer have any direct interest in each other...

The same applies to bad memories. If anything that could possibly remind us of bad experiences causes us to endlessly talk about them, we are extending the horror of the past and make it into the constant present. We produce similar unpleasant feelings and spread a negative energy similar to the one present within us and around us during the situation at that time. Instead of gladly noticing that things are so much better now, we think about what is equally bad in the present situation—or could become as bad. And then the joy in the here and now is long gone. Not because there is only suffering in our material existence but because we prefer our inner tragedy to the comedy available in the outside world.

The same also applies to not wanting to forgive. We are guaranteed to be the only ones suffering from our own hatred! Not wanting to forgive is one of the strongest blockages in the Heart Chakra.

The more time we spend in the dreamland of our fantasies and look at the shimmering soap bubbles, the less we can arrange the present so that it suits us—and the less we can enjoy the fruits of our life, letting them enrich us and motivate us anew. Why does the ego do this? Well, it attempts to protect us against what was in the past and it wants to fulfill our needs. But since it is a program, its possibilities for evaluating a situation are quite limited. The ego is also anything but wise. This is why it is advisable for us to take care of our mental health time and again and not let ourselves be taken for a loop by the screaming of the ego. Nothing tastes flatter than the champagne that was opened yesterday. And the fact that we were scared stiff ten years ago does not help us create a greater sense of security and more happiness today.[261]

The ego likes to fashion masks in order to have interfaces with other people—and their masks!. It also likes to talk about itself, what it believes it must be in order to be liked, perhaps even feared, admired, loved[262], desired, and respected. If we are not clear about the true function of our egos and restrain it when necessary, then we will believe at some point that *we are this mask*. If we think that we have to be a number of masks in order to survive, then the result is a large amount of conspicuous incongruence, inner tensions, stress, and psychosomatic complaints. In very severe cases, this can lead to one form or the other of a split personality. Above all, this can happen when our true identity powerfully strives for liberation from the constraints imposed by the ego. Examples of this may be living our sexuality in a truly pleasurable and loving way, relaxing lazily once in a while, or even allowing ourselves to get really mad on occasion.

Another very unpleasant thing also occurs quite frequently: When we identify with our mask and fall in love with someone else's mask—and vice versa—then two Punch and Judy figures are interacting instead of two living people. If we wake up at some point and learn to look behind our partner's mask and possibly even truly love what we see, this beautiful feeling that is absolutely important for the mutual path may be experienced as an existential threat by the person who is still confusing the mask with

---

[261] For those who would like to translate these insights in a practical way and free themselves of the corresponding problems: Other chapters of this book contain many appropriate techniques and methods for this purpose. In addition, the Bibliography includes many Reiki self-help books. When used in a knowledgeable way, the Usui System of Natural Healing has quite a bit to offer…

[262] Or what it considers this to be!

the ego. Fear and anger are stirred up and the beloved begins to engage in a battle against the truth that the state of being loved attempts to create. This is very sad—and it occurs so frequently.

And all of this happens just because of something that does not exist in reality. The ego is a working model, a little program on the hard disk of the PC (physical existence) that serves our soul. The ego is a figure of speech, an abstract concept in order to make certain behaviors more easily understandable. When we attempt to transform it, to delete it and get rid of it, we are assuming that the ego *actually exists.* And this means that we subject ourselves to it! It is simply just one of our ideas. If we think differently, then it changes automatically. The idea should not be confused with the brain.

We are actually the Creative Force—everything and nothing. We are the great magicians who perfectly create three universes before breakfast. When we accept ourselves and use our ego meaningfully, we can amuse ourselves after breakfast with the exciting game of "The Adventure of Being Human: The One Who Set Out to Love and to Learn!".

CHAPTER 22

Integrating Spiritual Experiences

This book provides information on how to create a close contact with the strong spiritual forces and extremely powerful and wise light beings who are connected with the spiritual life energy (Reiki) and the mystical tradition of the Usui Reiki System. In a much closer way than is possible with just the Reiki distant contacts, the meditations and other advanced techniques found here can guide us into the direct radiance, the personal light circle of the angels and deities.

All occupants of the spiritual spheres are filled with love for the other children of the Creative Force. They endeavor to help where they can and where it is permitted according to the rules of the Divine Order in order to make learning, love, and joy possible and create space for consciousness, meaning, and a self-determined life that serves the whole. Spiritual force fields and energies are the origins and regulators of the life forces that are at work on the material plane. On the basis of their state of existence, light beings can never be against life in thoughts or actions or be or do evil.[263]

And especially because the forces and beings of the spiritual realm are so uncompromisingly for liveliness, naturalness, and love, many people become very stressed and even frightened when they encounter them directly! Human beings make so many compromises—and many of these tend to be the lazy type! Human beings deny themselves so often—their physical nature, their true feelings and needs, their wonderful dreams and visions in which the divinity of our own soul is reflected like the sun on the ocean in the morning—shimmering and full of promise.[264]

Do we actually let our sun rise, radiant and proud?

Do we have the courage to develop our very own magical spells, spread our wings, and float toward the realization of our own potential

---

[263] Extensive explanations on this topic can be found in the chapter on Spiritual Cosmology.

[264] Incidentally, this is also the image from which the middle portion of the Master Symbol DKM was developed.

on the pinions of light and love with a happy heart—and do this even when so many other people see this as "dumb" and "crazy"? And do this even if there may be disappointments at some point on this path and the illusions burst like old soap bubbles?

It is very, very rare that we truly wake up completely from the dream of being a more or less isolated individual existing in total dependency upon the material world. The same applies to individuals who have been completely "normal" up to now and discover themselves with awe, completely accepting themselves with a happy smile. Of course, increasingly more people in our age are succeeding at finding this path that is really very apparent and yet so difficult to discover, and more than a few have risked the first steps. Yet, there are also extremely powerful countermovements from politics, culture, science, profession, family, education, and the dogmatic dogmas of the patriarchal religion. So it is not surprising when fear and sadness, anger and fright rise up within some people who directly encounter the light beings and experience their message of the divine truth within their own hearts. Then there would be so much to change. So much of the wisdom of the divine world stands in a crass contradiction to what we have experienced and learned in the parental home, everyday life, school, and our circle of friends. At the same time, the wonders that were seen can feed the ego if they are not correctly understood, not critically scrutinized in terms of what has reached consciousness. It is so easy to just leave out of the message what does not fit in with our self-image and view of life, then interpret the rest so that no problematic questions arise. This rarely occurs on a conscious level—in most cases this is an action taken by the powerful protection programs of the unconscious mind. These protection programs have the task of protecting against changes in learned behaviors and habits of thinking, feeling, and evaluating. Although this may be very important in childhood in order to become an accepted member of our respective family and the related social groups, at the latest with the onset of adulthood (puberty), a "major overhaul" of these programs becomes necessary so that we can truly build our own life instead of missing out on who we are, our happiness, and the unique potential that the Creative Force has given us at birth by living according to a more or less copied structure of our childhood situation. However, this important reorientation frequently just takes place in a partial, incomplete way because our outer and inner obstacles are too great and there is too little support in this situation. Then it remains up to the consciousness to recognize the ballast as such and learn to replace it with something more meaningful.

Among other things, important aids in this process can be seminars on personality development, appropriate literature, spiritual training courses, holistic psychotherapies, and meditation. And, obviously, close encounters with the light beings, who have already changed many lives in a thorough and lasting way—including my own.

The reason why direct contacts with spiritual creatures and forces can shake us up, confuse us, frighten us, or draw us into fascinating illusions when they are not used constructively is the resulting inner conflict, the clash between the ideas about the world and ourselves that we have learned in childhood and youth on the one hand and the influence of the light beings that is oriented upon pure liveliness, love, and naturalness on the other hand. In addition, the ego likes to get involved and attempts to avoid the collision with the truth and establish itself as our ruler.

The reactions triggered in the narrower sense by the spiritual experiences may relate to any of our levels and quite possibly also to more than one at the same time. Symptoms such as stomach cramps, headache, fatigue, fever, confusion, heart problems, shortness of breath, involuntary movements, panic attacks, fits of rage, and much more can be observed in the practice.[265]

Yet, if the conscious mind understands the situation, we can take simple countermeasures to quickly end the rearguard actions of the ego and the protective programs and harmonize their effects. *The symptoms do not indicate any problems that have been created through the encounter with spiritual beings and forces*, and also not the influence of "dark powers" or "negative energies," but just our struggles with the decision of wanting to enter into our divine legacy or continue to want to listen to the opinion of "society" and slavishly orient ourselves upon it.

From the experiences that I have had in my work with people striving for the divine, I (Walter) have summarized themes in this chapter that

---

[265] These obviously also includes relaxation, vitalization, feelings of happiness, and the like. But I think these symptoms are quite welcome.

occur quite frequently and cause problems, as well as what has proved to be truly effective for harmonizing them. The advice explained in this chapter not only saves us from having many unnecessary problems on our path to light and love, but can also allow us to provide some valuable help to our friends. When it is correctly prepared, the contact with spiritual beings and forces is something that is unbelievably enriching, deeply filled with happiness, that can change an entire life in a very positive way. It allows us to make the best out of our spiritual experiences. I wish you much joy with these experiences and with the tips explained in the following section.

A Reality Check

In my opinion, this is the most important advice: When we have an impressive, deeply touching spiritual experience, it is best to think about it in a thorough and, above all, very objective way, even if this is difficult. It is good to mediate on what we have experienced, speak with a qualified adviser or knowledgeable friend in order to separate illusion from reality and learn to differentiate between what can change our life for the better and the fog of feelings, memories, moral judgment and associations that may have been triggered.

Here are some questions we can use: What really happened? What are the useful aspects that I can use for my everyday life? How else can I understand what the experience might mean? Which literature, which competent adviser, which spiritual practice, which oracle (such as the *I Ching*, Tarot, *Chakra Energy Cards*, runes) could help me understand the experience in the clearest possible way and translate it into action for my path in the most meaningful way? Which risks could result for me if I translate the experience into action in the way that I now understand it?

These are important questions from my counseling practice that, I hope, can help anyone make the best out of a spiritual experience and avoid getting lost in illusions and destructive feelings.

When in doubt, I like to use oracles. They are the ideal uninvolved observers.

Grounding

After intensive spiritual experiences, thorough grounding is essentially important and helpful for essentially two reasons.

ॐ On the one hand, the energetic state of a human being is sometimes greatly shifted into the yang area through strong spiritual influences. But this is no surprise! After all, the greatest proximity to the spiritual is also found in this energy quality. The spiritual, heavenly per se is called *Tai Yang* in Chinese—the Great Yang. However, we tend to live in a more yin-oriented world and must attune ourselves to this once again after a profound spiritual experience in order to cope with our lives in the everyday world. The organism often succeeds in doing this quite well within a relatively brief amount of time (up to an hour) without any additional help. Yet, there are also many cases in which a person's energy would require many days or longer to accomplish the necessary switch to the natural life surroundings, the material world, without support.

ॐ On the other hand, many blockages are dissolved and their components should then be eliminated from the organism as soon as possible.

When used in a skilled way, Reiki is very good at helping in both of these situations.

In order to ground ourselves with Reiki, we should treat the front area of *the sole of the foot up to and including the middle of the foot* through the laying-on of hands or within the scope of a distant treatment. Those who are initiated into the 2nd Degree can additionally use several intensification symbols at these positions.

Healing stones that are very effective in supporting grounding are:

ॐ *Black tourmaline* (schorl). This can be placed under our hands when we treat the soles of the feet or at the coccyx. It very effectively draws off excessive energy, promotes a serene, unbiased mental attitude, and harmonizes negative thoughts and stress.

🕉 The *onyx* can be applied in the same positions as the tourmaline. The onyx helps greatly in not staying stuck in our feelings and not becoming overly active. It stimulates circumspection and discipline and imparts the pleasant feeling of standing on solid ground again.

🕉 The *hawk's eye* helps in getting to the bottom of the spiritual experience with the mind and feelings. It makes us serene and relaxed, helping us in the process to perceive the larger contexts. It works against dogmatic perspectives and judgments. It can be placed at the 1st major chakra, at the crotch, or held in the left hand.

🕉 *Petrified wood* also puts us back on solid ground and has a calming effect.

Bach Flowers that support grounding after intensive spiritual experiences are:

🕉 *Walnut* (strengthens the sense of identity and self-awareness);

🕉 *Crab Apple* (supports energetic and emotional purification);

🕉 *Clematis* (falling back to earth from the dream world of the illusions);

🕉 *Aspen* (to diffuse fears that have been triggered by what has been experienced).

A preceding Reiki treatment of the client's knees and ankles is often important since all types of life energies can easily become congested in these areas of the body and cause treatments on the soles of the feet to become less effective. When Reiki is given on the soles of the feet, the forces and information that are not appropriate for the body can flow out of it more easily. These are easily dissolved from the blockages through the intensive spiritual experiences because of the related increase in the vibrations of life energies if they had been previously "frozen" due to various types of trauma and blocked the material and the energetic metabolism. Through the energetic grounding with Reiki, symptoms that were produced by the dissolved disharmonious powers quickly disappear. In relation to grounding, an additional stabilizing measure is important...

Centering: The 3rd Chakra and the Hara

The 3rd chakra (Solar Plexus) is located in the stomach area about two fingerwidths beneath the sternum. This is where all of the information that flows into us from the outside, as well as the information that is released from our various parts such as memories, associations, perceptions of mood and the state of the body, is processed, classified, and translated into meaningful decisions of some form or another. This occurs both consciously and also, to a much larger degree, unconsciously through the so-called mental level.

The Hara is the energetic, psychic, and mechanical center of the body. Directing the attention of our consciousness to the Hara, which is located about two fingerwidths beneath the navel and somewhat on the inside of the body, creates calmness, energy, an expansion of consciousness, and inner peace.

We can direct our breath to it with the help of our imagination and give ourselves additional Reiki there. Little pauses between each inhale and exhale let us feel the energy.

The 3rd chakra can be strengthened and developed by giving it Reiki on a regular basis. Those initiated into the 2nd Degree can obviously also use the CR Symbol to intensify the flow of Reiki. In addition, the following healing stones are especially helpful if they are placed under the hands when treating the 3rd chakra:

> ॐ *Smoky quartz* is very de-stressing and relieves tension: When used regularly, it reduces the tendency of becoming stressed. Lets us become more resilient and helps overcome inner and outer resistance. It strengthens the nerves and is good for harmonizing the harmful effects of electro smog, which very much burdens the 3rd chakra.

ॐ *Citrine* is generally strengthening for the 3rd chakra. It improves the ability to set boundaries, increases self-confidence, strengthens the will to live, brightens the mood, and has an anti-depressive effect. It is good for the nerves, stomach, spleen, and pancreas. It improves digestion and helps against diabetes in the beginning stage.

ॐ *Lepidolite* has a healing and harmonizing effect on all types of trauma. It protects us against being influenced by the outside world, supports independence, self-discipline, actions based on personal responsibility, and making success possible through our own power.

ॐ *Aragonite* is the stone per se for development of the 3rd chakra. It stabilizes development processes on the mental-emotional level that occur too quickly. It works against excessive demands and disjointedness, promotes concentration, and has a calming effect.

ॐ *Amber* can be used when the disharmonies of the 3rd chakra tend to occur in the physical organs related to this energy center: the stomach, spleen, liver, and gallbladder.

Finding the Meaning

A genuine spiritual experience always has a practical meaning—something good that can clearly changes our everyday life for the better in some way. The process that is necessary to dig up this treasure is like washing gold: We sift through vast amounts of sand in the hopes of finding a few nuggets. However, in spiritual experiences it is guaranteed that we will discover something big, important, and very valuable for us.

The meaning is not always directly accessible to the objective mind. The wise teachings are frequently related to our emotional life in some way. Or the meaning may only become completely clear in the future. As always—each spiritual experience is somehow related to everyday life. When we truly make an effort to discover the meaning, we will find it. So we should never give up on it! Without our understanding of it, a spiri-

635

tual experience cannot do much for us: The path is the goal! When we forge ahead toward a clear understanding of a spiritual experience, every bit of progress is a victory. In my experience, deeply profound messages often require ten years or more. During that time, I continually come to understand and learn to use something important and useful from the message.

Healing Fears

In the context of intense spiritual experiences, fears often occur. For example, these may regard being threatened by "evil powers" or "negative energies." There is no devil, there are no fallen angels, nor any other astral creatures that want to do evil. The beings that are close to the Creative Force in the state of oneness have considerably more magical powers than human beings. But at the same time, their free will is limited because the closeness to the source of life, love, and oneness means that they are also more directly oriented upon these qualities. So we must take responsibility for whatever relates to us and take actions to master our problems step by step. In this way, the fear will also pass because we prove in practical terms that we are not helpless.

The Reiki mental-healing technique of the 2nd Degree can, in addition to the techniques of energy work explained in other sections of this book, be a very effective aid in harmonizing fears.

Translating Spiritual Experiences into Everyday Life

Spiritual experiences of any type must always be unconditionally translated into everyday life in a practical way. As already explained extensively in the chapter on Spiritual Cosmology, the material existence in individual form is very important from the divine perspective. Teachings and healing that are given to the occupants of the material world from the light beings, the servants of the Creative Force have the intention of not letting them forget their divine legacy. Instead, we should learn to deal with the demands of the material world in an increasingly better spiritual way and follow our vision and our very own spiritual path, develop our potential, be more and more in our hearts and dwell in love, and use the source of the joys that are here in great abundance for ourselves. And all of this in everyday life! This is the true path and the genuine challenge—not the secluded meditation alone in a remote cave somewhere in the Himalayas.

Since each of us here will die in any case[266], it is certainly not a problem to return back to the light worlds. We all have a round-trip ticket. A considerably greater challenge consists of walking our path in a meaningful way in this world according to the rules of the divine order, developing ourselves freely and simultaneously for the benefit of all, being happy, and spreading happiness.

Standing Up for Our Feelings and Not Letting Ourselves Be Ruled by Them

Strong feelings are often triggered by spiritual experiences. When we can cope with these dynamic energies, there are many useful things we can do with them. The following section is a brief explanation of how this works.

Our true feelings are part of our own truth. They are here and now—and can quickly change under the right conditions. Our feelings cannot and should not be the dictators of our life. And it is useful to learn to differentiate between genuine feelings and moods that we have been trained to have (secondary feelings). In the course of our childhood, we learn to show emotion-like reactions to which our social environment responds with positive feedback. These are the feelings that we should not orient ourselves upon—because they are not connected with our truth. Our true feelings are powerful, spontaneous, and cannot be continuously activated by similar stimuli like the secondary feelings—like a button that is pushed.

When we direct our attention to something, we will emotionally respond to it within a short period of time—always! This is also good

---

[266] One of the few things that can be guaranteed one-hundred percent in this world.

because the genuine feelings are intended to make the right type and amount of action energy available for the successful mastering of a present situation. And this comes out of the feelings, also called emotions, a word that is based upon the Latin word *exmovere*—which means to move out of something.

We are also not at the mercy of our feelings. When we assume responsibility for them and consciously focus our attention on the positive whenever this makes sense, we will soon feel an appropriate fundamental mood within ourselves. And this makes life worth living in the first place. It certainly is worth giving it a try.

Mental Healing and the Integration of Spiritual Experiences

The following affirmations are very useful within the scope of the Reiki mental-healing technique of the 2nd Degree for the constructive integration of spiritual experiences. They are especially effective when a selected affirmation is used up to two times a day for respective period of about 15 minutes each by means of mental healing.

1. *Everything that I am, is beautiful, true, and good.*

2. *My subconscious mind helps me in every moment of my life with all of its powers to be happy, healthy, and successful and serve the whole as a result.*

3. *Everything that enters into my consciousness is an important message of light and love and I will understand and put it into practice use at the right moment in the best possible way.*

4. *All of the energies that I do not require at this time will now collect in my Hara and are available to me when I need them.*

5. *I lovingly perceive myself, forgive myself for my mistakes, and praise myself for my successes.*

6. *Love and wisdom, feeling and mind, body and spirit come together within me in a harmony.*

7. *The power of my body follows the wisdom of my heart.*

8. *My mind opens itself widely for the love and wisdom of the Creative Force and its messengers.*

9. *With the desire of my body, I experience oneness with the divine.*

10. *I playfully follow the inspiration of my spiritual guides and spread goodness within me and around me.*

11. *Love permeates my entire being. Love is my whole existence.*

APPENDIX

Commentated Bibliography

The Complete Reiki Handbook by Walter Lübeck, Lotus Press/Shangri-La. Translated by Wilfried Huchzermeyer.

Comprehensive instructions for the practice of Reiki healing with a very extensive list of the special positions, notes about Reiki and medications, Reiki meditation, gemstone work, and aromatherapy. The focus of the book is on traditional hands-on healing. The chakra work with Reiki is precisely explained in theory and practice.

Reiki—Way of the Heart by Walter Lübeck, Lotus Press/Shangri-La. Translated by Christine M. Grimm.

Extensively describes the three degrees of the traditional Usui System, its spiritual meaning, the path of the Master, Reiki history, and special practices for supporting personality development with Reiki. Also explores the significance of Usui's Principles for the Reiki practice and everyday life, the Usui's birth chart, and Reiki Resonance Therapy.

Rainbow Reiki by Walter Lübeck, Lotus Press/Shangri-La. Translated by Christine M. Grimm.

Rainbow Reiki is an expansion of the Usui System the Natural Healing. Walter Lübeck has spent years thoroughly researching the possibilities of the three Reiki degrees and combined them with the thousand-year-old HUNA teachings and shamanic wisdom. This has created a complex system of highly developed energy work, based upon the traditional Reiki methods. Aura and chakra work with Reiki to achieve the highest level of effectiveness, power-place work, channeling, astral travels, journeys through time, crystal work, Reiki essences and energetic plant remedies—*Rainbow Reiki* opens the doors to a true wonderland for anyone traditionally initiated into Reiki.

The Pendulum Healing Handbook by Walter Lübeck, Lotus Press/Shangri-La. Translated by Christine M. Grimm.

Instructions on using the pendulum for both laypeople and pros. Includes an extensive collection of pendulum tables that are arranged in a type of oracle system so they can be consulted for holistically diagnosing deficiencies in the sense of well-being. Harmonizing remedies such as flower essences, aromas, and healing stones can also be determined.

The Aura Healing Handbook by Walter Lübeck, Lotus Press/Shangri-La. Translated by Christine M. Grimm. Precise instructions for perceiving and reading the auric and chakra fields. Additionally includes an extensive chapter on the human subtle energy system containing much valuable information.

The Chakra Energy Cards by Walter Lübeck, Lotus Press/Shangri-La. Translated by Christine M. Grimm.

This set of 126 specially designed affirmation cards is coordinated with the major and secondary chakras, as well as the four main fields of the aura. They can be used alone for holistic personality development, as well as in combination with Reiki and the Bach Flowers, healing stones, and aroma essences that are associated with each affirmation. The book explains all of the classifications in relation to their effects, with exact descriptions of their applications in individual chapters. The healing symbols of the Great Goddess and her angels are on each of the affirmation cards. These healing symbols can be used to easily make 126 highly effective spiritual essences and chakra oils in any desired amount. A special chapter provides an exact explanation of how to effectively do Feng Shui work for houses, apartments, and gardens with *The Chakra Energy Cards*. Dozens of well-test examples of questions provide valuable suggestions. The 126 affirmations are especially suitable for the Mental-Healing Technique of the 2nd Reiki Degree.

The Spirit of Reiki by Walter Lübeck/Frank Arjava Petter/William L. Rand, Lotus Press/Shangri-La. Chapters by Lübeck and Petter translated by Christine M. Grimm.

An extensive depiction of traditional Reiki according to Usui that includes precisely researched biographical information on Dr. Mikao Usui, Dr. Chujiro Hayashi, and Hawayo Takata. This book presents the classic treatment methods of Usui and Hayashi, the original Principles, the spiritual teacher-student relationship in Reiki, explanations on the Reiki symbols, the whole-body treatment with Reiki, and much more.

Reiki—Best Practices by Walter Lübeck/Frank Arjava Petter, Lotus Press/Shangri-La. Translated by Christine M. Grimm.

This book provides a multitude of Reiki techniques, some of which are published for the first time, with precise explanations for all degrees. Good suggestions for the treatment practice.

Reiki for First Aid by Walter Lübeck, Lotus Press/Shangri-La. Translated by Samsara Amato-Duex and Christine M. Grimm.

More than 40 different complex treatment techniques focused on specific health disorders are presented in this book. It also includes how to use healing stones, food supplements, and home remedies. The extensive atlas of the reflex zones supports the development of individual special positions. Other topics covered are comprehensive explanations on a healthier diet through the Reiki cure, well-tested tips on removing scars. and a description of the role water plays in maintaining good health.

The Original Reiki Handbook of Dr. Mikao Usui (edited by Frank Arjava Petter), Lotus Press/Shangri-La. Translated by Christine M. Grimm.

This is the knowledgably commented and beautifully illustrated seminar manual that Dr. Usui, the founder of the Reiki System, gave to his students. A must for every friend of Reiki.

Reiki Fire by Frank Arjava Petter, Lotus Press/Shangri-La.

This is the first book my friend Arjava wrote describing his discoveries about the teaching and life of the founder of the Reiki tradition of healing.

Reiki—The Legacy of Dr. Usui by Frank Arjava Petter, Lotus Press/Shangri-La. Translated by Christine M. Grimm.

Further discoveries about the life and work of Usui and Hayashi. In my opinion, both books are a must for friends of Reiki in order to truly understand the Usui System of Natural Healing. In addition, this book clarifies many confusions and delusions that arose in the time before there were reports directly from Japan on the origins of the Reiki System.

Sacred Calligraphy of the East by John Stevens, Shambala Pbl. (Boston & London).

A beautifully illustrated book on the spiritual calligraphy of Asia. It includes many important and hard-to-find details from the Asian treasure-chest of wisdom.

Mastering Your Hidden Self by Serge King, Quest Books.

Another book by a modern author on HUNA. S. King is a psychologist, has completed his training in NLP, and learned HUNA as a young man in a family tradition. Important insights into the human unconscious and many practical ideas for applying HUNA methods in everyday life make *Mastering Your Hidden Self* a useful companion on the individual path.

The Roots of Coincidence by Arthur Koestler, Vintage.

A high-quality marriage of modern scientific perceptions and spiritual knowledge takes place in this excellent book. Anyone who still believes that science and esotericism are mutually exclusive should take the time to study this informative tome.

Synchronicity by F. David Peat, Bantam.

The phenomenon of the meaningful meeting of occurrences that are not causally connected is explained and provided with many examples. This is also well-suited for providing background information on the topics of "oracles" and "subtle perception."

In Search of Schrodinger's Cat: Quantum Physics and Reality by John Gribbin, Bantam.

This summary of the history of quantum physic is exciting reading that is very well researched and full of surprises. In addition to the scientific aspect, I was especially captivated by the biographies of the scientists, the deeply human side of great genius. Many good things can be learned here as well.

The Character of Physical Law by Richard P. Feynman, Modern Library.

A professional describes the nature of physical laws to laypeople. After I read this book, I knew that physics can also be explained in an exciting way. I hope that this will become required reading for schoolteachers and university lecturers.

QED—The Strange Theory of Light and Matter by Richard P. Feynman, Princeton University Press.

The man who is probably the most significant theoretical physicist of the 20th Century explains his trailblazing theory here. Well-written, this book is also easily understandable and exciting for people without a background in science.

The Elegant Universe by Brian Greene, Vintage.
> Even easily readable and entertaining for those without a background in science. This book presents a very well-organized description of the superstring theory, the most significant contemporary theory of quantum physics.

A Dictionary of Gods and Goddesses, Devils and Demons by Manfred Lurker, Routledge.
> Almost any deity can be found in this well-researched dictionary. As for any book of this type, extremely profound information should not be expected. However, this work has been compiled in a reliable way and is without bias for the most part.

Tantra: Cult of the Feminine by André van Lysebeth, Weiser Books.
> This is an extensive treatise on classical Tantra with much background information on topics like the Age of the Goddess—but not one of the many fashionable books published today on Tantra. The author of this extremely informative classic knows his topic like the back of his hand.

Radical Awakening by Stephen Jourdain/Gilles Farcet, Inner Directions Foundation.
> An exciting book with a long interview conducted by the awakened journalist with a spiritually awakened man. Very entertaining, authentic, and witty.
> *The Medium, the Mystic, and the Physicist* by Lawrence LeShan, Ballantine.
> This is a well-told, knowledge-filled history of science from its modern beginnings to its (almost) close alliance with spiritual philosophy. Good reading for people who tend to see faith, science, and spirituality as two fundamentally different matters.

Yahweh's Wife by Arthur Frederick Ide, Monument Press.
> The renowned scientist Ide proves in detail that the Holy Ghost is a code name for the Great Goddess, who Solomon and many Jewish tribes worshipped directly until the very aggressive patriarchal fanatics in Judaism put a stop to this practice. The book shows how much the Bible has been falsified and provides abundant information on what really happened in Biblical times.

The Sacred Prostitute by Nancy Qualls-Corbett, Inner City Books (Toronto, Canada).
> A psychologist writes about the Holy Whore in history and within every woman. This book is unusual and knowledgeable.

Man and His Symbols by Carl Gustav Jung, Doubleday.
> A psychological treatise on symbols of all types. Worth reading because it helps us better understand what it means to be a human being.

I Ching—The Book of Changes, translated by Richard Wilhelm, Grange Books.
> This is a standard work around the world. Its writing is sometimes too complicated and burdened with Christian blinders. However, it is still an important book because of the immense wealth of information. As a sole source on the I Ching, it is too biased—but very useful as supplementary literature.

I Ching—The Book of Changes and the Unchanging Truth by Hua-Ching Ni, Seven Star Communications Group.
> In my opinion, this is currently by far the best version of the Chinese classic, the *I Ching*. This book is very extensive, precise, and written with much wisdom.

Woman's Dictionary of Symbols and Sacred Objects by Barbara G. Walker, Book Sales.
> An excellently researched treatise on well-known symbols of all types and their origins in the spiritual tradition of the Great Goddess. A treat for anyone who would like to have a more precise look at feminine spirituality.

The Woman's Encyclopedia of Myths and Secrets by Barbara G. Walker, Harper.
> Very extensive and, just like the previously mentioned work, precisely researched documentation on the history of the Goddess' spiritual path. In each of the world religions, Walker clears away the misinterpretations and falsifications of history. A magnificent book!

The Once and Future Goddess by Elinor W. Gadon, Harper.
> A comprehensive book on the religion of the Great Goddess from the Megalithic Age to today.

The Weaving of Mantras by Ryuichi Abé, Columbia University Press.
Kûkai Major Works by Yoshito S. Hakeda, Columbia University Press.
> Two highly recommended books for anyone who wants to learn more about *Kûkai*.

Index of Scientific Literature

Arai, Yûsei. *Kôyasan shingonshû danshinto hikkei.* Kôyasan: Kôyasan shuppansha, 1988.

Atsuji, Tetsuji. *Zusetsu kanji no rekishi (Fukyu han).* Tokyo: Taishukan shoten, 1996.

Books Esoterica No. 1. *Mikkyo no hon.* Tôkyô: Gakken, 1995.

Books Esoterica No. 10. *Koshintô no hon.* Tôkyô: Gakken, 2002.

Books Esoterica No. 19. *Shingon mikkyô no hon.* Tôkyô: Gakken, 2002.

Books Esoterica No. 2. *Shintô no hon.* Tôkyô: Gakken, 2002.

Books Esoterica No. 21. *Tendai mikkyô no hon.* Tôkyô: Gakken, 2002.

Books Esoterica No. 23. *Fûsui no hon.* Tôkyô: Gakken, 2002.

Books Esoterica No. 29. *Kobudô no hon.* Tôkyô: Gakken, 2001.

Books Esoterica No. 30. *Jujutsu no hon.* Tôkyô: Gakken, 2002.

Books Esoterica No. 4. *Dôkyô no hon.* Tôkyô: Gakken, 2002.

Books Esoterica No. 6. *Onmyôdô no hon.* Tôkyô: Gakken, 2002.

Books Esoterica No. 8. *Shugendô no hon.* Tôkyô: Gakken, 2001.

Books Esoterica. *Tôyô igaku no hon.* Tôkyô: Gakken, 2002.

Bunkachô, kanchô. *Juyô bunka zai 24. Kôgei hin 1. Kinkô.* Tôkyô: Mainichi Shinbunsha, 1976.

Bunkachô, kanchô. *Juyô bunka zai 29. Kôkô 2.* Tôkyô: Mainichi Shinbunsha, 1976.

Butsuzô wo arawashita kongôrei. Nara: Nara kokuritsu hakubutsukan, 1989.

Chandra, Lokesh. *Buddhist Iconography.* New Delhi: Aditya Prakashan, 1991.

Daigoji ten. Inori to bi no densho. Nara: Benrido, Nihon keizai shinbunsha, 1998.

Faure, Bernard. *The Rhetoric of Immediacy.* Princeton: Princeton University Press, 1991.

Faure, Bernard. *Visions of Power.* Princeton: Princeton University Press, 1996.

Franz, Heinrich Gerhard. *Das alte Indien (Ancient India).* Munich: Bertelesmann, 1990.

Fujiwara, Giichi. *Nihon sekizô ihô.* Vol.1. Tôkyô: Yamato shoinri, 1943.

Fukunaga, Mitsuji. *Dôkyô to nihon no bunka.* Jinbun Shôin. Kyôto. 1982.

Gakken. *Super Nihongo Daijiten.* Tôkyô, 1998.

Genshoku nihon no bijutsu. Vol. 20. Tôkyô: Shôgakukan, 1969.

Goepper, Roger. *Shingon. Die Kunst des Geheimen Buddhismus in Japan.* Museum fuer Ostasiatische Kunst der Stadt Köln: Köln, 1988.

Grewe, Gabriele. *Buddhistische Kultgegenstaende Japans. Ein Handbuch.* Wadakita: Goku Raku An, 1996.

Hanayama Shôyû. *Mikkyô no subete.* Tôkyô: PHP Kenkyû sho, 1994.

Hanayama Shôyû. *Zukai no subete.* Tôkyô: PHP Kenkyû sho, 1998.

Hane, M.. *Premodern Japan. A Historical Survey.* Boulder: Westview Press, 1991.

Hieizan—Koyasan Meihoten. *Nara kenritsu bijutsukan.* Nara: Nara Prefectural Museum, 1997.

Hosak, Mark. *Die Siddham-Schrift in der japanischen Kunst bis zum 14. Jahrhundert* (The Siddham Script in Japanese Art Up to the 14ᵗʰ Century). Heidelberg: Universitaet Heidelberg, 2002.

Hoshiba, Sekiho. *Butsuzoga nyumon.* Tokyo: Nichibo shuppansha, 1991.

Imamura, Kyujukju. *Jihi hozo.* Kyoto: Yamada insatsu, 1995.

Inoue Mitsusada. *Rekishi sanpo jiten.* Tôkyô: Yamagawa Shuppan, 1996.

Ishida Shige. *Mikkyô hôgu no kenkyû.* In: *Mikkyô hôgu.* Tôkyô: Kôdansha, 1965.

Itô, Toshiko. *Ise monogatari e.* Tôkyô: Kadokawa shoten, 1984.

Izumi, Takeo. *Ôchô no butsuga to girei.* Kyôto: Kyôto kokuritsu hakubutsukan, 1998.

Japan. An Illustrated Encyclopedia. Tokyo: Kodansha, 1994. S. 152

Jien, Shizuka. *Bonji de kaku hannya shingyô.* Ôsaka, Toki Shobô, 2001.

Kodama, Giryû. *Bonji hikkei. Shosha to kaidoku.* Ôsaka: Toki shobô, 1996.

Kodama, Giryû. *Bonji de miru mikkyo – sono oshie, imi, kakikata.* Tokyo: Taihô Rinkaku, 2002.

Kôbô Daishi to mikkyô bijutsu. Tôkyô: Asahi shinbunsha, 1984.

Kojien Daigohan CD-ROM. Tokyo: Iwanami shoten, 1998.

Kûkai to koyasan. Kobo Daishi nitto 1200 nen kenen. Osaka: NHK Osaka Hosokyoku, 2003.

Ladstätter, Linhart. *China und Japan. The Kulturen Ostasiens.* Vienna: Ueberreuter, 1983.

Ledderose, Lothar. *Some Taoist Elements in the Calligraphy of the Six Dynasties,* in: *T'oung Pao* 70, 1984.

Ledderose, Lothar. *Ten Thousand Things.* Princeton, New Jersey: Princeton University Press, 2000.

Louis, Frederic. *Buddhism – Flammarion Iconographic Guide.* Paris – New York: Flammarion, 1995.

Manabe, Shunshô. *Hakubyô shita e ise monogatari bonji kyô no bonji ni tsuite. Kômyô shingon no bunseki to sono kaidoku.* In: *Yamato bunka,* Vol. 53. Nara: Yamato Bunkakan, 1970.

Mikkyô bijutsu daikan. Vol. 4. Tôkyô: Asahi shinbunsha, 1984.

Mochizuki, Nobushige. *Kôryûji.* Kyôto: Wakôsha, 1963.

Mookerjee, *Ajit and Khanna, Madhu. The Tantric Way: Art, Science, Ritual.* New York: Thames and Hudson, 1977.

Nakamura, Hajime. *Bukkyô go daijiten.* Tôkyô: Shukusatsu, 1985.

Nara Kokuritsu hakubutsukan. *Busshari no sôgon.* Kyôto: Dôhôsha, 1983.

Nara kokuritsu hakubutsukan. *Busshari no bijutsu.* Nara: Tenriji hôsha, 1975.

Nara kokuritsu hakubutsukan. *Nara Saidaji ten.* Nara: Benridô,1991.

Nara rokudaiji taikan. Saidaji. Vol. 14. Tôkyô: Iwanami, 1973.

Nihon Bijutsukan. Tôkyô: Shôgakukan, 1997.

Nihon bijutsu. Busshari to kyô no sôgon. No. 280. Kyôto: Shibundô, 1989.

Nihon bijutsu. Butsugu. No. 16. Kyôto: Shıbundô, 1967.

Nihon bijutsukan. Tôkyô: Shôgakukan, 1997.

Nihon bukkyo bijutsu meiho ten—Nara kokuritsu hakubutsu kan hyakunen kinen – Tokubetsu ten. Nara: Nara National Museum, 1995.

Nihon kokuhô ten. Tôkyô: Tôkyô kokuritsu hakubutsukan & Yomiuri shinbunsha, 1990.

Nihon no Kokuhô. Tôkyô: Asahi Shinbunsha, 1998.

Nihon rekishi jinbutsu jiten. Tôkyô: Asahi shinbunsha, 1994.

Nishimura Kôchô. *Mikkyô nyûmon.* Tôkyô: Shinchô sha, 1996.

Okazaki Jôji. *Butsugu Daijiten.* Tôkyô: Kamakura shinsho, 1995.

Ôta, Masao. *Tendai mikkyô no hon.* Tôkyô: Gakken, 1998.

Ôyama, Kôjun. *Denju roku.* Ôsaka: Tôhô, 1997.

Petzold, Bruno. *Über Pagoden- und Tempelbau.* Tôkyô, 1935.

Ramm-Bonwitt, Ingrid. *Mudras—Geheimsprache der Yogis.* Freiburg: Hermann Bauer Verlag, 1998.

Ruppert, Brian Douglas. *Jewel in the Ashes. Buddha Relics and Power in Early Medieval Japan.* Harvard: Harvard University Asia Center, 2000.

Sawa, Ryûken. *Daigoji.* Tôkyô: Kôdansha, 1967.

Seckel, Dietrich. *Buddhistische Templenamen in Japan.* In: *Münchener Ostasiatische Studien.* Bd. 37. Franz Steiner Verlag Wiesbaden: Stuttgart, 1985.

Seckel, Dietrich. *Taigengû, das Heiligtum des Yuiitsu-Shintô.* in: *Monumenta Nipponica* Vol. VI. Sophia University, Tôkyô: 1943.

Sen-oku hakko kan—Sumitomo Collection. Kyoto: Sen-oku hakko kan, 1994.

Shakyo nyumon. Kyoto: Tankosha, 1992.

Sôga, Tetsuo. *Hôryûji no ihô.* Vol. 4. Tôkyo: Shôgakkan, 1985.

Sokura, T. *Nihon shiika no kigen ronsô, shukyô kigen setsu.* In: *Kôya nihon bungaku nosôten.* Vol. 1. Tôkyô, 1969.

Stevens, John. *Sacred Calligraphy of the East.* Boulder & London: Shambala, 1981.

Taisen, Miyata. *A Henro Pilgrimage Guide to the 88 Temples of Shikoku Island Japan.* Sacramento: Northern California Kôyasan Temple, 1984.

Takada, Takeyama. *Gotai jirui.* Tokyo: Saito shobo, 1998.

Takenishi, Hiroko & Miyagi, Hiroshi. *Byôdôin.* In: *Koji junrei.* Kyôto. Vol. 8. Tôkyô: Tankôsha, 1976.

Tanabe, George Jôji. *Myôe the Dreamkeeper: Fantasy and Knowledge in Early Kamakura Buddhism.* Harvard: Harvard University Press, 1992.

Tokuyama, Terusumi. *Bonji hannya shingyô.* Tôkyô: Kikuragesha, 1995.

Tokuyama, Terusumi. *Bonji tecchô.* Tôkyô: Kikuragesha, 1993.

Tsuboi Toshihiro. *Zukan kawara yane.* Tôkyô: Rikô gakusha, 1977.

Tucci, Giuseppe. *Teoria e pratica del mandala.* Tokyo: Kinkasha, 1992.

Wakasugi Satoshi. *Nihon no sekitô.* Tôkyô: Kikurage sha, 1970.

Yamada, Masaharu. *Koshintô no gyôhô to kagaku.* Tôkyô, BABJapan, 2002.

Yamashiro, Tôro. *Shinhan kihon gotai jiten.* Tôkyô, Tôkyôdô Shuppan, 1990.

Yoritomo, Motohiro. *Mandala no hotoketachi.* In: *Tokyo bijutsu sensho* Vol. 40. Tokyo: Tokyo bijutsu, 1985.

Zürn, Peter. *Erleuchtung ist überall,* Aitrang: Windpferd, 2002.

Index of Illustrations and Sources

Unless otherwise indicated, all of the calligraphies in this list are originals by Mark Hosak.

The illustrations of scenes from *Kûkai's* life (Ill. 2-9), as well as the mudrâs in ill. 62-66, 70, 74, 76, 78, 80, 82, 84, 86, 88, and 90 are by Peter Ehrhardt.

The illustrations 193-195, 197, 198, 200, 201, 203, 204, 207, and 208 were created by Marx Grafik & ArtWork on the basis of designs by Walter Lübeck.

The chakra illustrations in Chapter 20 were taken from *The Chakra Handbook* by Shalila Sharamon and Bodo J. Baginski, Lotus Press/Shangri-La, 1988. Translated by Peter Huebner.

Some of the illustrations come from very ancient, historical sources and therefore do not meet our contemporary quality standards in the printed reproduction.

The detailed bibliographical information for the quoted sources can be found in the Index of Scientific Literature, page 647ff.

The Biography of Mark Hosak, M.A.

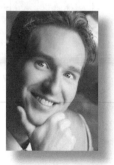

I enjoy life and this is why I live intensely. It has always been important to me to not stand still but to lead the way. As a result, I work in four different fields—I am a doctoral candidate in the subject of East Asian Art History, a Rainbow Reiki Master, a teacher of martial arts, and a calligrapher—in order to develop my potential. I am obviously especially happy when connections result between these topics. Of course, there have been and still are also times of uncertainty where it is difficult for me to find my path. But up to now I have always found a way to bring my great variety of interests together in my life and use them in my profession. This has taught me that life becomes increasingly fun the more we turn our hobbies into our profession. As in the life of any human being, it has also been necessary for me to grow into who I really am from the self-definition that I learned in childhood. Through spiritual methods and experiences—such as Reiki and meditation, pilgrimages, and mantra work—I have experienced great help on this journey to myself. When I no longer knew how to go on, the blessing came from above and opened doors for me where it had previously looked like there were just walls. After I had understood that life is much easier when the spiritual is given a solid place in everyday life, the wish awakened within me to also pass this beautiful gift on to others. Because of my various qualifications as a teacher in the above-mentioned areas, which I acquired in the following years, my life expanded in turn and I discovered the happiness of being able to walk the path to light and love together with my students.

Through my involvement with the inner martial arts since my childhood, I developed an understanding of how fear and the readiness to use violence can be transformed into love and the desire to heal and help. In the spiritual philosophy of the Asian inner martial arts, a central place is given to the goal of healing ourselves and relating meaningfully to life and our own potential. Many people of the Western world have learned to appreciate and use the great healing power of this philosophy in Taichi-chuan, the many forms of Qigong, and Aikido. According to the Hermetic Law of "as above, so below," spiritual philosophy can be experienced in a practical way through the body and the related everyday life. This also makes it much easier to differentiate between what really works, what has a meaning for us, and what does not. This is why bodywork in the form of Rei Ki Gong has been given an important place in this book. In my seminars, I use selected exercises from Qigong to impart a practical understanding of otherwise quite abstract spiritual laws and insights to my students. In a very natural way, the lotus flower in the love of the heart almost automatically develops when we peacefully rest in the Hara. Nature is the great textbook of the Creative Force. And through the spiritual tradition of shamanism, it is easy to study its concealed wisdom and apply it to healing and spiritual personality transformation. I like to walk in the forest and connect from my heart with the light-filled spirit beings of nature in ritual, prayer, and meditation. This is the necessary balance that I need when living and working in an urban environment and coping with the hectic pace of our age.

The strength of my heart that has grown through this contact with Mother Nature accompanies me in my seminars and consultations in order to help those who are suffering and seeking on their path to happiness. Especially at the beginning of this new time era, it is very important to let ourselves be inspired by nature in order to translate spiritual wisdom in a practical way for the necessary transformation of our lifestyle.

Japanese calligraphy involves bringing the spiritual power of the heart into the characters through the writing brush and the Chinese ink, which then stimulates our inspiration and meditation. Ever since my childhood, I have been fascinated by this spiritual tradition. Now I understand that writing a book like this is an additional aspect of my calligraphic work, which I have learned in many years of intensive studies with Asian masters in the traditional way. In the initial stage of my involvement with Reiki, I often came across the opinion that it was not correct to write spiritual insights in the script form. This made me sad because over thousands of years it has been the writings and calligraphies of the great masters that, in addition to oral instruction, have been the foundation of healing and of training the next generation of spiritual teachers. I see the script form as a meaningful and necessary addition to the mouth-to-ear form of transmitting information. Today I impart the deep calm and focusing of the mind and the opening of the heart to spiritual powers that can be brought about by calligraphy, within the scope of my Rainbow Reiki seminars and in special calligraphy courses. I would like to give other individuals in the West the opportunity to discover their potential in this area and enjoy it.

My childhood and youth held some very large and sometimes quite unusual challenges for me. As a result, I had to learn at a very young age to take care of myself and stand up for myself. It was only later that I understood how one part of my spiritual training takes place in the form of instruction and another one part is life itself. This is how I succeeded in overcoming the hardships of my early years with the help of spiritual beings to increase my willingness and live from my heart. Seen from the divine perspective, each experience offers a seed that can grow into a plant of happiness, beauty, and enlightenment. Instead of suffering because of our lives, each of us can distill our experiences into wisdom, meaning, and love. In keeping with the well-known rule of "the path is the goal," this does not mainly focus on attaining a certain level of development but the process of letting the disharmonious aspects become harmonious and always continuing to develop. In the Eastern spiritual tradition, this is described as a wonderful lotus flower that grows out of the mire of the swamp as it anchors itself with its roots and nourishes itself there. There is great wisdom in learning to respect and love both the flower and the swamp.

I got through my studies under difficult conditions. My entire free time was invested in several years of training to become a Rainbow Reiki Master. At the same time, I became financially independent. Then I very quickly aimed for an international scope of activity and now hold Rainbow Reiki seminars and consultations throughout the world. As a result of the many healing successes in Korea and Japan—the country where Reiki originated—I am welcome there as a spiritual adviser and teacher.

In addition to my obligations and training, I take the time to devote myself to art and work professionally as a calligrapher. This gives me a great deal and my heart blossoms. Because of this, I also integrate mantras and symbols in combination with calligraphy in my work.

Of course, there have also been doubts and difficulties on the path. Relatives and acquaintances wanted to persuade me : "The cobbler should stick to his last! This won't make something out of you. You won't succeed. That is much too difficult..." Despite this well-meant advice, I have always taken my own path. Even as a small child, I was enthusiastic about East Asian cultures—everything ranging from Chinese script, the Japanese language, energetic methods of healing, or inner martial arts. Everyone wanted to talk me out of it and many obstacles were placed in my way. Yet, I ultimately mastered it all and now orient my entire life upon it.

It was and is becoming increasingly important to me to do things and learn things instead of just thinking how complicated they are. I know that there are not many people who do this. I do it because the topics that touch my heart are so important to me. Whenever I feel that an idea corresponds with the path of my heart, nothing can keep me from it. I know of very few people who would dedicate half of their life to learning Japanese and finally go to Japan for several years in order to increase their knowledge by doing research there. But especially because this was so important to me, I searched for ways to make these seemingly impossible things possible for me.

In the process, I have also sometimes fallen flat on my face, but I always got up again and kept on going. I have learned that each problem on the path offers me a wealth of learning possibilities for growth. This theme runs through my life like a red thread. Since I am always on the ball, I have been able to win several speech competitions in Japanese in Japan and Europe, survive a 1500-kilometer pilgrimage through the Japanese primeval forest twice, learn several martial arts up to the degree of Master, become a teacher for calligraphy, simultaneously complete my course of studies at the University of Heidelberg and the two-level Rainbow Reiki Master Training with outstanding achievements, and virtually on the side earn my living with seminar, counseling, and interpreting.

I also place especially great value on my love live. After the delusions and confusions of various relationships, I met the woman of my dreams in Kyoto—Junghee from Korea. It was love at first sight, but I was still too shy at that time to approach her. In a dream during my pilgrimage, the monk *Kûkai* showed her to me once again as my companion for life. Years later, my Reiki Master Walter convinced me to bring her to Germany. Reiki has given me the power to overcome the cultural differences and large distances. For several years now, we have lived together happily in Heidelberg. Her immeasurable love and support in all areas of life give me the necessary warmth, sense of security, and creative power to progress on my path and help many people on their individual paths as well.

Concrete Experiences of My Life

First Contacts with Eastern Asian Culture

Whenever I saw a Chinese or Japanese character in my childhood, I was not only completely enthusiastic but also somehow felt at home with them. I had the impression that these signs radiate an energy that I had always longed for. One day, when I was six years old, I showed my father some of these signs and told him that I absolutely wanted to learn them. He said that this would probably take 12 years and was therefore completely unthinkable. Dissatisfied with this answer, I then secretly practiced these enchanting signs on my own without knowing what they meant and how to write them correctly. Unfortunately, this did not work out in the way that I had imagined.

My Path to the Inner Martial Arts

Because I was very slender by nature, actually thin, I became a target at school for the stronger students to let out their aggressions on a regular basis. No matter where I went, I was very soon subjected to physical abuse and teasing. For years, I did not receive any support from anyone. One day, I thought about how I could grow out of this on my own. In addition to the characters, I was also enthused about East Asian martial arts. However, I had no possibility at all to train in them. While on vacation with my parents, I was surrounded by about ten other children. One of them had a giant water pistol. He commanded me to raise my hands, which is what I did. Through my many years of experience, I thought that it almost didn't matter what I did in such a situation since I would be shot down in some way in the end by the children for their amusement. I do not know why to this day, but at this moment I had the idea to say: "Stop it! I know karate!," which was not at all the truth. In any case, the child with the water pistol became nervous. The other children called out: "That's a lie, shoot him down..." Once more, I repeated the sentence: "Stop it! I know karate!" This went back and forth for a while until I—involuntarily and without thinking about it—kicked the water pistol out of the other child's hand. All of the children were shocked. They suddenly respected me. Not only did they leave me alone after that, but also accepted me into their group. My decision was made at that point—the learning and mastering of a martial art is the path to peace.

My parents took a long time to allow me to do this. All of my efforts to convince them came to nothing. I should play golf instead and not always start something new, which I would soon give up anyway, was one of their arguments. So I secretly bought myself books on karate and *Ninjutsu*. When walking my dog, I practiced the techniques from the book. At night, after my parents had gone to bed, I frequently snuck out of the house to the forest to practice some more. I made the best of every free minute. I was not especially successful at it since it is obvious that we learn less from books than directly from a master. So the wish to find a master—at best, a Japanese one—grew within me.

About one-and-a-half years later, a Japanese boarding school for Japanese children whose parents live in Europe opened close to my home in Bremen. My mother told me that I would be allowed to train if I could find a master there. At the time, I still believed that all Japanese are great masters of the martial arts. When I inquired about a master at the Japanese school, I soon learned differently. There was only one karate master. He gave me private lessons in karate and I taught him German. It was a fair exchange and the fulfillment of my big dream. I had my own master and it did not take long until I became inviolable at school.

But there was something else in the martial arts. To be precise, I soon learned that there are phenomena that cannot be explained so simply. My teacher went jogging with me barefoot in glass shards on a regular basis. There were no injuries. Even without muscle power, I was soon able to smash granite stones. At that time, I still had no idea that this was just the beginning, that martial arts would at some point save my life on more than one occasion, and that they were related to the healing arts.

663

The masters at the Japanese School changed from time to time, which meant that I was also able to learn several styles and even full contact without protectors. My numerous visits to the hospital sent me on a search for a martial art form that was better suited to me. I finally came upon *Ninjutsu*, which includes all areas of fighting without and with weapons like the stick and sword, as well as healing, meditation, and magic.

After I had already trained several times in Japan, I finally came across the *Ninjutsu* Master Taguchi in Osaka, whose style I still teach today in the areas of *Ninjutsu*, *Kenjutsu,* and *Bojutsu*.

My First Trip to Japan

Through the martial arts and training with Japanese, my interest grew in the Japanese culture and language. In my childhood, I had already been enthused by the script but had never seen the connection with the language. The script affected me like sacred symbols.

At the age of 18, I traveled to Japan for the first time. These six weeks of my life were so inspiring that I swore to myself that I would one day also have a profession that had something to do with Japan. For the first time in my life, I felt at home. The country was wonderful, the food delicious and agreeable, and the people were very friendly. The Buddhist temples especially impressed me.

This trip gave me the strength to complete my very difficult and painful school years. My grades at school had never been very good. The eighth grade appealed to me so much that I even repeated it. I was very happy to discover that the school began to offer the languages of Japanese and Chinese when I reached the upper grades. I immediately learned both. My grades were better here than those of the native speakers. They helped me graduate. Otherwise, things would have been very difficult for me.

My Path to Reiki

After I completed school, I became a conscientious objector and did community service instead. For the most part, my work consisted of going to the homes of old, helpless people and caring for them or talking to them. Most of them were very depressed about the world and the state of their health. But my worst case, an 88-year-old woman who was paralyzed on her entire right side, was completely different. She was always in a good mood, content, and tried to do as much as possible for herself. Even her house appeared to me to be much more alive than all of the others. Even on the very dismal and rainy November days in Bremen, I had the impression that the sun always shone there. But I could not explain this. When I gave her flowers for her birthday, these remained just as fresh as on the first day after many weeks. Full of amazement and half in fun, I asked what she did with the flowers because this actually could not be happening. Without words and with a friendly smile, she held her left hand—which she could still move—above the flowers. I had no idea what this gesture meant. From her son—a former NASA physicist—I learned that she gave her flowers Reiki. Up to that time, I had never heard of anything like that. From the perspective of physics, he explained to me what Reiki is, how it functions, and even presented me with scientific proof for Reiki from his experience with NASA in the rain forest.

It did not take long for me to become initiated into the 1st Degree by his Reiki Master. I was also skeptical but wanted to find out the truth about it through my own experience. My skepticism soon vanished through the many wonderful experiences and healing successes with Reiki.

The 2nd Degree and My Introduction to Symbol Calligraphy
In order for me to do the 2nd Degree with her, my teacher asked me to write the Reiki-characters very large with the writing brush in the manner of calligraphy. She explained to me that I should not worry about not yet having learned calligraphy. She was quite certain that I would draw the sign to her complete satisfaction. That was a big challenge. So just like at the beginning of my martial arts career, I practiced day after day without a teacher. I used the writing brush to draw the Reiki characters until they were perfect.

Studies of East Asian Art History and Japanology as a Basis
After the community service, I went to Heidelberg to study East Asian Art History and Japanology there. I soon broke all the records at the University of Heidelberg. After just three semesters, I completed the intermediate examination with outstanding grades. Despite the short amount of time, I earned more than twice the usual amount of credits. My next goal was to get to Japan as quickly as possible.

Studies in Calligraphy with a Zen Monk

On the bulletin board at the Department of Japanology, one day I saw a slip of rice paper with a wonderful script written on it. Together with my Japanese teacher, we deciphered the text. In it, a Japanese man wrote in a very polite and somewhat old-fashioned language that he was looking for a private teacher for German. My Japanese teacher advised me against contacting this person because he was definitely not normal based on his strange language and script that was somewhat too beautiful. The very same day, I called him and was able to fulfill another wish in this way. He was not only Japanese but also a Zen master and well-known in Buddhist circles as a master of Chinese calligraphy. So in addition to Reiki, *Ninjutsu,* and my course of studies, I also practiced calligraphy every day.

Japan—Reiki Symbols—Pilgrimage

Soon I received two scholarships (DAAD and Rotary International), which allowed me to go to Japan for several years. I researched Buddhist rituals at the University of Kyoto and in the temples. Time and again, I came across correlations with the Reiki symbols. Every answer resulted in many new questions. When my Japanese professor told me about a pilgrimage of Esoteric Buddhism, I felt something like a flash of lightening through my heart. The monk *Kûkai* is said to have meditated for a long time in the forest on the island of Shikoku. He laid the foundation stones at Shikoku's power places for many temples, which then became the pilgrimage of the "88 Temples of Shikoku." I knew that I had to make this pilgrimage in order to progress on my own path. A few weeks later, I set out on foot on my pilgrimage from temple to temple through the Japanese primeval forest. After about ten days, I had to end the pilgrimage at temple no. 24 because of exhaustion. One year later, I set out again on the path and went on a pilgrimage to all 88 of the temples in several weeks time. Every day, I experienced true miracles. One day, a Bodhisattva disguised as a dog showed me the path, and then disappeared in front of my eyes. He later appeared again when I wanted to go in the wrong direction. Eagles or butterflies the size of a human head traveled with me for long periods of time as true companions. In a dream, my future wife appeared to me. The monk *Kûkai* transformed himself from a bronze statue in the forest into his true to life form as a pilgrim and gave me the advice to follow the path of my heart. In response to the question as to what the path of my heart is, he said: "You will experience it when you continue on your pilgrimage with me." Then he dissolved in light and disappeared. These are just some examples. Even long after the pilgrimage, I still felt his wonderful energy.

The path of my heart is Reiki. The monk *Kûkai* brought the roots of Reiki to Japan with Esoteric Buddhism.

The pilgrimage was the greatest experience of my life. I have written a book about it in the Japanese language. In Japan and Europe, I won two speech competitions in Japanese on this topic.

Thanks to the inspiring meeting with Frank Arjava Petter in Japan, I was soon able to meet Walter Lübeck after my return to Germany and began my Reiki Master Training in 1999.

In the meantime, I have completed my course of studies. In my master's thesis, I discussed the *Siddham* script in Japan, to which the Reiki Symbols also belong. A dissertation about the same script within the context of healing rituals will follow.

Contact Address and Seminar Information for Mark Hosak

König-Heinrich-Strasse 42
69412 Eberbach
Germany
Tel: 011-49l- (0)6271-947957
Email: office@markhosak.com
Website: www.markhosak.com

My website has a forum for reader questions about the topics covered in this book. It requires a simple registration.

The Biography of Walter Lübeck

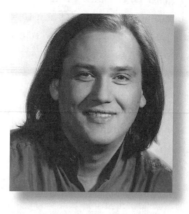

Walter Lübeck, born on February 17, 1960 (Aquarius, Asc. Sagittarius) has been active as a spiritual teacher since 1988. Throughout the world, he teaches the Rainbow Reiki System that he has developed, the Three Rays Meditation, the shamanic White Feather Path, Angel Light Work, Feng Shui, Spiritual NLP, mantra work, Heavenly Dragon Qi Gong, Lemurian Crystal Healing, Reincarnation Therapy, and Lemurian Tantra in the German and English language.

The three principles of personal responsibility, love, and consciousness are important spiritual guidelines for him in his private and professional life.

With his work, he would like to contribute to the dawning of a new Golden Age on Earth as soon as possible, in which nature, human beings, and light beings live with each other in peace and happiness.

In 25 books, 8 of which are on the topic of Reiki and have been translated into 20 languages, in diverse articles in specialized magazines, teaching videos, and personal counseling software, he makes the results of his research available to the public. He finds it very important for spiritual knowledge to be used for increasing the holistic quality of life and for healing our planet.

He is trained in the Western and Japanese Reiki tradition (Western lineage/Master/Teacher: Usui – Hayashi – Furumoto – Brigitte Müller * Japanese lineage/Master/Teacher: Usui – Hayashi – Chiyoko Yamaguchi) and has intensively researched the Usui System of Natural Healing, together with its roots and possibilities, since he first became acquainted with Reiki in 1987.

Through his great diversity of trainings, personal research, and memories of past lives as a high priest and healer in places like Lemuria, India, Egypt, and Mesopotamia, his teachings have a unique character and convey deep spiritual experiences and insights. It is very important to him to impart the various spiritual paths and their wisdom as meaningful teachings that complement and are related to each other in order to help his students optimally progress on their individual paths.

Numerous research trips on the topic of Reiki have taken him to Japan, India, Bali, Hong Kong, and the USA.

He likes to spend his free time with family, friends, and animals. Walter also enjoys hiking, cooking, playing computer games, running cross-country, and practicing Qi Gong.

Since the turn of the millennium, another emphasis of his work has been Goddess Radionic, which he founded. This is a spiritual technology that can be used to prepare flower essences and homeopathic remedies and energetically purify and upgrade water, for example. It can also neutralize the dangerous effects of electro smog.

As an enthusiastic musician, he likes to use drums, didgeridoo, singing, and dance in rituals and spiritual healing. He has composed many spiritual songs, which he releases from time to time in music productions, such as the CD "Power Reiki"

He lives in the Weser Mountains of North Germany in the middle of a wonderful landscape that is full of ancient power places and mystical sites.

Contact Address and Seminar Information for Walter Lübeck

E-Mail: info@rainbowreiki.net

Website (German/English/Portuguese): www.rainbowreiki.net

www.rainbowreikiUSA.net

How the Book Cover Was Created

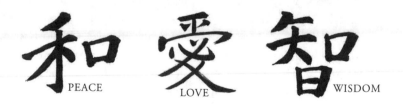

和　　愛　　智
PEACE　　LOVE　　WISDOM

I (Mark) would like to briefly tell you in conclusion how the cover for this book was created. This story is a beautiful example of how the techniques described in this book can be applied in practice. In addition, it shows the wondrous „coincidences" and experiences with Reiki and the light beings that we can also have when we use them.

Walter initially had the idea of transforming the words love, wisdom, and peace into calligraphies for the book cover because they are appropriate for the spiritual content. So I began to search for the suitable characters. There are actually many associated symbols with a similar meaning and different nuances.

The symbol on the left represents peace and is called *wa* in Japanese. At the same time, it means harmony and is also an old name for Japan.

The symbol on the right stands for wisdom and called *chi* in Japanese. Without its lower portion, this symbol represents pure knowledge. The sun beneath it turns the knowledge into wisdom. Since this is a light-filled and spiritual form of wisdom, it is very frequently employed within the Buddhist context. Another Japanese meaning of it is *satoru*. Even if it is actually a different character, this word is closely related to enlightenment in Zen Buddhism, which is called *satori*.

Finally, the word love *ai*, which unites peace and wisdom and all beings with each other, stands in the middle. This is the love that works for the highest good of all those who are involved, which truly includes every being and naturally also ourselves. It is the love that is expressed through the 4th chakra. At the same time, ai is a symbol that is used for all things that are important to us.

670

When I had found these three symbols, I once again began searching for masters of calligraphy to serve as an inspiration. I landed in the ancient China of the *Tang* era with the great calligrapher *Ouyang Xun* (557-641), whose style I copied on paper in the traditional way with a brush and Indian ink.

The Paradise Buddha *Amida Nyorai* offered to support me in the creation of the calligraphies for the book cover. As described in this book, I then established contact with him. This allowed me to transfer his power through my body by means of the brush in the Indian ink onto the paper. I would like to once again express my heartfelt gratitude to him at this point!

As I drew the calligraphies with his help, I was not aware that the Paradise Buddha would once again appear on the cover. Ms. Jünemann, of the Windpferd Verlag publishing company, and I had long deliberated about what we could select as a worthy background. She ultimately came across the photo of a temple door from Frank Arjava Petter's art collection. And this door is the entrance to a temple—that of the Paradise Buddha! It is located on Mt. Hiei, directly across from the Mt. Kurama, where Dr. Usui was initiated into Reiki.

So the symbols for love, peace, and wisdom were placed on the door into the Pure Land of the Paradise Buddha. Anyone who passes through this door and uses all the good things in love, harmony, and wisdom can truly reach this place. It is open to all of us. This book is the key to the door. But each of us must walk the path on our own.

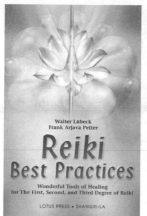

Walter Lübeck · Frank Arjava Petter

Reiki–Best Practices

Wonderful Tools of Healing for the First, Second and Third Degree of Reiki

Western Reiki techniques–published and presented in great detail for the first time

The internationally renowned Reiki Masters Walter Lübeck and Frank Arjava Petter introduce primarily Western Reiki techniques and place a valuable tool in the hands of every Reiki practitioner for applying Reiki in a specific and effective way for protection and healing. A total of 60 techniques, such as: aura massage with Reiki, deprogramming of old patterns, karma clearing, protecting against energy loss, Tantra with Reiki are exclusively presented and described in detail for the first time in this fascinating guide. With black&white drawings

296 pages · $19.95 · ISBN 978-0-9149-5574-0

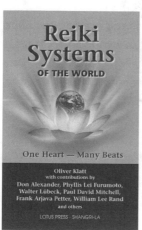

Oliver Klatt

Reiki Systems of the World

One Heart · Many Beats

With contributions by the leading Reiki Masters of the world: Phyllis Lei Furumoto, Don Alexander, Walter Lübeck, William Lee Rand, Paul David Mitchell, Frank Arjava Petter

An inspiring and fascinating reference guide offering an overview of the development of the world's Reiki systems. For the first time anywhere, you obtain fundamental information about internationally known and recognized Reiki schools and lineages. You can also understand their similarities and especially their differences on the basis of practical examples and exercises. The author's warmhearted and sincere style is supported by his respect for, and great knowledge of Reiki.

with 51 black&white drawings · 352 pages
$19.95 · ISBN: 978-0-9149-5579-5